The Smallpox Vaccination Program

Public Health in an Age of Terrorism

Committee on Smallpox Vaccination Program Implementation

Board on Health Promotion and Disease Prevention

Alina Baciu, Andrea Pernack Anason, Kathleen Stratton, and Brian Strom, Editors

INSTITUTE OF MEDICINE
OF THE NATIONAL ACADEMIES

THE NATIONAL ACADEMIES PRESS
Washington, D.C.
www.nap.edu

THE NATIONAL ACADEMIES PRESS 500 Fifth Street, NW Washington, DC 20001

NOTICE: The project that is the subject of this report was approved by the Governing Board of the National Research Council, whose members are drawn from the councils of the National Academy of Sciences, the National Academy of Engineering, and the Institute of Medicine. The members of the committee responsible for the report were chosen for their special competences and with regard for appropriate balance.

This study was supported by Contract No. 200-2000-00629, Task Order No. 10 between the National Academy of Sciences and the Centers for Disease Control and Prevention. Any opinions, findings, conclusions, or recommendations expressed in this publication are those of the author(s) and do not necessarily reflect the view of the organizations or agencies that provided support for this project.

Library of Congress Cataloging-in-Publication Data

The smallpox vaccination program : public health in an age of terrorism / Committee on Smallpox Vaccination Program Implementation, Board on Health Promotion and Disease Prevention ; Alina Baciu ... [et al.], editors.
p. ; cm.
Supported by contract no. 200-2000-00629, task order no. 10 between the National Academy of Sciences and the Centers for Disease Control and Prevention.
Includes bibliographical references and index.
ISBN 0-309-09592-1 (pbk.)—ISBN 0-309-54877-2 (pdf)
1. Smallpox—Vaccination—Government policy—United States. I. Baciu, Alina. II. Institute of Medicine (U.S.). Committee on Smallpox Vaccination Program Implementation.
[DNLM: 1. Immunization Programs—organization & administration—United States. 2. Smallpox—prevention & control—United States. 3. Bioterrorism—prevention & control—United States. 4. Government Programs—organization & administration—United States. 5. Health Policy—United States. 6. Smallpox Vaccine—United States. WC 588 S635 2005]
RA644.S6S59 2005
614.5′21′0973—dc22 2005010062

Additional copies of this report are available from the National Academies Press, 500 Fifth Street, NW, Lockbox 285, Washington, DC 20055; (800) 624-6242 or (202) 334-3313 (in the Washington metropolitan area); http://www.nap.edu.
For more information about the Institute of Medicine, visit the IOM home page at **www.iom.edu.**

Printed in the United States of America.

The serpent has been a symbol of long life, healing, and knowledge among almost all cultures and religions since the beginning of recorded history. The serpent adopted as a logotype by the Institute of Medicine is a relief carving from ancient Greece, now held by the Staatliche Museen in Berlin.

"Knowing is not enough; we must apply.
Willing is not enough; we must do."

—Goethe

INSTITUTE OF MEDICINE

OF THE NATIONAL ACADEMIES

Adviser to the Nation to Improve Health

THE NATIONAL ACADEMIES

Advisers to the Nation on Science, Engineering, and Medicine

The **National Academy of Sciences** is a private, nonprofit, self-perpetuating society of distinguished scholars engaged in scientific and engineering research, dedicated to the furtherance of science and technology and to their use for the general welfare. Upon the authority of the charter granted to it by the Congress in 1863, the Academy has a mandate that requires it to advise the federal government on scientific and technical matters. Dr. Bruce M. Alberts is president of the National Academy of Sciences.

The **National Academy of Engineering** was established in 1964, under the charter of the National Academy of Sciences, as a parallel organization of outstanding engineers. It is autonomous in its administration and in the selection of its members, sharing with the National Academy of Sciences the responsibility for advising the federal government. The National Academy of Engineering also sponsors engineering programs aimed at meeting national needs, encourages education and research, and recognizes the superior achievements of engineers. Dr. Wm. A. Wulf is president of the National Academy of Engineering.

The **Institute of Medicine** was established in 1970 by the National Academy of Sciences to secure the services of eminent members of appropriate professions in the examination of policy matters pertaining to the health of the public. The Institute acts under the responsibility given to the National Academy of Sciences by its congressional charter to be an adviser to the federal government and, upon its own initiative, to identify issues of medical care, research, and education. Dr. Harvey V. Fineberg is president of the Institute of Medicine.

The **National Research Council** was organized by the National Academy of Sciences in 1916 to associate the broad community of science and technology with the Academy's purposes of furthering knowledge and advising the federal government. Functioning in accordance with general policies determined by the Academy, the Council has become the principal operating agency of both the National Academy of Sciences and the National Academy of Engineering in providing services to the government, the public, and the scientific and engineering communities. The Council is administered jointly by both Academies and the Institute of Medicine. Dr. Bruce M. Alberts and Dr. Wm. A. Wulf are chair and vice chair, respectively, of the National Research Council.

www.national-academies.org

COMMITTEE ON SMALLPOX VACCINATION PROGRAM IMPLEMENTATION

BRIAN STROM, M.D., M.P.H., (Chair), George S. Pepper Professor of Public Health and Preventive Medicine, Professor of Biostatistics and Epidemiology, Professor of Medicine and Professor of Pharmacology, University of Pennsylvania School of Medicine, Philadelphia

KRISTINE GEBBIE, Dr.P.H., R.N., (Vice Chair), Elizabeth Standish Gill Associate Professor and Director of Center for Health Policy, Columbia University School of Nursing, New York, NY

ROBERT WALLACE, M.D., M.Sc., (Vice Chair), Irene Esminger Stecher Professor of Epidemiology and Internal Medicine, University of Iowa

E. RUSSELL ALEXANDER, M.D., Professor Emeritus of Epidemiology, School of Public Health and Community Medicine, University of Washington

RONALD BAYER, Ph.D., Professor of Sociomedical Sciences, Mailman School of Public Health, Columbia University, New York, NY

R. ALTA CHARO, J.D., Associate Dean for Research and Faculty Development, University of Wisconsin Law School and Elizabeth S. Wilson Professor of Law and Bioethics, University of Wisconsin Law School and Medical School

THOMAS COATES, Ph.D., Professor, Division of Infectious Diseases, David Geffen School of Medicine, University of California, Los Angeles

PENELOPE H. DENNEHY, M.D., Professor, Division of Pediatric Infectious Diseases, Brown Medical School, Providence, RI

VINCENT FULGINITI, M.D., M.S., Professor Emeritus of Pediatrics, University of Arizona Health Sciences Center

JAY HARPER, M.D., M.B.A., M.P.H., Medical Director of Employee Health Services, University of Pittsburgh Medical Center, Pittsburgh, PA

COLEEN KIVLAHAN, M.D., M.S.P.H., Medical Director, Ambulatory Primary Care, Fantus Health Center, Bureau of Health Services, Cook County, IL

JEFFREY LEVINE, M.A., Senior Vice President of Healthcare Media Relations, Hill & Knowlton, Washington, DC

KENNETH MCINTOSH, M.D., Professor of Pediatrics, Harvard Medical School and Professor of Immunology and Infectious Diseases, Harvard School of Public Health, Boston, MA

ELIZABETH MURANE, B.S.N., M.A., Public Health Nurse and Retired Director of Public Health Nursing, Shasta County, CA

PETER ROSEN, M.D., Attending Emergency Medical Physician, Beth Israel Deaconess Hospital, Boston, MA; Professor Emeritus of Clinical Medicine and Surgery, University of California, San Diego
WILLIAM WESTON, M.D., Professor of Dermatology and Pediatrics, University of Colorado School of Medicine
ROBERT WOOLSON, Ph.D., Professor of Biostatistics, Bioinformatics and Epidemiology, Medical University of South Carolina

Health Promotion and Disease Prevention Board Liaison

GEORGE ISHAM, M.D., Medical Director and Chief Health Officer, HealthPartners, Inc., Minneapolis, MN

Consultant

WILLIAM H. FOEGE, M.D., M.P.H., Presidential Distinguished Professor, Department of International Health, Emory University, Atlanta, GA, and Health Advisor, Bill and Melinda Gates Foundation

Staff

KATHLEEN STRATTON, Ph.D., Study Director
ANDREA PERNACK ANASON, M.P.H., Program Officer
ALINA BACIU, M.P.H., Program Officer
NICOLE AMADO, M.P.H., Research Associate (until December 2003)
AMBER CLOSE, M.F.S., Research Associate
ROSE MARIE MARTINEZ, Sc.D., Director, Board on Health Promotion and Disease Prevention

Reviewers

This report has been reviewed in draft form by persons chosen for their diverse perspectives and technical expertise, in accordance with procedures approved by the National Research Council Report Review Committee. The purpose of this independent review is to provide candid and critical comments that will assist the institution in making its published report as sound as possible and to ensure that the report meets institutional standards for objectivity, evidence, and responsiveness to the study charge. The review comments and draft manuscript remain confidential to protect the integrity of the deliberative process. We wish to thank the following for their review of this report:

John R. Ball, M.D., J.D., American Society for Clinical Pathology
Kenneth I. Berns, M.D., Ph.D., University of Florida
Edward N. Brandt, M.D., Ph.D., University of Oklahoma
William K. Chiang, M.D., New York University
Thomas N. Denny, M.Sc., New Jersey Medical School
Lawrence O. Gostin, J.D., Johns Hopkins University and Georgetown University Law Center
Peter Jensen, M.D., VA Medical Center, San Francisco
Michael Katz, M.D., March of Dimes
Stanley M. Lemon, M.D., University of Texas at Galveston
Paul Light, Ph.D., Brookings Institution
John Lumpkin, M.D., M.P.H., Robert Wood Johnson Foundation
Nicole Lurie, M.D., M.S.P.H., RAND Corporation
Tener Goodwin Veenema, R.N., Ph.D., M.P.H., M.S., CPNP, University of Rochester

Although the reviewers listed above have provided many constructive comments and suggestions, they were not asked to endorse the conclusions or recommendations, nor did they see the final draft of the report before its release. The review of this report was overseen by **Bernard Lo, M.D.,** University of California, San Francisco, who was appointed by the Report Review Committee. He was responsible for making certain that an independent examination of this report was carried out in accordance with institutional procedures and that all review comments were carefully considered. Responsibility for the final content of this report rests entirely with the author committee and the institution.

The committee's letter reports released between January 2003 and July 2004 (in Appendixes B-G) were also subject to independent review.

Letter Report #1

Susan Allan, M.D., J.D., M.P.H., Arlington County Health Department, VA
John G. Bartlett, M.D., Johns Hopkins University School of Medicine
Doug Campos-Outcalt, M.D., M.P.A., Maricopa County Department of Public Health, AZ
Richard T. Johnson, M.D., Johns Hopkins University School of Medicine
J. Michael McGinnis, M.D., M.P.P., Robert Wood Johnson Foundation
John M. Neff, M.D., Children's Hospital and Regional Medical Center, Seattle, WA
Tara O'Toole, M.D., M.P.H., Johns Hopkins University
David Ropeik, M.S., Harvard Center for Risk Analysis
Thomas W. Valente, Ph.D., University of Southern California

Monitor appointed by NRC and IOM: **Ronald Estabrook, Ph.D.,** University of Texas Southwestern

Letter Report #2

Ruth Berkelman, M.D., Emory University
Bobbie Berkowitz, Ph.D., R.N., University of Washington
Mary Gilchrist, Ph.D., D(ABMM), University of Iowa
Michael Katz, M.D., March of Dimes Birth Defects Foundation
John Lumpkin, M.D., M.P.H., Illinois Department of Health
Hugh H. Tilson, M.D., Dr.P.H., University of North Carolina
Tener Goodwin Veenema R.N., Ph.D., M.P.H., M.S., CPNP, University of Rochester

Monitor appointed by NRC and IOM: **Elaine Larson, Ph.D., R.N.,** Columbia University

Letter Report #3

John Ball, M.D., J.D., American Society for Clinical Pathology
Ruth Berkelman, Emory University
Bobbie Berkowitz, Ph.D., R.N., University of Washington
R. Gordon Douglas, Jr., M.D., Cornell University Medical College
Mary Gilchrist, Ph.D., D(ABMM), University of Iowa
Peter Jensen, M.D., University of California, San Francisco
Michael Katz, M.D., March of Dimes Birth Defects Foundation
Fitzhugh Mullan, M.D., *Health Affairs*
Tener Goodwin Veenema R.N., Ph.D., M.P.H., M.S., CPNP, University of Rochester
Robert A. Weinstein, M.D., John Stroger Hospital of Cook County, IL

Monitor appointed by NRC and IOM: **Ronald Estabrook, Ph.D.,** University of Texas Southwestern

Letter Report #4

Bobbie Berkowitz, Ph.D., R.N., University of Washington
John Conte, M.D., University of California, San Francisco
Michael Katz, M.D., March of Dimes Birth Defects Foundation
John Lumpkin, M.D., M.P.H., Robert Wood Johnson Foundation
Nicole Lurie, M.D., M.S.P.H., The RAND Corporation
Hugh H. Tilson, M.D., Dr.P.H., University of North Carolina

Monitor appointed by NRC and IOM: **Ronald Estabrook, Ph.D.,** University of Texas Southwestern

Letter Report #5

Mary Gilchrist, Ph.D., D(ABMM), University of Iowa
Peter Jensen, M.D., VA Medical Center, San Francisco, CA
John Lumpkin, M.D., M.P.H., Robert Wood Johnson Foundation
Nicole Lurie, M.D., M.S.P.H., RAND Corporation
Scott Ratzan, M.D., M.P.A., Johnson & Johnson
Helen Smits, M.D., Eduardo Mondlane University
Tener Goodwin Veenema R.N., Ph.D., M.P.H., M.S., CPNP, University of Rochester
Robert Weinstein, M.D., John Stroger Hospital of Cook County, IL

Monitor appointed by NRC and IOM: **Ronald Estabrook, Ph.D.,** University of Texas Southwestern

Letter Report #6

John R. Ball, M.D., J.D., American Society for Clinical Pathology
Mary Gilchrist, Ph.D., D(ABMM), University of Iowa
Peter Jensen, M.D., VA Medical Center, University of California, San Francisco
John Lumpkin, M.D., M.P.H., Robert Wood Johnson Foundation
Nicole Lurie, M.D., M.S.P.H., RAND Corporation
Kimberley Shoaf, Dr.P.H., University of California, Los Angeles
Hugh H. Tilson, M.D., Dr.P.H., University of North Carolina

Monitor appointed by NRC and IOM: **Ronald Estabrook, Ph.D.,** University of Texas Southwestern

Acknowledgments

This report and the series of brief, timely reports that preceded it represent the collaborative efforts of many organizations and individuals.

The committee wishes to thank its liaison panel, drawn from the leadership of multiple public health, health care, and professional associations and organizations. Liaison panel members responded to committee queries and provided helpful information at the committee's public meetings. Their diverse perspectives and expert input contributed in important ways to the committee's work. The liaison panel included the following:

American Academy of Dermatology, Connie J. Tegeler
American Academy of Family Physicians, Herbert F. Young
American Academy of Neurology, Richard T. Johnson
American Academy of Ophthalmology, James Sprague
American Academy of Pediatrics, Julia McMillan
American Ambulance Association, Larry Wiersch
America's Health Insurance Plans,[1] Carmella Bocchino
American College of Occupational and Environmental Medicine, Rosemary Sokas
American Federation of State, County and Municipal Employees, John A. Bonnage

[1]Formerly American Association of Health Plans.

American Hospital Association, Roslyne D.W. Schulman
American Medical Association, James J. James
American Nurses Association, Cheryl A. Peterson
American Organization of Nurse Executives, Jo Ann Webb
American Public Health Association, Georges C. Benjamin
American Society for Clinical Pathology, Karen C. Carroll
Association of State and Territorial Directors of Nursing, Prue Albright
Association of State and Territorial Health Officials, George E. Hardy
Council of State and Territorial Epidemiologists, Gianfranco Pezzino
Emergency Nurses Association, Cheryl A. Smart
Immune Deficiency Foundation, Jonathan C. Goldsmith
International Association of Fire Chiefs, David Fischler
National Association of County and City Health Officials, Patrick M. Libbey
National Association of Emergency Medical Technicians, Paul M. Maniscalco
National Association of Emergency Medical Technicians, John Roquemore
National Association of EMS [Emergency Medical Services] Physicians, Robert O'Connor
National Association of Public Hospitals and Health Systems, Edward L. Martinez
National Association of State EMS [Emergency Medical Services] Directors, Margaret Trimble
Service Employees International Union, William Borwegen

The committee is grateful to the numerous individuals who generously shared their knowledge and expertise in their presentations to the committee at information-gathering meetings (agendas provided in Appendix H).

Larry Anderson, Centers for Disease Control and Prevention
Ron J. Anderson, Parkland Health & Hospital System, Texas
Kris Arnold, International Association of Chiefs of Police
Erik Auf der Heide, Agency for Toxic Substances and Disease Registry, Department of Health and Human Services
Brad Austin, Health Resources and Services Administration
Georges Benjamin, American Public Health Association
Luciana Borio, Department of Health and Human Services
Eddy Bresnitz, State of New Jersey Department of Health and Senior Services
Shepard Cohen, National Association of Local Boards of Health
Yehuda L. Danon, Professor of Pediatrics at Tel Aviv University, Israel
Van Dunn, National Association of Public Hospitals and Health Systems

Michael Edmond, Virginia Commonwealth University Health System Authority
COL Renata Engler, Department of Defense
Commissioner David Fischler, International Association of Fire Chiefs
David Fleming, Centers for Disease Control and Prevention
COL John Grabenstein, Department of Defense
Franklyn Judson, Denver Health
George Hardy, Association of State and Territorial Health Officials
Joseph Henderson, Centers for Disease Control and Prevention
Jon Mark Hirshon, American College of Emergency Physicians
Katherine Kelley, Association of Public Health Laboratories
Kelvin Kelkenberg, Department of Homeland Security
Vicky Kipreos, Centers for Disease Control and Prevention
Patrick Libbey, National Association of County and City Health Officials
Yvonne Madlock, Memphis and Shelby County Health Department, Tennessee
Gina Mootrey, Centers for Disease Control and Prevention
John Neff, Vice-Chair of the Advisory Committee for Immunization Practices Working Group
Karen Nikolai, Hennepin County Community Health Department, Minnesota
Glenn Nowak, Centers for Disease Control and Prevention
Robert O'Connor, National Association of EMS [Emergency Medical Services] Physicians
Cheryl Peterson, National Nurses Association
Gianfranco Pezzino, Kansas Department of Health and Environment and Council of State and Territorial Epidemiologists
Alonzo Plough, National Association of County and City Health Officials
Maggie Potter, University of Pittsburgh, Graduate School of Public Health
Enrico (Henry) Quarantelli, Disaster Research Center, University of Delaware
Linda Quick, Centers for Disease Control and Prevention
William Raub, Department of Health and Human Services
Bob Rehm, America's Health Insurance Plans
John Roquemore, National Association of Emergency Medical Technicians
Lisa Rotz, Centers for Disease Control and Prevention
Sandra Santa, Department of Homeland Security
Roslyne D.W. Schulman, American Hospital Association
Robert Schweitzer, Department of Homeland Security
Mary Selecky, Washington State Department of Health

Skip Skivington, Kaiser Permanente
Dan Sosin, Department of Health and Human Services
Lynn Steele, Centers for Disease Control and Prevention
Ray Strikas, Centers for Disease Control and Prevention
Jonathan Temte, American Academy of Family Physicians
Kathleen Toomey, Division of Public Health, Georgia Department of Human Resources
Margaret Trimble, National Association of State EMS [Emergency Medical Services] Directors
Margaret VanAmringe, Joint Commission on Accreditation of Healthcare Organizations
Donald Williamson, Association of State and Territorial Health Officials
The Honorable William Winkenwerder, Assistant Secretary of Defense for Health Affairs, Department of Defense
David J. Witt, Kaiser Permanente

The committee would like to thank the numerous staff members of the Institute of Medicine, the National Research Council, and the National Academies Press who contributed to the development, production, and dissemination of this report, including study staff Kathleen Stratton, Andrea Pernack Anason, Alina Baciu, Nicole Amado, Amber Close, and Rose Marie Martinez, other staff in the Board on Health Promotion and Disease Prevention, Janice Mehler, Bronwyn Schrecker, Jennifer Bitticks, Christine Stencel and the Office of News and Public Information, and Norman Grossblatt.

Preface

On December 13, 2002, the president of the United States announced that smallpox vaccination would be offered to some categories of civilians and administered to members of the military and government representatives in high-risk areas of the world. The events that precipitated that historic announcement included a series of terrorist attacks during the 1990s, which culminated in the catastrophic events of 2001. Deliberate releases of microbial and chemical agents had occurred in the past (for example, *Salmonella* in an Oregon salad bar, sarin gas in the Tokyo subway) but the juxtaposition of the September 2001 terrorist attacks in New York, Washington, and Pennsylvania and the October 2001 anthrax bioterrorism attacks represented a watershed; it provided a glimpse of the scale and devastation possible in an attack with biologic weapons. Speculation and concern among policy-makers and in the mass media about specific types of threats (such as the use of low-flying aircraft to spread biologic agents) compelled the general public to acknowledge the potential of bioterrorism on a large scale.

Although preparedness for deliberate attacks with biologic weapons was already the subject of much public health planning, meetings, and publications as the twentieth century neared its end, the events of 2001 led to a steep rise in bioterrorism-related government policies and funding, and in state and local preparedness activities, for example, in public health, health care, and the emergency response and public safety communities. The national smallpox vaccination program is but one of many efforts to improve readiness to respond to deliberate releases of biologic agents.

The Institute of Medicine (IOM) Committee on Smallpox Vaccination Program Implementation was convened in October 2002 at the request of the Centers for Disease Control and Prevention (CDC), the federal agency charged with implementing the government's policy of providing smallpox vaccine first to public health and health care workers on response teams, then to all interested health care workers and other first responders, and finally to members of the general public who might insist on receiving the vaccine. The committee was charged with providing "advice to the CDC and the program investigators on selected aspects of the smallpox program implementation and evaluation." The committee was asked to review and make recommendations to CDC to improve

- The informed consent process for vaccine recipients
- Professional education and training materials
- Communication plans developed by CDC for public health and medical professionals and the public
- State smallpox vaccination implementation plans
- CDC guidelines and instruments to identify potential vaccine recipients at high risk of vaccine adverse events and complications
- CDC measures to ensure the early recognition, evaluation, and appropriate treatment of adverse events and complications of smallpox vaccination
- CDC plans for collecting and analyzing data on vaccine immunogenicity, adverse events, complications, and vaccine coverage
- The achievement of overall goals of the smallpox vaccination program, such as vaccine coverage rate, equity of access, and adverse reaction rates

The IOM committee faced some unusual challenges in its work, given the rapidly changing nature of the program and the need for multiple reports in a short period. The committee's task was to review the implementation of the policy, not to comment on the policy itself. However, the committee has since recognized that the broader context in which the policy was developed and implemented may have created some unusual challenges within the program and may have affected its progress and outcomes.

In public health practice, the success of implementation of any program depends in part on how convinced constituencies are of the correctness of a policy decision. In the case of pre-event vaccination, the committee has found evidence that many key actors had an unfavorable perception of the policy. They questioned the unknown rationale used in decision-making and requested information and clarification that were not made available, presumably because of national security concerns. The lack of clarity and the confusion and concern on the part of public health partners are further reflected in the committee's being asked for advice on the program by individuals involved in its implementation. In the end, those factors led to poor participation in the program.

The committee met six times over 19 months and wrote a series of brief "letter" reports. This volume constitutes the committee's seventh and final report, and the committee hopes that it will fulfill three purposes:

- To serve as an archival document that brings together the six reports addressed to Julie Gerberding, director of CDC, and previously released on line and as short, unbound papers.
- To serve as a historical document that summarizes milestones in the smallpox vaccination program.
- To comment on the achievement of overall goals of the smallpox vaccination program (in accordance with the last item in the charge), including lessons learned from the program.

The committee is grateful for the opportunity to be of service to CDC as the agency and its state and local counterparts implemented a challenging program, and it hopes that this final report will support CDC and the public health community as they use the lessons learned from the program to strengthen the nation's public health preparedness.

Brian Strom, *Committee Chair*
Kristine Gebbie, *Committee Vice Chair*
Robert Wallace, *Committee Vice Chair*

Contents

Executive Summary

The national smallpox vaccination program announced on December 13, 2002, was the result of an extraordinary policy decision: to vaccinate people against a disease that does not exist with a vaccine that poses some well-known risks. The rationale for such a decision can be considered only against the backdrop of the terrorist and bioterrorist attacks of 2001.

The vaccination program is a case study at the intersection of public health and national security, two fields brought together by the threat of bioterrorism. The vaccination campaign has involved government entities (such as homeland security) and required considerations (such as classified information) generally not encountered in typical public health programs.

Bioterorrist attacks epitomize "low-likelihood, high-consequence" events.[1] Preparing for such events is challenging—efforts to prepare for an event that may never occur are likely to come under criticism if the threat never materializes. Also, such events are accompanied by uncertainty, including an unclear ratio of risk to benefit. For this reason, implementing a program of preparedness for bioterrorism and similar types of events requires careful consideration of information and communication needs. In the smallpox vaccination program, the uncertainty surrounding the threat created a great need for information among key constituencies.

[1]"Low-likelihood, high-consequence" is a term used in the insurance, emergency management, and other industries to describe events that are infrequent or have a low probability of occurring but would have potentially catastrophic consequences.

Before the beginning of the smallpox vaccination program, the Centers for Disease Control and Prevention (CDC) asked the Institute of Medicine (IOM) to convene an expert committee to advise it on the implementation of a pre-event smallpox vaccination program. The committee was charged with providing "advice to the CDC and the program investigators on selected aspects of the smallpox program implementation and evaluation," including the informed consent process for recipients of smallpox vaccine; professional education and training materials; communication plans developed by CDC for public health and medical professionals and the public; state smallpox vaccination implementation plans; CDC guidelines and instruments to identify potential vaccine recipients at high risk of vaccine adverse events and complications; CDC measures to ensure the early recognition, evaluation, and appropriate treatment of adverse events and complications of smallpox vaccination; CDC plans for collecting and analyzing data on vaccine immunogenicity, adverse events, complications, and vaccine coverage; and the achievement of overall goals of the smallpox vaccination program, such as vaccine coverage rate, equity of access, and adverse reaction rates. The IOM agreed to provide advice through a series of reports responding to CDC's original charge and to new requests that would arise in the course of program implementation.

In a series of six brief timely reports released over 19 months, the committee presented its findings and offered recommendations to help guide the program and, later, its integration into the broader public health preparedness effort. In its first four reports, the committee's recommendations focused on staff training and education, the informed consent and contraindications screening processes, the collection of data, follow-up and conduct of research related to vaccine adverse events, public communication, and the need for vaccine injury compensation. The committee also recommended evaluating all program components (including issues related to cost), defining smallpox preparedness to help establish a baseline or standard against which preparedness efforts could be measured, and using scenarios, including multithreat scenarios, to sharpen national and local plans to respond to smallpox and other threats. In its fifth and sixth reports, the committee responded to CDC's request to comment on its draft indicators of smallpox preparedness (in the context of a larger set of public health preparedness indicators), on the value of using scenarios, and on the state of the science (across other disciplines, such as disaster response) on the conduct of exercises as a strategy for evaluating and testing preparedness. The six individual letter reports have been gathered into a larger archival work that also responds more substantively on the last item in the charge, the achievement of overall goals of the smallpox vaccination program.

This final report consists of four newly written chapters and seven appendixes that contain the committee's body of prior work. The first appendix contains a summary of the recommendations in the committee's six previous reports. The remaining appendixes contain the complete text of the committee's first six reports, released from January 2003 to July 2004 in response to CDC's requests for specific and timely advice, and they reflect in part information gathered at the committee's public meetings held from December 2002 to March 2004.

The report's first chapter, "Smallpox and Smallpox Control in the Historical Context," provides a brief summary of the history of smallpox and its eradication. The historical narrative explains the near-mythic status of smallpox among other dangerous diseases, but it also tells the hopeful story of a disease that was vanquished thanks to an effective vaccine and the coordinated and capable efforts of public health and health care workers around the world.

The second chapter, "Policy Context of Smallpox Preparedness," outlines policies that predated the 2002 smallpox vaccination policy and describes key events and people that contributed to the decision to vaccinate selected groups in advance of a potential smallpox virus release. The chapter is intended to provide some background information about the complex circumstances (such as the high level of public, congressional, and media interest) surrounding the federal government's decision to revive smallpox vaccination. The committee believes that its summary of the program's policy context is consistent with its charge because it highlights early factors that the committee asserts influenced the implementation and outcomes of the vaccination program. Specifically, CDC's difficulties in communicating about the smallpox vaccination policy and program and in securing the participation of public health and medical professionals (the third item in the committee's charge) may be traced to the way the policy and its rationale were communicated to key constituencies.

In the report's third chapter, "The Implementation of the Smallpox Vaccination Program," the committee provides a loosely chronological account of the program's implementation structured around major events, from the president's program announcement in December 2002 to the enactment of a compensation plan for injuries resulting from smallpox vaccination in April 2003 and the June 2003 Advisory Committee on Immunization Practices (ACIP) recommendation to bring pre-event smallpox vaccination to a close. The committee also explores congressional interest in the program and the relationship between the civilian and military smallpox vaccination programs. The chapter includes a discussion of vaccination program challenges. The committee found that the implementation of the program was compromised by operational factors related to broader, strategic issues (examined in Chapter 4). For example, some of the program's challenges were due to its extraordinarily rapid implementation; there was little time to identify and resolve potential difficulties (such as the lack of a compensation plan) or to plan carefully for crucial program components, including materials for prospective vaccinees and the data system. Although rapid implementation would be justified in a crisis, the public and program participants were repeatedly assured that there was no evidence of imminent attack with smallpox virus. Chapter 3 also includes a discussion of favorable outcomes and concludes with a detailed chronology, from events that paved the way for the program through the time of this writing. In this chapter, the committee cites mass media references that document the perspective of key constituencies and their perceptions of the program and the federal government's role. Although media sources are limited in some ways, they provide important insight into the implementation of the program, and the committee has found them concordant with information gathered during the committee's public meetings.

The report's fourth and final chapter, "Lessons Learned from the Smallpox Vaccination Program," constitutes the core of the report, and in that chapter the committee discusses two additional sets of findings from its review of the program and provides a conclusion and a recommendation based on the findings (see Figure ES-1). Trust is a unifying theme among the committee's findings. The committee asserts that a relationship of trust between CDC and the public health and health care communities is a critical requirement in the implementation of biopreparedness programs.

The committee recognized that CDC requested IOM's guidance on the implementation of the program, not on the smallpox vaccination policy itself. Therefore, in its deliberations the committee made every effort to separate the program from the policy-making that preceded it. In Chapter 4, the committee continues its work within the boundaries of the charge by not commenting on the substance of the policy itself. However, the committee's interpretation of its charge is broadened somewhat, allowing it to examine the way the policy and its rationale were communicated and the effects that appeared to have had on the implementation of the program and on the achievement of overall goals of the program (as stated in the last item of the charge).

The smallpox vaccination program involved the implementation of a public health strategy that required the buy-in and participation of numerous public health and health care administrators and personnel. It is a well-documented principle of health promotion planning that the commitment and attitudes of staff who will implement a program are critical to its success, and that they are shaped in the process of communication and information-sharing (Green and Kreuter, 1991). Also, public health practitioners have long known that the activities of community health improvement require "buy-in from those who control what is to be changed" (Nolan, 2004). Smallpox vaccination has been implemented as a public

Key Findings		
Program rationale unclear to key constituencies	**Implementation compromised due to**	**Unknown effect on preparedness**
- Rationale for policy and for program structure not explained clearly - No reiteration or update of the rationale during implementation - No review of program's course or reassessment of starting assumptions - Apparent constraints on CDC's ability to communicate to key constituencies (discussed in Chapter 4)	- Barriers (such as the lack of compensation plan) not removed promptly - Program components (forms, data system) not ready, leading to logistical and practical problems - No revision or clarification of program structure and goals despite confusion and need for clarity (discussed in Chapter 3)	- Are we prepared for a smallpox attack? - Are we prepared to mount another public health biopreparedness program? - Did we learn all we could scientifically about smallpox vaccine? (discussed in Chapter 4)

Conclusion	Recommendation
Based on the lessons learned from the smallpox vaccination program, the committee concludes that a policy strategy and a mechanism are needed to balance the need for scientific evidence and public health analysis with the imperatives of national security, ensuring in the process that the authoritative voice of CDC, the nation's public health leader, will be preserved.	**The committee recommends that, in collaboration with its state and local partners and in the context of broad bioterrorism preparedness, CDC define smallpox preparedness; set goals that reflect the best available scientific and public health reasoning; conduct regular, comprehensive assessments of preparedness at the national level and by state; and communicate to the public about the status of preparedness efforts.**

FIGURE ES-1 Key findings, conclusion, and recommendation.

health component of a national security program, so the principles outlined above apply. It was important to ensure that the people who would implement the program understood and supported the rationale for the program. However, the committee found that the key constituencies expected to play vital roles in the implementation of the vaccination program did not receive sufficient information about the reasoning that led to the program and remained skeptical of the need for pre-event vaccination.

The vaccination policy set expectations for numbers of vaccinees to be reached in three phases beginning with rapid implementation of the first phase, but no explanation for that overall strategy was offered to those who would implement it. For example, when the smallpox vaccination policy ultimately developed by top officials of the executive branch (of which CDC is a part) diverged from the recommendations of ACIP, the panel that advises the government on immunization policy, only vague explanation was given. Although it is understandable that the policy for the public health component of a national security program would be shaped by information from both fields, the national security assessment informing it was not available (except for the caveat that there was no information to suggest that an attack was imminent), and the public health reasoning behind the smallpox vaccination policy and program was never fully explained. Skepticism among key constituencies was followed by a lack of buy-in. Despite their expressed willingness to strengthen preparedness for bioterrorism in general, and their desire to serve their communities, many public health and health care workers were ultimately unwilling to accept the well-known risks of smallpox vaccine in the context of limited information about the risk of smallpox. The lack of buy-in led to poor participation in the vaccination program.

In addition to the fact that the rationale for the program and its structure was not explained, communication with key constituencies created confusion and concern. The typically open and transparent communication from CDC—the nation's public health leader that generally provides guidance for science-based decision-making—seemed constrained by unknown external influences. Furthermore, as the program was experiencing difficulties and appeared to fall short of initial expectations, goals were not clarified or revised in any substantial way. For example, if it was important to vaccinate specific numbers rapidly, what was the effect of the low vaccinee numbers on readiness for a release of smallpox virus? This question went unanswered, as did the larger questions about the definition and requirements of smallpox preparedness.

Based on the lessons learned from the smallpox vaccination program, the committee concludes that a policy strategy and a mechanism are needed to balance the need for scientific evidence and public health analysis with the imperatives of national security, ensuring in the process that the authoritative voice of CDC, the nation's public health leader, will be preserved.

Finally, the committee found that the program's outcomes (for example, the status of smallpox preparedness in each jurisdiction and nationally) are unknown because there has been no systematic assessment of smallpox preparedness, no review of administrative lessons learned, and no accounting of what has been done with the opportunities for scientific research. At the time of this writing, the status of efforts to develop measures and indicators for smallpox (and bioterrorism) preparedness is unknown.

The committee recommends that, in collaboration with its state and local partners and in the context of broad bioterrorism preparedness, CDC define smallpox preparedness; set goals that reflect the best available scientific and public health reasoning; conduct regular, comprehensive assessments of preparedness at the national level and by state; and communicate to the public about the status of preparedness efforts.

The trust of the general public in government's ability to protect the public's health also is a critical requirement for responding to bioterrorism. Conducting and disseminating assessments of national and state preparedness will inform and reassure Americans about the public health system's ability to protect their health and will help jurisdictions continuously improve and learn from the process of preparing for public health emergencies, including a possible smallpox virus release.

It is an unfortunate reality that bioterrorism continues to be a threat. Therefore, future programs to prepare for this type of low-likelihood, high-consequence event will be needed, and the lessons learned from the smallpox vaccination program may help to ensure successful implementation.

REFERENCES

Green L, Kreuter M. 1991. Health Promotion Planning: An Educational and Environmental Approach. Mountain View, California: Mayfield Publishing Company.

Nolan P. 2004. The choice of the public in public health policy and planning: the role of public judgment. *Journal of Public Health Policy* 25(2):209-210.

1

Smallpox and Smallpox Control in the Historical Context

On December 13, 2002, President George W. Bush announced that the United States would begin two programs of smallpox vaccination: a military program, and a voluntary civilian program. The president stated:

> We know, however, that the smallpox virus still exists in laboratories, and we believe that regimes hostile to the United States may possess this dangerous virus. To protect our citizens in the aftermath of September the 11th, we are evaluating old threats in a new light. Our government has no information that a smallpox release is imminent. Yet it is prudent to prepare for the possibility that terrorists would kill indiscriminately—who kill indiscriminately would use diseases as a weapon (White House, 2002).

The president's announcement revived a program of civilian vaccination that the United States discontinued in 1972, after the eradication of naturally occurring smallpox in the Western hemisphere (CDC, 2004).

Smallpox is a highly infectious disease caused by the large and complex variola virus (one of the largest viral genomes known), a member of the family Poxviridae and the genus Orthopoxvirus (WHO, 2001). Although the disease was eradicated over two decades ago and live samples remain in only two known locations, there are concerns that in the wake of the fall of the Soviet Union, samples of the smallpox virus may have fallen in the wrong hands, with the potential of being used as weapons of terror (Henderson et al., 1999). Smallpox virus can be transmitted from person to person, a characteristic that makes it relatively unique among bioterror threats. Given these concerns and recent terror attacks, there has been a surge in interest in the smallpox virus and vaccine and in the history of the disease and its eradication. The potential use of smallpox virus in bioterrorism challenges public health and health care systems in many ways. Smallpox is a disease unfamiliar to most current health care providers, the population of the United States is relatively immunologically naïve since vaccination was discontinued more than thirty years ago, and much of the clinical and epidemiologic data on the virus and the vaccine is decades-old.

A BRIEF HISTORY OF SMALLPOX

The modern history of smallpox disease begins in the seventeenth century, with detailed records of cases and epidemics, as well as the earliest accounts of variolation, a precursor to contemporary immunization which involved inserting particles obtained from smallpox lesions under the skin or into the nostrils of a person who had never had smallpox. In the late eighteenth century, Edward Jenner discovered that dairy maids who had suffered and recovered from the less serious cowpox were not susceptible to smallpox infection, and he subsequently developed and refined the technique of removing material from a human cowpox lesion and transferring it to another person. Jenner vaccinated his own child as a test case, to give confidence in his technique (Fenner et al., 1988).

Jenner published a monograph on the causes and effects of cowpox, in which he speculated about the safety and efficacy of vaccination, the former confirmed by the much milder resulting disease, smaller lesions, and fewer fatalities than variolation, and the latter proven by challenge inoculations with smallpox (Fenner et al., 1988; Radetsky, 1999). Using human sources of cowpox virus presented some technical and medical challenges. Therefore, in 1864, the use of calves as a continuous source of vaccine was expanded from its origins in Italy to the rest of Europe, and then the world (Fenner et al., 1988).

Toward the end of the nineteenth century, vaccination became widespread across Europe and the world, and in the 1920s and 1930s, smallpox cases across Europe and North America dropped to a few dozen per year. The Second World War interrupted many public health efforts, including vaccination, and major epidemics again appeared in Asia and Africa. The World Health Organization (WHO) initiated a program of global smallpox eradication at the 11th World Health Assembly meeting in 1958, and revived it at the 18th World Health Assembly meeting in 1965. The Intensified Smallpox Eradication Program was established in 1967, and the invention of the bifurcated needle allowed for improved and efficient immunization against smallpox in the coordinated mass vaccination and surveillance and containment activities (for example, ring vaccination, described in Chapter 2) that followed (IOM, 1999; Radetsky, 1999). The combined extraordinary efforts of health care and public health workers from across the world led to the eradication of smallpox, officially acknowledged by the WHO in 1980 (Barquet, 1997).

The last endemic case of smallpox in the world occurred in 1977 in Somalia. Since that time, the virus has ceased to exist in the wild, with official repositories for live variola virus remaining only at two secure locations in Atlanta, Georgia, in the United States, and in Novosibirsk, Russia. Subsequently, the WHO Committee on Orthopoxvirus Infections planned a coordinated destruction of all existing stocks of smallpox virus, all stored clinical material containing virus, and all intact virus DNA in June 1999. However, by the late 1990s, the scientific and public health communities had found both scientific and civil defense reasons for retaining the stocks of live virus. In 1998, an Institute of Medicine committee was convened "to assess the scientific and medical information that might be lost were live variola virus no longer available for research purposes" (IOM, 1999). The *Assessment of Future Scientific Needs for Variola Virus* found that "much scientific information, particularly concerning the human immune system, could be learned through experimentation with live variola virus," but "the most compelling need for long-term retention of live variola virus is for the development of antiviral agents or novel vaccines to protect against a reemergence of smallpox due to accidental or intentional release of variola virus" (IOM, 1999). After international dialogue on the fate of the known smallpox virus stocks, the WHO did not proceed with the planned destruction of the virus but resolved to temporarily retain variola stocks for future use in specific scientific endeavors and in research activities related to the preventing and responding to bioterrorism. Variola research accomplishments and outcomes would be reviewed periodically (WHO, 2002, 2003).

UNDERSTANDING THE DISEASE

The last endemic case of smallpox in the United States was in 1949, and vaccination of the general public in this country ended in 1972 (DHHS, 2003). The reintroduction of civilian smallpox vaccination in 2003 called on the public health and health care communities to recall and prepare to fight a mostly forgotten microbe.

Variola virus is a specifically human pathogen, and there are no known animal reservoirs for the disease (Fenner et al., 1988). There are two types of the disease: variola major and variola minor. The latter has been found to cause a much milder form of the disease, with a fatality rate of 1 percent, compared to the 30 percent rate of variola major (Henderson et al., 1999). Five clinical types of variola major have been identified: the ordinary type, the modified type, variola sine eruptione, flat type, and hemorrhagic type (Fenner et al., 1988). Before the eradication of the variola virus, ordinary type smallpox accounted for approximately 90 percent of cases in unvaccinated individuals and 70 percent in previously vaccinated individuals whose immunity had weakened over time (CDC, 2002b).

The variola virus spreads relatively slowly (Fenner et al., 1988). Its transmission generally occurs through aerosols or respiratory-droplet nuclei that settle on the nasal or oropharyngeal mucosal membranes or on the alveoli of the lungs, and also (though less frequently) through infected bedding or clothing. The disease is less infectious than measles or influenza, requiring considerable exposure to an infected person, such as that found in the household or in the health care setting (Breman and Henderson, 2002; Henderson et al., 1999). Furthermore, a person infected with smallpox is not infectious during the incubation stage of the disease, which may range from 7 to 17 days (19 days has also been reported), with a mean of 10-12 days (Breman and Henderson, 2002; Fenner et al., 1988; Henderson et al., 1999; IOM, 1999). Although this stage is free of observable symptoms, it is a period of intense viral replication and spread to internal organs. The disease's prodromal (initial symptoms) stage, which lasts 2 to 4 days, is characterized by the sudden onset of severe headache, backache, and fever, sometimes vomiting, and less frequently, diarrhea (Breman and Henderson, 2002; CDC, 2002a). Individuals in the prodromal stage may be contagious. The prodromal stage is followed by eruption into a rash with lesions on the skin and lesions of the oral mucosa, which shed large amounts of the virus. The early rash stage is followed by the progression of the lesions simultaneously from macules, to papules, which become vesicles, then pustules, and finally, crusts or scabs (CDC, 2002a). Individuals remain infectious, though less so, until the last scab has separated from the skin, 3 to 4 weeks after the onset of the rash (CDC, 2003e).

Smallpox infection leads to a generally distinctive rash. However, smallpox has not been part of the diagnostic experience of most currently practicing health care providers, and smallpox disease could be confused with certain drug reactions and other diseases (such as chickenpox) or skin conditions. The smallpox rash may be distinguished by its centrifugal distribution—lesions are found in greater concentration at the extremities, on the face, hands, and feet, but as the disease progresses, they generally cover the entire body—and the fact that all pustules in a given area develop and progress at the same time rather than in crops (Fenner et al., 1988). Definitive diagnosis can be confirmed in the laboratory; the shape of the variola virus is different from that of varicella-zoster, the cause of chicken pox, and a polymerase-chain-reaction assay is the definitive method for identifying variola virus (Breman and Henderson, 2002).

Controlling and Eradicating Smallpox

The smallpox virus, while a formidable historic threat to health, was eradicated as a result of characteristics of the smallpox virus, the disease, and the vaccine. These characteristics include: a highly effective and very stable vaccine, a noninfectious incubation stage and a disabling prodromal stage that limited the mobility of infected individuals, a distinctive rash that made smallpox cases readily identifiable and helped to facilitate limiting the spread of the disease, and the fact that humans are the only known reservoir for variola virus (IOM, 1999).

At the time smallpox was endemic in much of the world, smallpox vaccination proved to be highly effective in preventing smallpox infection, and in the rare cases where symptoms of the disease occurred, they were milder, and the disease was far less likely to be fatal. In addition to vaccination's prophylactic value, there is historic evidence that administering the vaccine within three days of a suspected exposure to smallpox virus can prevent the onset of the disease or significantly lessen its severity (Breman and Henderson, 2002; Lane and Goldstein, 2003). Although the smallpox vaccine is very effective, it was its use in conjunction with surveillance and containment that ultimately brought the disease under control and culminated in the eradication of the disease (Fenner et al., 1988).

Vaccine Efficacy

Experience documented during the global smallpox eradication campaign has shown that smallpox vaccine is highly effective, but its efficacy has not been measured with precision in controlled studies (CDC, 2003a). The Dryvax® vaccine (used in the vaccination campaign begun in 2003) was used successfully to eradicate smallpox in West and Central Africa and other areas during the global campaign. The scar showing previous vaccination signified that an individual was protected against smallpox, and in household contact studies, there was a 90 percent reduction in smallpox among contacts with a vaccine scar, compared to those without (CDC, 2003a).

The need for vaccination disappeared along with the disease itself. By 2002, some Americans had not been vaccinated against smallpox in over three decades, and the remainder had never been vaccinated. It is unclear what level of vaccine-induced immunity remains in previously vaccinated Americans; past evidence on the efficacy and durability of protection provided by vaccination is limited (Henderson, 1988). According to one estimate, fewer than 20 percent of persons vaccinated before 1972 retain immunologic protection (CIDRAP and IDSA, 2004). Other twentieth-century data show that vaccinated individuals have a high level of protection for up to 5 years, and some level of immunity, while diminishing over time, may persist for up to 10 years, and perhaps even longer (CDC, 2001; Cohen, 2001; WHO, 2001; Eichner, 2003). Current research is still in its early stages and takes place in the absence of actual smallpox disease, relying instead on three surrogate measures of immunity: neutralizing antibody, cellular immunity, and skin reactions. There is some evidence that significant immunity may be maintained beyond five to ten years after vaccination. Crotty and colleagues (2003) found that smallpox-vaccine–specific memory B cells may persist for longer than 50 years after immunization. Also, Hammarlund and colleagues (2003) found that more than 90 percent of volunteers vaccinated 25-75 years ago exhibited stable levels of vaccinia-specific antibody, and persisting, though diminishing antiviral T-cell response. There is little agreement whether these findings can be interpreted to mean that individuals vaccinated before 1972 would have any significant level of protection against smallpox (Roos, 2003). Additional research is needed to shed more light on this complex matter.

Smallpox Vaccine and Vaccination

Dryvax vaccine is a highly stable, live-virus vaccine containing the vaccinia virus, another orthopoxvirus. Vaccinia's origins are unclear, as it differs from Jenner's "variolae vaccinae," but vaccinia has been widely studied, and much of what is known about orthopox viruses was first learned from this species (Fenner et al., 1988).

Immunization with vaccinia-based vaccines involves inoculation of the skin using a bifurcated needle that holds a dose of the vaccine (a small drop) in its fork, and that is first used to release the liquid on the skin and then, held perpendicular to the skin, to rapidly and vigorously puncture the skin in an area of about 5 mm diameter, making a trace of blood appear (CDC, 2003c).[1] Reaction to the vaccine, or "vaccine take," can be evaluated based on the appearance of the skin lesion that develops after vaccination. There are two types of reactions: major and equivocal. A major reaction, proof of successful vaccination, consists of "a pustular lesion or an area of definite induration or congestion surrounding a central lesion, which might be a scab or an ulcer" (CDC, 2003d). The size of lesions peaks between days 8 and 12, and the infection is sometimes accompanied by mild fever and malaise. Three weeks after vaccination, the scab falls off, leaving a small

[1]CDC recommended 15 punctures for secondary vaccinees and 3 punctures for primary vaccinees (CDC, 2003c).

pitted scar (IOM, 1999). Any type of reaction that is not a major reaction is considered equivocal and indicates that revaccination is necessary.

In 1999, the Working Group on Civilian Biodefense, an expert panel convened by the Center for Civilian Biodefense Studies at Johns Hopkins University (now the Center for Biosecurity at the University of Pittsburgh Medical Center) acknowledged that a deliberate release of smallpox virus was in the realm of possibility and that such an event would require widespread vaccination (Henderson et al., 1999). However, until the fall of 2001, smallpox vaccine had FDA approval only for use in a very small group of laboratory workers, and a limited supply of smallpox vaccine existed under the control of the Centers for Disease Control and Prevention (CDC), containing the New York City Board of Health (NYCBH) vaccinia virus strain grown on scarified calves, and produced by Wyeth laboratories under the trade name Dryvax (Henderson et al., 1999).

The policy changes that revived civilian smallpox vaccination and vaccine research, development, and production in the United States are discussed in Chapter 2.

The Vaccine Supplies Available in the United States

At the time the military and civilian smallpox vaccination programs began in late 2002 and early 2003, respectively, the federal government had access to two stores of smallpox vaccine: 15 million doses of Dryvax in government storage since 1982, and 70-90 million doses of Aventis Pasteur vaccine available from the company (Lueck, 2002; Roos, 2002; CDC, 2003b). Both vaccines were derived from the NYCBH strain of vaccinia virus, but Dryax was stored frozen in dry form, while the Aventis vaccine was stored frozen as a liquid. A clinical trial of Dryvax conducted by the National Institute of Allergy and Infectious Disease (NIAID) showed that the vaccine was viable and could be diluted fivefold and even tenfold and retain its efficacy, as shown by high "take" rates (Fauci, 2003; Frey et al., 2002; NIH, 2002). A later dilution study of Aventis Pasteur (also derived from the NYCBH strain) vaccine showed similarly high vaccination success rates among the three dilution groups (Talbot et al., 2004). Diluting existing vaccine and efforts to develop new vaccines provided assurance that enough vaccine would soon be available to protect all Americans in case of an attack with smallpox virus.

In 2002, changes to the diluent used for Dryvax required that the vaccine be relicensed by the Food and Drug Administration (FDA). On October 25, 2002, FDA approved a new 100-dose kit for Dryvax that included a new supply of diluent (to be mixed with the dried vaccine before it is administered) and bifurcated needles for vaccine administration (FDA, 2004). Each available lot would be approved separately. At the time civilian vaccination began, 6.7 million doses of the undiluted Dryvax vaccine were approved for distribution as a licensed vaccine: 1 million doses for use in the military vaccination program, and the remaining 5.7 million doses for the Department of Health and Human Services to be used for smallpox preparedness vaccination activities. New vaccine then under production was not expected to be available as a licensed product until 2004, but in the event of a smallpox release, the government planned to use available vaccine under Investigational New Drug protocol for mass vaccination.

In September 2000, CDC awarded Acambis Inc. a contract for a stockpile of 40 million doses of smallpox vaccine, and the contract was later increased to 54 million doses (DHHS, 2001). In November 2001, a second contract was awarded by DHHS to Acambis in partnership with Baxter Healthcare Corporation to produce an additional 155 million doses of vaccine for the U.S. government (DHHS, 2001). Although the Acambis vaccines, ACAM1000 and ACAM2000, are also derived from the NYCBH strain, they are grown in two types of cell culture rather than on the skin of a calf (Dryvax) (FDA, 2004). The Department of Defense is also supporting the clinical development of a cell culture vaccine by DynPort Corporation (PRNewswire, 2002).

Vaccine Safety

Vaccination is an effective public health tool in cases where the known risks of the vaccine are weighed against the known benefits of the vaccine and the risk of disease. Smallpox vaccination is known to cause generally mild symptoms and only rarely has resulted in more severe infection or death. Given the remarkable severity of smallpox disease, and the high effectiveness of the vaccine, the risk-benefit ratio was very clear while the disease was endemic. Historic objections to vaccination were made on moral or philosophical grounds and not on the basis of vaccine safety. It had always been known that smallpox vaccine was not innocuous, and as smallpox cases dropped to zero in industrialized nations, the adverse outcomes related to vaccination became more worrying. The case-fatality rate for smallpox vaccines in 1968 was one per one million primary vaccinations, and children had higher rates (number of events per million primary vaccinees) of severe vaccine-related complications when compared with primary vaccinees age 20 and older (Breman and Henderson, 2002). This was part of the reason the United States halted vaccination of the general public in 1972. At the end of the century, analysis of the risks posed by the vaccine could only be assessed in the context of a disease presenting no cases, leading to a significantly different risk-benefit balance.

Vaccine safety findings must also be viewed in the context of differences between the experience of developing nations and that of developed nations. The reaction rate of vaccinees in developing countries may be confounded by malnutrition, co-infections, and other factors. Furthermore, experience with smallpox vaccine in the United States was largely in infants, and adequate surveillance among adults may have been lacking. Specific events, such as the New York smallpox outbreak in 1947 provide some evidence about vaccinating adults. Four main complications may be associated with vaccination; three complications are in the form of skin eruptions (eczema vaccinatum, progressive vaccinia, and generalized vaccinia) and a fourth, and the most serious, is postvaccinial encephalitis (CIDRAP and IDSA, 2004). Two studies conducted in 1968, a national study and a 10 state study of these complications, provide somewhat different estimates of vaccine adverse event rates, reflecting differences in methods and case definitions (for example, the case definition of generalized vaccinia). In the national survey, 14 million people were vaccinated, leading to a total of 9 deaths, 11 cases of progressive vaccinia, 74 cases of eczema vaccinatum, 143 cases of generalized vaccinia, and 16 cases of encephalitis (WHO, 2001). Based on such historic data, 1,000 per million primary vaccinees would experience severe adverse events, and 14 to 52 individuals per million primary vaccinees would experience life-threatening reactions to the vaccine (i.e., eczema vaccinatum, progressive vaccinia, and post-vaccinal encephalitis), and 1 or 2 people would die (CDC, 2003g). Although recent smallpox vaccination has been associated with adverse events affecting the heart (discussed in Chapter 3), studies of death certificates of vaccine-associated deaths were conducted in 1959-1966 and in 1968 did not find deaths associated with cardiac complications (CDC, 2003f).

The vaccine's side effects are known to include malaise and fever that could interfere with a person's ability to work, therefore raising questions about the need for time off, with implications for the workforce and for staff scheduling. In the dilution study of Aventis Pasteur vaccine, 25 percent of volunteers missed regularly scheduled duties due to vaccine-related symptoms (Talbot et al., 2004).

Because of those safety concerns and the changed risk-benefit balance in the face of the limited number of cases of disease, the United States ceased general vaccination in 1972, several years before smallpox was officially declared eradicated. After the terrorist attacks of 2001, the safety of the vaccine came into focus as one of the most significant factors in decision-making (see below). Smallpox vaccination plans included vaccinia immune globulin (available in very limited quantity in 2002) and cidofovir as first- and second-line therapies, respectively, for treatment of serious vaccine-related complications (CIDRAP and IDSA, 2004; CDC, 2003h).

Surveillance and Containment

Although vaccination was responsible for the dramatic drop in smallpox deaths during the first decades of the twentieth century, its success was at least in part due to the use of vaccination in conjunction with public health strategies of surveillance and containment. Even compared to mass vaccination, surveillance and containment are thought to have provided the more effective means of controlling the spread of smallpox disease (Fenner et al., 1988).

Epidemiologic study of the spread of smallpox in Pakistan and Bangladesh in the 1960s demonstrated that the disease was not widely disseminated, but occurred in clusters, transmitted through close personal contact (Fenner et al., 1988). To cope most effectively with this type of disease distribution, smallpox eradication teams emphasized the identification of cases and the containment of outbreaks, a strategy termed surveillance and containment. A critical component of this strategy was the program known as ring vaccination. When a smallpox case was identified, all immediate contacts and their households were identified and vaccinated (ACIP, 2002). Any individuals who then developed a fever were isolated. In this way, an initial case was effectively surrounded with (or ringed by) vaccinated individuals, virtually stopping transmission to others in the population (CIDRAP and IDSA, 2004). Historic evidence also suggests that surveillance and containment worked well not only in populations with a high level of immunity, but also in areas where population immunity was relatively low (e.g., due to lack of vaccination) (IOM, 1999).

Contemporary Circumstances

A smallpox release in today's world would present new clinical and epidemiologic challenges. For example, a significant proportion of the population in the United States (most individuals born after 1972) has never been vaccinated against smallpox. This means that there is little or no herd immunity, and previously identified patterns of disease spread may not apply (Gani and Leach, 2001). Furthermore, the current population includes more very elderly people and individuals with immune systems impaired due to chemotherapy, preparation for organ transplantation, or HIV infection.

Vaccination strategies that were successful in the past might be less successful in the contemporary context. Ring vaccination that was an effective means of controlling disease transmission among developing country populations that may have been significantly less mobile may not work for today's highly mobile populations. There are further concerns about ways in which the deliberate introduction of smallpox virus could differ from naturally occurring smallpox (for example, multiple points of simultaneous introduction or repeated attacks) (Fauci, 2002). There has also been speculation about the existence of weaponized smallpox, a pathogen with some different characteristics from naturally-occurring Variola virus, including potentially less protection afforded by existing vaccine.

Although epidemiologic data about smallpox disease is substantial, one of the difficulties of relying on historic data to assess smallpox infectivity is the fact that these data were collected in a context of significant population immunity. As smallpox vaccination was discontinued, successive generations of children were born and grew to adulthood without vaccination, gradually decreasing the immunity of the population. This means that whereas past findings showed that an initial case of smallpox could infect at most 5 others, a case caused by a contemporary deliberate release of the disease could potentially infect more, perhaps as many as 10 additional persons (WHO, 2001).

Concluding Observations

Smallpox disease has been unknown for over two decades. Routine immunization has been discontinued for many years, new generations of clinicians have little knowledge of the disease, and the United States population is characterized by significant numbers of people with weakened immune systems (e.g., due to cancer chemotherapy, HIV infection). As the nation's public health and health care systems contemplated the possibility of a deliberate release of smallpox virus by terrorists, these factors were reasons for concern, subjects of research, and considerations for vaccination plans and other types of preparedness activities.

REFERENCES

ACIP (Advisory Committee on Immunization Practices). 2002. Record of the Meeting of the Advisory Committee on Immunization Practices, June 19-20, 2002. Centers for Disease Control and Prevention, National Immunization Program, Atlanta, GA.

Barquet NDP. 1997. Smallpox: the triumph over the most terrible of the ministers of death. *Annals of Internal Medicine* 127:635-642.

Breman JG, Henderson DA. 2002. Diagnosis and management of smallpox. *New England Journal of Medicine* 346(17):1300-1308.

CDC (Centers for Disease Control and Prevention). 2001. Vaccinia (Smallpox) vaccine: recommendations of the Advisory Committee on Immunization Practices (ACIP), 2001. *Morbidity and Mortality Weekly Report* 50(RR-10):1-25.

CDC. 2002a. Smallpox Fact Sheet: Smallpox Disease Overview. [Online] Available at http://www.bt.cdc.gov/agent/smallpox/overview/disease-facts.asp. Accessed September 13, 2004.

CDC. 2002b. Smallpox Response Plan and Guidelines (Version 3.0). [Online] Available at http://www.bt.cdc.gov/agent/smallpox/response-plan/. Accessed January 9, 2003.

CDC. 2003a. Course: "Smallpox: Disease, Prevention, and Intervention." Module 5: Smallpox Vaccine Overview.

CDC. 2003b. Questions and Answers: Smallpox Vaccination Program Implementation. [Online] Available at http://www.bt.cdc.gov/agent/smallpox/vaccination/vaccination-program-qa.asp. Accessed March 10, 2003.

CDC. 2003c. Smallpox Fact Sheet—Information for Clinicians: Smallpox Vaccination Method.

CDC. 2003d. Smallpox Vaccination Status and Procedures—Guidelines for Grantees Using Licensed Undiluted Wyeth Dryvax Vaccine.

CDC. 2003e. Smallpox Response Plan and Guidelines. Executive Summary. (Updated).

CDC. 2003f. Cardiac adverse events following smallpox vaccination—United States, 2003. *Morbidity and Mortality Weekly Report* 52(12):248-250.

CDC. 2003g. Smallpox Fact Sheet: Side Effects of Smallpox Vaccination. [Online] Available at http://www.bt.cdc.gov/agent/smallpox/vaccination/reactions-vacc-public.asp. Accessed September 7, 2004.

CDC. 2003h. Smallpox vaccination and adverse reactions: guidance for clinicians. *Morbidity and Mortality Weekly Report Dispatch* 52:1-29.

CDC. 2004. Smallpox Fact Sheet: Vaccine Overview. [Online] Available at http://www.bt.cdc.gov/agent/smallpox/vaccination/facts.asp. Accessed January 26, 2005.

CIDRAP (Center for Infectious Disease Research and Policy) and IDSA (Infectious Disease Society of America). 2004. Smallpox: Current, Comprehensive Information on Pathogenesis, Microbiology, Epidemiology, Diagnosis, Treatment, and Prophylaxis. [Online] Available at http://www.cidrap.umn.edu/cidrap/content/bt/smallpox/biofacts/smllpx-summary.html. Accessed August 2004.

Cohen J. 2001. Smallpox vaccinations: how much protection remains? *Science* 294(5544):985.

Crotty S, Felgner P, Davies H, Glidewell J, Villarreal L, Ahmed R. 2003. Cutting edge: long-term B cell memory in humans after smallpox vaccination. *Journal of Immunology* 171(10):4969-4973.

DHHS (Department of Health and Human Services). 2001. News Release: HHS Awards $428 Million Contract to Produce Smallpox Vaccine. Acambis/Baxter Will Produce 155 million Doses by End of 2002. [Online] Available at http://www.hhs.gov/news/press/2001pres/20011128.html. Accessed January 26, 2005.

DHHS. 2003. FAQs About Smallpox: The Disease and the Vaccine. [Online] Available at http://www.smallpox.gov/QuestionsAnswers.html. Accessed August 1, 2004.

Eichner M. 2003. Analysis of historical data suggests long-lasting protective effects of smallpox vaccination. *American Journal of Epidemiology* 158:717-723.

Fauci A. 2003. NIH's Role in Implementing a Smallpox Vaccination Program. Testimony before the Senate Committee on Appropriations: Subcommittee on Labor, HHS, Education and Related Agencies, January 30, 2003.

Fauci AS. 2002. Smallpox vaccination policy—the need for dialogue. *New England Journal of Medicine* 346(17):1319-1320.

FDA (Food and Drug Administration). 2004. Smallpox Vaccines: Questions and Answers. [Online] Available at http://www.fda.gov/cber/vaccine/smallpox.htm#lic. Accessed November 14, 2004.

Fenner F, Henderson D, Arita A, Jezek Z, Ladnyi I. 1988. Smallpox and Its Eradication. Geneva: World Health Organization.

Frey SE, Couch RB, Tacket CO, Treanor JJ, Wolff M, Newman FK, Atmar RL, Edelman R, Nolan CM, Belshe RB. 2002. Clinical Responses to Undiluted and Diluted Smallpox Vaccine. *New England Journal of Medicine* 346(17):1265-1274.

Gani R, Leach S. 2001. Transmission potential of smallpox in contemporary populations. *Nature* 414(6865):748-751.

Hammarlund E, Lewis M, Hansen S, Strelow L, Nelson J , Sexton G, Hanifin J, Slifka M. 2003. Duration of antiviral immunity after smallpox vaccination. *Nature Medicine* 9(9):1131-1137.

Henderson D. 1988. Smallpox and Vaccinia. In: Plotkin SA, Mortimer EA, eds. *Vaccines*. Philadelphia: WB Saunders Company, Harcourt Brace Jovanovich, Inc., pp. 8-30.

Henderson DA, Inglesby TV, Bartlett JG, Ascher MS, Eitzen E, Jahrling PB, Hauer J, Layton M, McDade J, Osterholm MT, O'Toole T, Parker G, Perl T, Russell PK, Tonat K, for the Working Group on Civilian Biodefense. 1999. Smallpox as a biological weapon: medical and public health management. *Journal of the American Medical Association* 281(22):2127-2137.

IOM (Institute of Medicine). 1999. Assessment of Future Scientific Needs for Live Variola Virus. Washington, DC: National Academy Press.

Lane J, Goldstein J. 2003. Evaluation of 21st-century risks of smallpox vaccination and policy options. *Annals of Internal Medicine* 138(6):488-493.

Lueck S. 2002, March 29. Drug Maker Finds Millions of Doses of Smallpox Vaccine in Storage. *Wall Street Journal*.

NIH (National Institutes of Health). 2002, March. Press Release: NIAID Study Results Support Diluting Smallpox Vaccine Stockpile to Stretch Supply. [Online] Available at http://www2.niaid.nih.gov/newsroom/releases/smallpox.htm. Accessed January 30, 2005.

PRNewswire. 2002, April 26. DynCorp Company Enters Phase I Smallpox Vaccine Clinical Trial. [Online] Available at http://www.prnewswire.com/gh/cnoc/comp/260725. Accessed January 3, 2005.

Radetsky M. 1999. Smallpox: a history of its rise and fall. *Pediatric Infectious Disease Journal* 18(2):85-93.

Roos R. 2002, March 28. Aventis has cache of up to 90 million doses of smallpox vaccine. *CIDRAP News*.

Roos R. 2003, August 21. D.A. Henderson critiques report on duration of smallpox immunity. *CIDRAP News*.

Talbot T, Stapleton J, Bready R, Winokur P, Bernstein D, Germanson T, Yoder S, Rock M, Crowe J, Edwards K. 2004. Vaccination success rate and reaction proficle with diluted and undiluted smallpox vaccine: a randomized controlled trial. *Journal of the American Medical Association* 292(10):1205-1212.

White House. 2002. President Delivers Remarks on Smallpox. [Online] Available at http://www.whitehouse.gov/news/releases/2002/12/20021213-7.html. Accessed January 8, 2003.

WHO (World Health Organization). 2001. WHO Fact Sheet on Smallpox. [Online] Available at http://www.who.int/emc/diseases/smallpox/factsheet.html. Accessed July 23, 2004.

WHO. 2002. Smallpox Eradication: Destruction of Variola Virus Stocks. Executive Board 111th Session, Provisional agenda item 5.3. WHO Document EB111/5.

WHO. 2003. WHO Advisory Committee on Variola Virus Research: Report of the Fifth Meeting. Geneva: World Health Organization. Global Health Security, Epidemic Alert and Response.

2

Policy Context of Smallpox Preparedness

In 1980, the World Health Organization (WHO) declared smallpox eradicated, three years after the last endemic case of smallpox and after two years of effective surveillance that enabled the certification of a final few nations as smallpox-free. With eradication came a series of policy changes that brought to an end general vaccination against smallpox and the production of smallpox vaccine in the United States. In 1980, the Advisory Committee on Immunization Practices (ACIP),[1] the federal advisory body that develops guidance and recommendations for national immunization policy, recommended smallpox vaccination only for particular groups of laboratory workers (CDC, 2001). In 1982, Wyeth ceased production of smallpox vaccine for general use, and a Centers for Disease Control and Prevention (CDC) notice in *Morbidity and Mortality Weekly Report* informed readers that smallpox vaccine would no longer be available to civilians (CDC, 1983). Military smallpox vaccination from 1984 was limited to recruits entering basic training, and it was finally discontinued in 1990 (DOD, 2002).

[1]ACIP is a federal advisory body consisting of 15 experts in fields associated with immunization. ACIP members are selected by the Secretary of Health and Human Services to provide advice and guidance to the secretary, the assistant secretary for health, and the Centers for Disease Control and Prevention on the most effective means to prevent vaccine-preventable diseases. ACIP develops written recommendations for the routine administration of vaccines to the pediatric and adult populations and schedules regarding the appropriate periodicity, dosage, and contraindications applicable to the vaccines (CDC, 2004a).

In 1991, ACIP updated its recommendations regarding the use of smallpox vaccine for occupational exposures to include "health-care workers involved in clinical trials using recombinant vaccinia virus vaccines" and lengthened to 10 years the recommendation for revaccination of relevant groups of laboratory workers (CDC, 2001). A series of domestic and international terrorist attacks occurred over the decade that followed, ranging from sarin gas attacks on the Tokyo subway to anthrax attacks by mail in the United States. Those developments stimulated robust discussion of the need for new public health policy and legislation to confront the possibility of bioterrorist attack. When the 1991 ACIP recommendations were updated in June 2001, they included "recommendations for the use of vaccinia vaccine if smallpox (variola) virus were used as an agent of biological terrorism or if a smallpox outbreak were to occur for another unforeseen reason" (CDC, 2001). ACIP concluded that recommendations regarding pre-exposure vaccination should be on the basis of a calculable risk assessment that considers the risk for disease and the benefits and risks regarding vaccination. Because the current risk for exposure is considered low, benefits of vaccination do not outweigh the risk regarding vaccine complications. If the potential for an intentional release of smallpox virus increases later, pre-exposure vaccination might become indicated for selected groups (e.g., medical and public health personnel or laboratory workers) who would have an identified higher risk for exposure because of work-related contact with smallpox patients or infectious materials.

After the events of 2001, the possibility of future bioterrorism and the specter of deliberate exposure to the smallpox virus, a dangerous category A pathogen,[2] caused CDC to reconsider smallpox vaccination as a tool for preparedness. CDC requested that ACIP provide an update of recommendations for the use of smallpox vaccine. The Department of Health and Human Services (DHHS) began to assess the status of smallpox vaccine stocks and initiated planning and activities for increasing the vaccine stocks, and CDC, the National Institutes of Health, and the Department of Defense intensified their work in the development of new vaccines (such as safer or less reactogenic smallpox vaccines) to prepare effectively for a potential smallpox virus release (Cohen and Marshall, 2001). The Public Health Security and Bioterrorism Preparedness and Response Act of 2002, signed into law on June 12, 2002, included provisions for supporting smallpox vaccine development.

[2]This CDC classification denotes biologic agents that: are easy to disseminate or transmit person-to-person; cause high mortality; might cause public panic and social disruption; and require special action for public health preparedness (CDC, 2000, 2002a).

STEPS TOWARD READINESS FOR A SMALLPOX VIRUS RELEASE

Role of Public Health Organizations

Over the 15 months between September 11, 2001, and the announcement of the smallpox vaccination policy on December 13, 2002, CDC, other government agencies, public health organizations, and other interested professional groups had extensive and productive interactions that led to the development of smallpox response plans and the discussion of strategies to prepare for a potential smallpox threat (Alliance for Health Reform, 2002; ASTHO, 2001; McIlroy, 2002). For example, the Association of State and Territorial Health Officials (ASTHO), the National Association of County and City Health Officials, the American Public Health Association, the Association of Public Health Laboratories, and the Council of State and Territorial Epidemiologists (CSTE) interacted regularly to discuss needs and strategies for bioterrorism (including smallpox) preparedness and urged the federal government to focus on increasing bioterrorism preparedness and to improve public health infrastructure funding (ASTHO, 2002). ASTHO also testified about public health preparedness on October 3, 2001, before the Senate Subcommittee on Labor, Health and Human Services, and Education Appropriations (ASTHO, 2001). At that hearing, ASTHO recommended that a national plan be developed for responding to a smallpox virus release, including vaccine delivery and administration.

CDC's Smallpox Vaccination and Preparedness Activities

Shortly after the 2001 attacks, CDC took steps to strengthen its internal smallpox response capacity by forming 20 multidisciplinary smallpox response teams of 10 persons each and vaccinating them (ACIP, 2002; Altman, 2002a). CDC also adopted a two-pronged approach to strengthening the ability of the nation's state and local public health agencies to respond effectively to a smallpox virus release: pre-event planning and activities (largely involving the advance vaccination of specific types of personnel who would respond to an attack) and post-event planning and activities, pertaining to the personnel, resources, facilities, and capabilities necessary for effective response. The present Institute of Medicine (IOM) committee was charged with providing guidance to CDC on subjects related to the pre-event smallpox vaccination program, and this task has been the committee's main focus. Therefore, the present report briefly mentions post-event planning only as part of the setting for the smallpox vaccination program and smallpox preparedness in general.

On November 21, 2001, CDC published the federal Post-Event Smallpox Response Plan and Guidelines and forwarded it to state and local public health agencies. In the October 2002 version[3] of the Post-Event Response Plan and Guidelines, CDC asked states and the District of Columbia, the territories, and the nation's three largest municipalities (all CDC grantees under the Cooperative Agreement on Public Health Preparedness and Response for Bioterrorism) to develop their own post-event plans and to submit them to CDC by December 12, 2002 (CDC, 2002f). The Post-Event Response Plan and Guidelines included a description of a model smallpox vaccination clinic and provided instruction on all aspects of planning, setting up, and operating voluntary vaccination clinics on a large scale. On November 22, 2002, CDC issued Supplemental Guidance for Planning and Implementing the National Smallpox Vaccination Program; this guidance added specific smallpox vaccination and planning requirements to the Cooperative Agreement on Public Health Preparedness and Response for Bioterrorism. States, territories, three municipalities and the District of Columbia were asked to submit their pre-event vaccination plans by December 9, 2002 (CDC, 2002e). In addition to the pre-event and post-event programmatic guidance, CDC provided a series of smallpox-related training opportunities to help to develop the knowledge and skills of public health workers and clinicians, including video training, webcasts, slide sets, and other training materials on topics from vaccine administration to the clinical diagnosis of smallpox (CDC, 2004b). It is important to note that training and education activities occurred in an unusual context, in preparation for responding to a disease unfamiliar to most health care providers and public health workers, and a disease for which the evidence base is decades old.

Evolution of the Smallpox Vaccination Policy

The policy for pre-event smallpox vaccination was developed while discussion was occurring and guidance was being issued at several different levels: CDC gave ACIP several options and questions to consider and asked it to make recommendations about smallpox vaccination; federal officials considered the various strategies for pre-event vaccination; the White House was debating vaccination approaches; IOM was asked by CDC to hold a forum for discussing vaccination options; and an array of public health partners and others contributed recommendations and advice. The minutes and recommendations of ACIP, the variety of public opinion on the matter, and the perspectives of public health organizations are documented in this and subsequent chapters. There is little information, however, about the

[3]The Post-Event Smallpox Response Plan and Guidelines also underwent several updates from December 2003 to June 2004.

decision-making process at the highest levels of government. A lack of information about the development of health policy does not always provoke concern. However, the nature of the decisions about the smallpox vaccination program use of a vaccine with known potential complications to protect against an eradicated disease has brought into question the evidence, data, and reasoning that contributed to the fashioning of the final policy.

Rationale for the Policy

The smallpox vaccination policy announced in December 2002 was unusual in bringing together a national security program with a public health strategy. The president stated on December 13, 2002, that "we believe that regimes hostile to the United States may possess this dangerous virus" (White House, 2002). The initial policy announcement and later clarifications by DHHS provided little information about the threat assessment other than reassuring the public that there was no information to suggest that a smallpox virus release was imminent. The combination of known vaccine-related problems and unmeasurable disease threat was deeply problematic, and was reminiscent of the challenges faced by decision makers who planned the swine influenza campaign of 1976 discussed in Chapter 4.

The intelligence considered in the development of the policy was not shared with the public or with those who would be called upon to respond to a smallpox event. However, coverage in the print and broadcast media provided fragments of information about intelligence and speculation about the suspected location of smallpox virus around the world. In 2002, the mass media reported that two unnamed U.S. government officials who had received classified briefings revealed that the federal government had information about Iraq's possession of smallpox virus. Other news reports suggested that North Korea, Iraq, Russia, and France might possess stocks of smallpox, and reported on the smallpox vaccination status of Iraqi prisoners of war, and reported on other possible indications that the Iraqi bioweapons program included smallpox (Boyle, 2002; Gellman, 2002).

In fall 2002, the possibility of war with Iraq loomed, owing in part to fears that Iraq possessed weapons of mass destruction. At the same time, the federal government named Iraq as one of the nations suspected of possessing smallpox stocks that could be used in a bioterrorist attack (Manning and Sternberg, 2002; Meckler, 2002b; National Journal Group, 2002). This may help to explain the perception of many in the public health and health care communities that the government's decisions about the Iraq war and some of the considerations leading to the smallpox vaccination policy were associated in some way, and this perception later influenced the course of the vaccination program (Krupnick, 2003; Kuhles and Ackman, 2003; Manning, 2003; McNeil, 2003). The comments of legislators and other officials that may have contributed to this perception are discussed in Chapter 4.

June 2002 ACIP Meeting

In 2001, CDC asked ACIP to review the recommendations for smallpox vaccination in light of the recent anthrax attacks. ACIP met in June 2002 to review and discuss vaccination needs for smallpox readiness. At the time of the meeting, the vaccination policy options being considered (see Box 2-1) revolved around two key issues: in the pre-event scenario, identifying who, if anyone, should be vaccinated before a smallpox virus release (issue is addressed by questions 1 and 2), and in the post-event scenario, identifying what vaccination strategy should be used (that is, ring vs. mass vaccination, addressed by a third question not included in Box 2-1). The second issue, in the post-event scenario, is outside this IOM committee's charge and will not be discussed here. ACIP achieved consensus on Option 1 for Question 1 (against recommending vaccination of the general public in the absence of a confirmed smallpox case or attack) and on Option 2 for Question 2 (for restricting pre-event vaccination of designated persons who would have direct contact with or be called upon to investigate initial cases of smallpox) (ACIP, 2003). The groups targeted for such limited vaccination were later defined in greater detail as smallpox public health response teams and smallpox health care teams, or people who would conduct public health investigation and implement other public health activities and those who would provide medical care to people infected with smallpox virus (CDC, 2002c). Although ACIP did not provide a target number of vaccinees at its meeting, ACIP Chairperson John Modlin suggested in a CDC telebriefing that up to 20,000[4] designated smallpox response team members with specific functional roles (health care and public health response) would be an appropriate target for pre-event vaccination (Brown, 2002b; CDC, 2002b; Roos, 2002; Maguire, 2003). That recommendation reflected the most limited of the pre-event vaccination options that ACIP considered. ACIP members explained that risks related to the vaccine and what was known about the risk of attack were factors used in making the recommendation (Brown, 2002a).

---

[4]The ACIP chairperson provided an estimate of 10,000-20,000. Media reports have cited the figure as either 20,000 or 15,000, the midpoint of the range. To avoid confusing the reader, "up to 20,000" will be used in this report in referring to ACIP's initial target number for pre-event smallpox vaccination.

BOX 2-1
CDC's Draft Policy Options

CDC asked ACIP to consider three questions and develop options under each. The results of its deliberations, presented as options, follow each question. The following two questions refer to pre-event vaccination. A third question about post-event vaccination options is not provided below.

Question 1: With no known cases of smallpox worldwide, should there be any change in the current recommendation for not vaccinating members of the general public?

Option 1: In the absence of a confirmed smallpox case or a confirmed smallpox bioterrorism attack, ACIP does not recommend vaccination of members of the general public (i.e., no change from the current recommendation).

Option 2: In the absence of a confirmed smallpox case or a confirmed smallpox bioterrorism attack, ACIP does not recommend that members of the general public be vaccinated; however, members of the general public may choose to be vaccinated. (This is a negative recommendation by ACIP, but there is choice by members of the public.)

Option 3: In the absence of a confirmed smallpox case or a confirmed smallpox bioterrorism attack, ACIP recommendations for smallpox vaccine do not now include members of the general public; however, members of the general public may choose to be vaccinated. (ACIP is neutral, and there is choice by the public.)

Option 4: In the absence of a confirmed smallpox case or a confirmed smallpox bioterrorism attack, ACIP recommends vaccination for those members of the general public who decide to receive the vaccination.

Question 2: In addition to laboratory workers who work with viruses related to smallpox, are there other individuals in specific occupational groups who should be vaccinated to enhance smallpox preparedness? If so, what guidelines should be used to determine which individuals should be vaccinated?

Option 1: In the absence of a confirmed smallpox case or a confirmed smallpox bioterrorism attack, ACIP does not recommend pre-exposure vaccination for any individuals other than laboratory or medical personnel who work with non-highly attenuated orthopox viruses.

Option 2: In the absence of a confirmed smallpox case or a confirmed smallpox bioterrorism attack, ACIP recommends smallpox vaccination of persons predesignated by the appropriate bioterrorism and public health authorities who have responsibility for direct contact or investigation of the initial cases of smallpox.

Option 3: In the absence of a confirmed smallpox case or a confirmed smallpox bioterrorism attack, ACIP recommends extending Option 2 above to include smallpox vaccination of "essential" medical and non-medical service personnel predesignated by the appropriate bioterrorism and public health authorities.

SOURCES: ACIP (2002); IOM (2002b).

ACIP further developed the primary strategy for controlling and containing a smallpox outbreak. Its recommendations, developed in consultation with the DHHS National Vaccine Advisory Committee and CDC's Hospital Infection Control Practices Advisory Committee, were forwarded to the acting CDC director and to the Secretary of HHS for review and consideration.

Reported Viewpoints of Top Officials

As ACIP deliberated and DHHS and CDC discussed pre-event vaccination options and their ramifications, information about the discussion and debate occurring within the administration was also relayed in the mass media. President Bush expressed concern about immunizing the general public before a smallpox virus release (pre-event) and risking fatal complications, and he stated he would consider all available options before making a decision (Altman, 2002a; Federal Document Clearing House, 2002). Perhaps in part because of the advice of D. A. Henderson, who was opposed to widespread smallpox vaccination on safety grounds (U.S. Senate, 2001), the president reportedly planned to wait to see the results of the first phases of vaccinations before deciding how to proceed with a wider offering of the vaccine (National Journal Group, 2002). Vice President Dick Cheney reportedly preferred widespread vaccination before a smallpox virus release, due to concerns about the ability of DHHS to stop an outbreak with efficient mass vaccination (Cohen and Enserink, 2002; McKenna, 2003). DHHS Secretary Tommy Thompson reportedly supported a delayed voluntary program with an improved, safer vaccine (Altman, 2002a; CDC, 1983; CDC, 2001, 2002c; Gellman, 2002; IOM, 2002a; Meckler, 2002b; National Journal Group, 2002). CDC Director Julie Gerberding stated that the agency favored waiting until a new vaccine was licensed before offering it to the public (Meckler, 2002b) but recognized that individual citizens may, after evaluating the risks and benefits of the vaccine for themselves, choose to receive the existing vaccine and should have the opportunity to make such a choice (Meckler, 2002a). Others, including some governors and legislators, favored making the vaccine available to the public (Frist, 2002; Gregg, 2002; Hallow, 2002). The reported arguments for offering the vaccine to the public included these: people need to have options and the ability to decide whether they want to choose vaccination for themselves and their families rather than having the decision made for them, and people should not have to depend on the government to deliver the vaccine in a crisis (Bicknell, 2002; Frist, 2002; Gregg, 2002; Hallow, 2002; Kemper, 2002).

CDC's Efforts to Inform Government Policy

Elsewhere in this report, the committee discusses its concerns about CDC's independence to speak authoritatively about the scientific and public health rationale for the smallpox vaccination program. However, it must be noted that CDC made substantial efforts to involve its public health partners and the general public in a national discussion about the risk of smallpox, the smallpox vaccine, and vaccination options. In May 2002, CSTE presented its recommendations on smallpox vaccination to an ACIP working group (Pezzino, 2003). The organization opposed large-scale immunization of all first responders and advocated limiting vaccination to personnel who would be likely to come into contact with an index case of smallpox.

In June 2002, CDC held a series of public forums in New York, San Francisco, St. Louis, and San Antonio, to inform health professionals and the general public about smallpox and smallpox vaccine, to discuss the risks and benefits of reviving smallpox vaccination, and to solicit opinions on the use of smallpox vaccine before and after a potential smallpox virus release (Serafini, 2002). A total of five hundred people participated; many spoke on the CDC-developed options the ACIP would consider in its meeting later that month (see Box 2-1). The informal consensus favored Option 1 for Question 1: no vaccination of members of the general public in the absence of a confirmed smallpox case or a confirmed smallpox bioterrorism attack. Forum attendees were divided with regard to Question 2. Both Option 2 (vaccinate members of designated state smallpox response teams) and Option 3 (vaccinate, in addition, essential medical and non-medical personnel designated by authorities) seemed acceptable to various constituencies.

CDC also asked IOM to hold a workshop to consider the scientific, clinical, administrative, and procedural aspects of various smallpox immunization options (IOM, 2002a). The June 15, 2002, IOM workshop provided a forum for discussion of the array of options being considered by ACIP were discussed and debated. A workshop summary, titled *Scientific and Policy Considerations in Developing Smallpox Vaccination Options*, was later published.

Early News of the DHHS Plan

On July 7 and 8, 2002, the *New York Times* reported for the first time on the federal government's plans to vaccinate a half-million health care and emergency workers against smallpox, a much higher number than the maximum of 20,000 recommended by ACIP in June (Broad, 2002; Connoly, 2002). Government officials emphasized that the secretary of DHHS had not yet approved a plan to be forwarded to the White House, but details about the probable outline of the plan continued to circulate (Connolly, 2002). According to the *New York Times*, D.A. Henderson, then principal science adviser to the DHHS secretary for public health preparedness, explained the federal government's tentative new plan for a larger number of vaccinees (Broad, 2002): "We could easily be at a half-million without too much difficulty. . . . Wide peacetime vaccinations," he said, "would help educate not only the nation's medical community on the practical aspects of smallpox immunization but also the public." The pre-event smallpox vaccination plan, believed to reflect to some extent ACIP's June 2002 recommendations, was sent by DHHS to the White House in August 2002 (Moscoso, 2002).

By fall 2002, the administration was beginning to build a case for war against Iraq and, as discussed later in this report, that fact may have provided some of the context within which decisions regarding smallpox vaccination were made. At an October 4, 2002, news conference,[5] DHHS officials reportedly outlined the program's three-part structure, beginning with vaccination of up to 500,000 designated personnel, continuing with the vaccination of other health care workers and first responders, and finally, offering vaccination to the public using a new vaccine yet to be developed (Altman and Stolberg, 2002; Meckler, 2002a; Meckler, 2002b). The *Associated Press*, the *New York Times* and the *Washington Post* reported on October 5 and 6, 2002, that the federal government's smallpox vaccination plans were near completion and appeared to call for vaccinating millions of health care workers (Manning and Sternberg, 2002; McGlinchey, 2003; Meckler, 2002b). On October 7, 2002, an article in *USA Today* quoted CDC Director Gerberding's explanation of why the federal government was planning to vaccinate a number much greater than that recommended by ACIP in June. She reportedly stated: "We were in an environment where we were confident the threat was low. Where we are right now is still an environment where we have no imminent threat . . . but we recognize that we are in the process of considering war on our enemies. The context has changed a bit" (Manning and Sternberg, 2002). The *New York Times* also reported that at the October 4, 2002, news conference at DHHS, members of the press learned that the federal government was planning to make the smallpox vaccine available eventually to all Americans who wanted it (Altman, 2002b) as part of a program that would provide "ongoing and ever-expanding access to immunization" (Meckler, 2002a).

---

[5]A transcript was unavailable.

October 2002 ACIP Meeting

In September 2002, CDC asked ACIP to provide additional guidance on eight smallpox vaccination implementation issues: types of health care workers to be included in smallpox health care response teams, vaccination site care, need for administrative leave, screening for atopic dermatitis, screening for HIV, screening for pregnancy, simultaneous administration of smallpox vaccine and other vaccines, and the vaccination of smallpox vaccinators (CDC, 2002d).

ACIP responded to CDC's request at its October 17, 2002, meeting. It recommended the vaccination of smallpox vaccinators (who would then vaccinate the public health and health care response teams) to reduce the possibility of inadvertent inoculation (and to contribute to the development of a cadre of experienced vaccinators who could be deployed immediately in the event of a smallpox virus release), provided guidance on vaccination site care, confirmed that smallpox vaccination could be administered together with other immunizations except chickenpox and concluded that administrative leave would not be required for vaccinated health care workers but recommended phasing in vaccination in participating hospitals, beginning with a small number of hospitals and staggering vaccination to minimize the impact on workforce.

ACIP developed contraindications screening guidelines for the conditions identified by CDC and recommended that previously vaccinated people be preferentially targeted for vaccination, given the decreased incidence of adverse events in revaccinees (CDC, 2002d). ACIP also provided specific guidance to CDC on the type of health care staff and support personnel to be included in the composition of smallpox health care teams, and the potential number of vaccinees was noted later on October 17, 2002, during a CDC press telebriefing. The ACIP chairperson estimated that if each of about 5,100 acute-care hospitals in the United States participated in the program of precautionary, pre-event smallpox vaccination, and each hospital had a team of approximately 100, that would add up to about 500,000 health care workers (CDC, 2002c). However, both the ACIP chairperson and CDC officials participating in the call emphasized the importance of the composition of response teams and the adequacy of coverage within a given hospital rather than the number of vaccinees. In the same telebriefing, the timeframe of 30 days was given as a rough goal for the first phase of vaccination.

One member of ACIP, Paul Offit, dissented from ACIP's endorsement of the new, larger number of vaccinees (500,000) and observed that "the sense was that the course was already set and we wouldn't make any difference" (ACIP, 2002; Manning, 2002; McCullough, 2003). The timing of ACIP's revision of its recommendation, after news of the federal government's intention to vaccinate 500,000, seemed oddly coincidental to observers concerned about undue pressure on the federal advisory panel (Cohen and Enserink, 2002). However, ACIP Chairperson John Modlin and members of ACIP explained that the first, smaller number was based on the assumption that only staff at designated "smallpox hospitals" would be vaccinated (in addition to public health response teams). Later discussion with various stakeholders indicated that hospitals would resist a "smallpox" designation, and at a more practical level, smallpox victims would be more likely to go to the nearest emergency department rather than to a specific hospital (Brown, 2002b; Cohen and Enserink, 2002; Kemper, 2002; Maguire, 2003; Manning and Sternberg, 2002). ACIP had therefore changed its basic assumptions and expanded the number of prospective vaccinees to account for the participation of more hospitals. However, ACIP did not endorse any vaccination beyond the 500,000 response team members and was explicit in its opposition to offering vaccine to the general public, given the vaccine-related risks and the smallpox threat assessment at that time (Brown, 2002b, 2002c; Maguire, 2003).

The Policy

With the exception of phase I (vaccination of 500,000 volunteers), the federal government's final policy decision was an unprecedented departure from the ACIP recommendations (Altman, 2002a). As announced by the president on December 13, 2002, and further elaborated in DHHS and CDC communications and telebriefings, the policy called for resuming military vaccinations and in the civilian sector first vaccinating smallpox response team members (a target of about 500,000 was provided by DHHS officials after the president's announcement). This would be followed by an even larger number of health care and emergency personnel (up to 10 million), and finally, members of the general public who insisted on receiving the vaccine would be vaccinated (although with the caution that the government does not recommend smallpox vaccination for the general public, and with the caveat that the public would be given a new smallpox vaccine not yet developed at the time) (CDC, 2002g; White House, 2002).

Funding for Bioterrorism and Smallpox

In 1999, DHHS launched a bioterrorism initiative that had six goals: preventing bioterorrism, strengthening infectious disease surveillance, enhancing medical and public health readiness for mass casualty events, the National Pharmaceutical Stockpile (renamed the Strategic National Stockpile on March 1, 2003), conducting research on and development of new drugs and vaccines, and strengthening the information technology infrastructure (Redhead et al., 2002). In the wake of the terror attacks of 2001, the DHHS budget for bioterrorism preparedness increased from $305 million for FY 2001 to $2.98 billion for FY 2002 (DHHS, 2002b).

In 2002, Congress appropriated $940 million to CDC, which made $918 million available to 62 state, territorial, and local public health agencies as part of its Cooperative Agreement on Public Health Preparedness and Response (DHHS, 2002a). Twenty percent of the award was available for immediate use, and 80 percent was contingent on approval of plans submitted to CDC. In FY 2003, funding for CDC's cooperative agreement was $870 million; in FY 2004, funding had decreased to $849 million (DHHS, 2003a, 2003b). Proposed funding for FY 2005 is $829 million (ASTHO, 2004).

The smallpox vaccination program began as an agent-specific effort somewhat linked with other bioterrorism preparedness activities. When the smallpox vaccination program was announced, there was no specific funding linked with it; the November 2002 planning guidelines provided by CDC stated that the vaccination program would be funded by the already disbursed bioterrorism funds provided to grantees under the CDC cooperative agreement. After state and local public health agencies began to express concerns about the costs of the smallpox vaccination program and about their having to absorb a substantial proportion of funding earmarked for more general bioterrorism preparedness, in addition to other resources, the federal government provided $100 million in one-time supplemental funding for smallpox-related activities (DHHS, 2003b).

CONCLUDING OBSERVATIONS

The federal government's decision to reintroduce smallpox vaccination was unprecedented and emerged at the challenging intersection of public health with national security considerations related to potential terrorism. A public health immunization program against a nonexistent disease was an unusual step initiated in the context of concern about the possible existence and whereabouts of illegal smallpox virus stocks and the recent bioterrorist attacks on U.S. soil. The smallpox vaccination policy emerged at the intersection of public health with national security considerations related to potential terrorism.

ACIP has long served as a key advisory body to the federal government in all vaccination policy, and ACIP filled this role as it provided recommendations regarding specific aspects of the smallpox vaccination program. Little information has been made public about the other advisory groups and individuals most intimately involved in fashioning the actual policy. However, information available in the news media and in government communications shows that multiple opinions were considered at various levels and that the formulation of the policy captivated public and mass media interest for some time.

Greatly increased federal funding was made available to help states with bioterrorism preparedness, and additional funding was allocated for smallpox vaccination and related activities several months after the vaccination program began.

REFERENCES

ACIP (Advisory Committee on Immunization Practices). 2002. Record of the Meeting of the Advisory Committee on Immunization Practices, June 19-20, 2002. Centers for Disease Control and Prevention, National Immunization Program, Atlanta, GA.

ACIP. 2003. Advisory Committee on Immunization Practices (ACIP) Statement on Smallpox Preparedness and Vaccination. [Online] Available at http://www.bt.cdc.gov/agent/smallpox/vaccination/pdf/acipjun2003.pdf. Accessed July 17, 2003.

Alliance for Health Reform. 2002. *Preparing for Smallpox: Who to Vaccinate? How Soon?* Washington, DC.

Altman L. 2002a, August 25. Health Workers Await Official Smallpox Policy. *New York Times*.

Altman L. 2002b, October 8. The Doctor's World: At the Health Department, the Messengers Still Stumble. *New York Times*.

Altman LK, Stolberg SG. 2002, October 5. Smallpox Vaccine Backed for Public. *New York Times,* A1.

ASTHO (Association of State and Territorial Health Officials). 2001. Bioterrorism Preparedness. Testimony Before the Senate Committee on Appropriations: Subcommittee on Labor, Health and Human Services, and Education Appropriations, October 3, 2001. [Online] Available at http://www.astho.org/templates/display_pub.php?u=JnB1Yl9pZD0zMTQ=. Accessed August 1, 2004.

ASTHO. 2002. 2002 Government Relations Committee Annual Report—September. [Online] Available at http://www.astho.org/?template=government_relations_committee.html. Accessed January 30, 2005.

ASTHO. 2004. Preparedness Policy Fact Sheet: Public Health Preparedness FY 2005 Appropriations. [Online] Available at http://www.astho.org/pubs/FactSheetBioT Appropriations.pdf. Accessed January 30, 2005.

Bicknell WJ. 2002. The Case for voluntary smallpox vaccination. *New England Journal of Medicine* 346(17):1323-1325.

Boyle A. 2002, December 13. The How and Why of Smallpox Shots. *Bioterror* News. [Online] Available at http://msnbc.msn.com/id/3076449. Accessed February 6, 2003.

Broad W. 2002, July 7. US to Vaccinate 500,000 Workers Against Smallpox. *New York Times*.

Brown D. 2002a, June 21. Limited Smallpox Vaccine Use Eyed; Expert Panel Rejects Mass Inoculations. *Washington Post*.

Brown D. 2002b, October 17. Panel Alters Advice on Smallpox Shots: Wider Use for Health Workers Backed. *Washington Post,* A3.

Brown D. 2002c, October 17. Panel Leery of Mass Smallpox Doses; Major Risks Outweigh Benefits of Immunizing the General Public, Experts Say. *Washington Post*.

CDC (Centers for Disease Control and Prevention). 1983. Notice to readers smallpox vaccine no longer available for civilians—United States. *Morbidity and Mortality Weekly Report* 32(29):387.

CDC. 2000. Biological and chemical terrorism: strategic plan for preparedness and response. *Morbidity and Mortality Weekly Report* 49(RR04):1-14.

CDC. 2001. Vaccinia (smallpox) vaccine: recommendations of the Advisory Committee on Immunization Practices (ACIP), 2001. *Morbidity and Mortality Weekly Report* 50(RR-10):1-25.

CDC. 2002a. Frequently Asked Questions About Smallpox. [Online] Available at http://www.bt.cdc.gov/agent/smallpox/disease/faq.asp. Accessed January 30, 2005.

CDC. 2002b. CDC Telebriefing Transcript Smallpox Vaccine, June 20, 2002. [Online] Available at http://www.cdc.gov/od/oc/media/transcripts/t020620.htm. Accessed August 9, 2004.

CDC. 2002c. CDC Telebriefing Transcript: ACIP Smallpox Vaccine Meeting Briefing, October 17, 2002. [Online] Available at http://www.cdc.gov/od/oc/media/transcripts/t021017.htm. Accessed July 31, 2003.

CDC. 2002d. Summary of October 2002 ACIP Smallpox Vaccination Recommendations. [Online] Available at http://www.bt.cdc.gov/agent/smallpox/vaccination/acip-recs-oct2002.asp. Accessed January 9, 2003.

CDC. 2002e. Supplemental Guidance for Planning and Implementing the National Smallpox Vaccination Program (NSVP). [Online] Available at http://www.bt.cdc.gov/agent/smallpox/vaccination/pdf/supplemental-guidance-nsvp.pdf. Accessed December 15, 2002.

CDC. 2002f, December 12. Press Release: CDC Initial Review of State Smallpox Vaccination Plans Complete. [Online] Available at http://www.cdc.gov/od/oc/media/pressrel/r021212.htm. Accessed July 7, 2004.

CDC. 2002g. CDC Telebriefing Transcript: HHS Teleconference on Smallpox Policy. [Online] Available at http://www.cdc.gov/od/oc/media/transcripts/t021214.htm. Accessed January 10, 2003.

CDC. 2004a. Advisory Committee on Immunization Practices (ACIP) Website. [Online] Available at http://www.cdc.gov/nip/ACIP/default.htm. Accessed January 30, 2005.

CDC. 2004b. Smallpox: Training. [Online] Available at http://www.bt.cdc.gov/agent/smallpox/training/index.asp. Accessed January 30, 2005.

Cohen J, Enserink M. 2002. Rough-and-tumble behind Bush's smallpox policy. *Science* 298:2312-2316.

Cohen J, Marshall E. 2001. Vaccines for biodefense: a system in distress. *Science* 294: 498-501.

Connolly C. 2002, July 8. Smallpox Vaccine Program Readied: Inoculations May Surpass 500,000 Under US Plan. *Washington Post.*

DOD (Department of Defense). 2002, December 13. News Release: DOD Details Military Smallpox Vaccination Program. [Online] Available at http://www.dod.gov/releases/2002/b12132002_bt634-02.html. Accessed January 30, 2005.

DHHS (Department of Health and Human Services). 2002a, June 6. News Release: HHS Approves State Bioterrorism Plans so Building Can Begin. States, Cities to Receive Additional Funds for Strengthening Public Health Systems. [Online] Available at http://www.hhs.gov/news/press/2002pres/20020606c.html. Accessed January 30, 2005.

DHHS. 2002b. News Release: Highlights of 2002. [Online] Available at http://www.hhs.gov/news/press/2002pres/20021227.html. Accessed January 30, 2005.

DHHS. 2003a, March 20. News Release: HHS Announces Bioterrorism Aid for States, Including Special Opportunity for Advance Funding. [Online] Available at http://www.os.dhhs.gov/news/press/2003pres/20030320.html. Accessed January 30, 2005.

DHHS. 2003b, May 9. News Release: Guidelines for Bioterrorism Funding Announced. [Online] Available at http://www.hhs.gov/news/press/2003pres/20030509.html. Accessed January 30, 2005.

Federal Document Clearing House. 2002. Transcript: George W. Bush Holds News Conference.

Frist B. 2002, August 9. Deciding Who Is Protected Against Smallpox. *New York Times.*

Gellman B. 2002, November 5. Findings Spur New Smallpox Concerns. *Albany (NY) Times Union.*

Gregg J. 2002, October 6. Let the Public Choose on Smallpox Vaccine. *Washington Post.*

Hallow R. 2002, November 24. Governors Seek Access to Smallpox Vaccine. *The Washington Times,* A4.

IOM (Institute of Medicine). 2002a. Biological Threats and Terrorism: Assessing the Science and Response Capabilities. Washington, DC: National Academy Press.

IOM. 2002b. Scientific and Policy Considerations in Developing Smallpox Vaccination Options: A Workshop Report. Washington, DC: The National Academies Press.

Kemper V. 2002, October 5. Public Access to Smallpox Vaccine Is Urged; People Should Be Allowed to Opt in After Emergency Workers Are Inoculated, Officials Say. The White House Is Undecided. *Los Angeles Times.*

Krupnick M. 2003, January 24. CNA Calls Smallpox Program "Political"; Nursing Union Offical Says Bush's Plan Carries More Risks Than Benefits. *Contra Costa Times,* A1.

Kuhles D, Ackman D. 2003. The federal smallpox vaccination program. Where do we go from here? *Health Affairs* (Web Exclusive) W3:503-510.

Maguire P. 2003, January. As the Country Gears Up for Smallpox Vaccinations, Physicians Find Themselves on the Front Lines. *ACP-ASIM Observer,* American College of Physicians-American Society of Internal Medicine. [Online] Available at http://www.acponline.org/journals/news/jan03/smallpox.htm. Accessed January 30, 2005.

Manning A. 2002, October 17. Advisory Panel Expands Smallpox Vaccine Plan. *USA Today.*

Manning A. 2003, April 22. Second Round of Smallpox Vaccinations Begins. *USA Today.*

Manning A, Sternberg S. 2002, October 7. Officials Ponder Timing, Sequence of Immunizations. *USA Today.*

McCullough M. 2003, February 7. Americans Aren't Rolling Up Their Sleeves for Smallpox Inoculation. *The Salt Lake Tribune.*

McGlinchey D. 2003, February 26. CDC Says It Never Aimed for 500,000 Smallpox Vaccinations. *Global Security Newswire.*

McIlroy C. 2002. HHS to Formulate Smallpox Vaccination Strategy. *Front & Center, Newsletter of the National Governors' Association Center for Best Practices.*

McKenna M. 2003, February 15. No Vaccination for Nation's Fear, Unease Hinders Smallpox Program. *Atlanta Journal-Constitution.*

McNeil D. 2003, February 7. Many Balking at Vaccination for Smallpox. *New York Times.*

Meckler L. 2002a, October 4. US Health Officials Say Smallpox Vaccine Should Be Rolled Out Slowly. *Associated Press.*

Meckler L. 2002b, October 5. US Divided on Smallpox Policy. *Associated Press.*

Moscoso E. 2002, August 28. Smallpox Plan in White House Hands. *Atlanta Journal-Constitution,* 9A.

National Journal Group. 2002, November 25. Smallpox: Bush Favors Extensive Immunization. *Global Security Newswire.*

Pezzino G. 2003. Transcript from the IOM's Committee on Smallpox Vaccination Program Implementation Meeting Three on May 1, 2003, Washington, DC:106-122.

Redhead C, Vogt D, Tiemann M. 2002. Bioterrorism: Legislation to Improve Public Health Preparedness and Response Capacity. Report for Congress. Congressional Research Service, Library of Congress.

Roos R. 2002, June 21. ACIP Urges Smallpox Shots Only for Response Teams, Some Hospital Workers. *CIDRAP News.*

Serafini MW. 2002. Smallpox vaccinations: who should decide? *National Journal* 34(24):1800.

U.S. Senate. 2001. U.S. Senator Edward Kennedy (D-MA) Holds Hearing on Bioterrorism. Senate Health, Education, Labor and Pensions Committee: Health Subcommittee.

White House. 2002. President Delivers Remarks on Smallpox. [Online] Available at http://www.whitehouse.gov/news/releases/2002/12/20021213-7.html. Accessed January 8, 2003.

3

The Implementation of the Smallpox Vaccination Program

As described in Chapter 2, a long chain of events and policy decisions led to the revival of civilian smallpox vaccination in the United States. Plans to implement pre-event vaccination of a limited number of health care and public health personnel began to take shape in late 2002.

A detailed timeline of the vaccination program is provided at the end of this chapter (Table 3-2). The chapter does not address every event in the timeline, but in the first section highlights a short list of relevant events and program milestones. Each subsection begins with a description of an event and then moves on to a broader discussion of its significance. For example, the monkeypox outbreak that occurred several months into the implementation of the program is summarized, and then there is a discussion of the outbreak as a proxy event that tested public health preparedness in general and smallpox preparedness specifically.

Major markers on the civilian smallpox vaccination program timeline include the following (see Figure 3-1 for a graph of weekly vaccination numbers in January–September 2003, with several key events):

- December 13, 2002—National smallpox vaccination policy is announced.
- January 24, 2003—Civilian pre-event smallpox vaccination begins.
- March 19, 2003—War with Iraq begins. Both the buildup to the war and the declared end of major combat appeared to have an effect on the smallpox vaccination program.

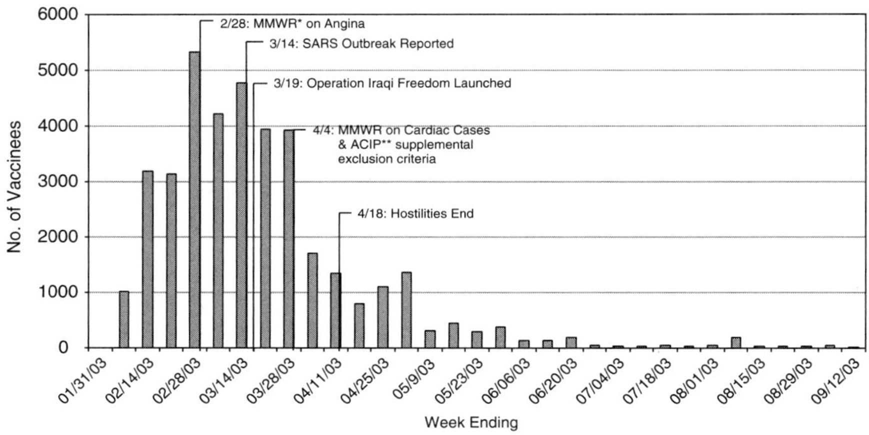

FIGURE 3-1 Timeline of smallpox vaccination program with number of weekly vaccinations and key events.
SOURCE: Henderson (2003b).
*MMWR = Morbidity and Mortality Weekly Report.
**ACIP = Advisory Committee on Immunization Practices.

- Late March and early April 2003—Concerns about vaccine and program safety reach high point in response to reported fatal cardiac adverse events and cases of heart inflammation, known as myo/pericarditis.
- April 2003—Smallpox vaccination compensation plan is enacted in response to widespread concern about vaccine-related injuries.
- April 2003—General Accounting Office (GAO, now Government Accountability Office) report provides first systematic assessment of vaccination program progress and highlights challenges.
- May 2003—Department of Health and Human Services (DHHS) makes supplemental funding available for smallpox vaccination program.
- May and June 2003—Monkeypox outbreak tests public health (and smallpox) preparedness.
- June 2003—Advisory Committee on Immunization Practices (ACIP) recommends ending smallpox vaccination after completing vaccination of response teams; vaccination continues, very slowly approaching 40,000 vaccinees.

The section on program milestones is followed by a discussion of two noteworthy features of the program (congressional interest and involvement, and the significance of the parallel military smallpox vaccination program). The chapter's third section focuses on the committee's findings about challenges that arose in the course of the vaccination program and about which the committee has written in previous reports, included here as Appendixes B-G. The fourth and final section highlights some of the favorable outcomes of the smallpox vaccination program.

In this chapter and elsewhere in this report, the committee has cited multiple articles from the mass media on the smallpox vaccination policy and on the program implementation. Using news media references was necessary because of the limited scientific peer-reviewed and other formal literature available on the newly initiated and continuing program. Although newspaper articles may capture events in a manner that is incompletely documented, subjective, and even out of context, the committee found that some themes emerged consistently from diverse media sources and provided useful information about how the program was perceived in the public health and health care communities. More important, mass media coverage of the program was concordant with the information presented at committee meetings by state and local public health officials and health care administrators, with the congressional testimony of public health leaders, and with findings from qualitative surveys that became available later in the course of the program. Mass media reports reflected the perceptions of key constituencies and the public; their perceptions of CDC, the program, and the federal government's role may provide insight into the lessons to be learned from this program.

MAJOR MILESTONES AND RELEVANT EVENTS

The Policy Is Announced

> On December 13, 2002, President George W. Bush announced that smallpox vaccine would be administered to selected civilians and members of the military. The announcement was the culmination of planning and decision-making that spanned the latter half of 2002. The president explained that "government has no information that a smallpox release is imminent. Yet it is prudent to prepare for the possibility that terrorists would kill indiscriminately" with biologic weapons (White House, 2002b).

To prepare the nation for the threat of smallpox, the military vaccination program would provide mandatory[1] vaccination to selected members

[1]For designated military personnel without contraindications.

of the military and offer vaccination to others who "serve America in high-risk parts of the world," and a civilian smallpox vaccination program would make the vaccine "available on a voluntary basis to medical professionals and emergency personnel and response teams that would be the first on the scene in a smallpox emergency" (White House, 2002b). Although the president's announcement acknowledged and reiterated that there was no imminent danger and that pre-event vaccination would therefore be limited to specified groups, he stated that vaccination would be offered to members of the general public "who insist on being vaccinated" (White House, 2002b).

The program's general structure and timeline were only sparsely outlined in the president's announcement and the White House news release. Additional details were conveyed in later telebriefings, program guidance, and other communications from the secretary of Health and Human Services and from Centers for Disease Control and Prevention (CDC) officials (CDC, 2002a, 2002b, 2002d; Connolly and Milbank, 2002; McGlinchey, 2003a). In the joint CDC–DHHS telebriefing on December 14, 2002, the number of prospective vaccinees was discussed in some detail (CDC, 2002d). DHHS Secretary Tommy Thompson said that state pre-event vaccination plans designated a total of 439,584 people to be offered the vaccine.[2] State plans included 1,100 public health smallpox response teams, adding up to 20,000 personnel that would be vaccinated, and 4,500 health care teams, adding up to 400,000 personnel that would be vaccinated; and DHHS officials also gave the figure of 10 million as a secondary target to include all health care workers and other first responders who would volunteer to be vaccinated (CDC, 2002d; Connolly and Milbank, 2002; McGlinchey, 2003a).

The public health and health care communities came to understand that the program would progress in three stages or phases:

- Phase I would involve the vaccination of designated members of health care and public health smallpox response teams with a goal of about 500,000 and a timeline of 30 days.
- Phase II would involve the expansion of vaccination to up to 10 million health care personnel and other first responders, such as firefighters and police.
- In Phase III, intended to begin in 2004, vaccination with a new, not yet approved, vaccine would be offered to members of the public who in the absence of a smallpox release insisted on being vaccinated.

---

[2]Recipients of CDC funding for bioterrorism preparedness who developed smallpox plans include not only states, but also the U.S. territories, the District of Columbia, and three metropolitan jurisdictions. *State* is used here to include all those entities.

The Program Begins

The program did not begin immediately after the president's announcement, because government coverage of liability (of vaccine manufacturers, hospitals, and health departments that would operate vaccination clinics) in the provision of bioterrorism countermeasures (vaccine) would not go into effect until weeks later. On January 22, 2003, CDC began shipping smallpox vaccine from its vaccine stockpiles to the 11 states that had requested it. On January 24, 2003, the secretary of Health and Human Services declared that the smallpox vaccination program could begin under the authority of an amendment to the Public Health Service Act by Section 304 of the Homeland Security Act[3] (DHHS, 2003a). The secretary's declaration marked the true beginning of the smallpox vaccination program, in that states, territories, and municipalities chose to defer program implementation until the protections conferred by the Homeland Security Act went into effect (Kemper, 2003a).

[3]The Homeland Security Act was signed by the president on November 25, 2002.

Vaccination programs in the 62 states, territories, and municipalities began gradually. Some jurisdictions ordered vaccine stocks as soon as CDC made them available and began vaccinating immediately after the program was authorized. Other jurisdictions delayed ordering vaccine and initiating vaccination in order to finalize their plans, or in expectation of CDC's completion of program components (such as the safety system and informational materials), or to await the settlement of the unresolved vaccine injury compensation issue for people injured by the vaccine or the accidental, inadvertent transmission of vaccinia from a vaccination site.

The vaccination program was generally supported by the public health and health care communities in recognition of the need for biopreparedness (ANA, 2002; Hardy, 2002; Libbey 2003). A survey of state health officials in June 2002 found that a majority (77 percent of 44 respondents) favored smallpox vaccination of designated response teams (Banks and Hannan, 2002). Two surveys of physicians, nurses, and other health care personnel largely working in emergency departments, conducted in late 2002, found that that a majority of respondents (61 percent of 1,165 respondents in one survey, 73 percent of 1,701 respondents in the other) expressed a willingness to receive smallpox vaccination as part of a pre-event program (Everett et al., 2002; Yih et al., 2003). However, support of the program by the public health and health care communities was qualified because of questions and concerns about several aspects of the program; these contributed to implementation delays and to other challenges. Subjects of concern ranged from the scientific—such as the reliability of historical measures for estimating transmission rates, and the relevance and accuracy of historical adverse events data—to the procedural and administrative, including the structure of the vaccination program and its effect on overall bioterrorism preparedness, the actual and opportunity costs of the program, the adequacy of measures to address compensation and liability, and the safety of the vaccine. Questions and concerns were communicated in open letters to DHHS and to the White House, in press releases and policy statements, at congressional hearings, and at meetings of the present committee (ANA, 2002; Baker, 2003; Libbey, 2003; NGA, 2003; Rosado, 2003).

This committee's first report recognized that the smallpox vaccination program was an atypical vaccination campaign that was neither a research study nor an ideal public health program, but a public health component of bioterrorism preparedness (IOM, 2003a). The committee also emphasized the program's voluntary nature and the need for a focus on safety, requiring active monitoring of side effects related to vaccination.

Unlike the views and input of national organizations, which were made public through press releases and other formal communications, the perspectives of individual hospitals and those of health care and public health workers were captured largely in mass media reports. In late January and early February 2003, people involved in the program were interviewed or cited in newspaper articles and news broadcasts; their comments reflected a wide array of feelings and opinions. They included commitment to doing what was needed to protect the public's health, confusion and suspicion about the rationale for the program, confidence in the usefulness of vaccination, concern about the vaccine's safety and about potential loss of wages because of non-life-threatening but important postvaccination symptoms, and criticism of or worry about the reluctance of many public health and health care workers to be vaccinated (Bavley and Dvorak, 2003; Kemper, 2003a; Marchione, 2003; McKenna, 2003; Meckler, 2003a). The net results of individual and institutional concerns were hesitation and low participation among public health and health care workers and great variability in hospital participation.

Hospitals differed greatly in their anticipated degree of participation in the smallpox vaccination program. Some hospitals planned to participate, at least by having a small number of staff members vaccinated to serve later as vaccinators, but others (DHHS Secretary Thompson estimated about one-third of hospitals) planned to opt out (Bavley and Dvorak, 2003; Ornstein and Richardson, 2003). Some of the hospitals that did not plan to participate in vaccination chose to hold training sessions and to educate their staff on smallpox disease and smallpox vaccination (Judson, 2003; Toomey, 2003). Hospitals that chose not to participate in pre-event vaccination cited various reasons: the desire to avoid infecting immunosuppressed patients, concerns about strain on their workforce (due to sick time necessary because of complications or to prevent patient exposure), and questions about liability if nonstaff (families and patients) were inadvertently infected with the vaccinia virus (*Associated Press*, 2003; McCullough, 2003; McNeil, 2003; Ornstein and Bonilla, 2003; Pasternack, 2003). Some newspaper editorials described hospital decisions against implementing vaccination as "deplorable" and characterized workers who opted out as "refuseniks" and "vaccine-dodgers" (*New York Times*, 2002; *Washington Post*, 2002; *Boston Herald*, 2003; *Washington Times*, 2003). Physicians spoke of being criticized as "unpatriotic" for not being willing to receive the vaccine (Connolly, 2003a). Despite such tensions, CDC guidelines and the efforts of public health agencies sought to ensure that the voluntary nature of the program was preserved while the implementation of the biopreparedness policy continued.

Confusion About the Program Goals and Timeline

The program goals and timetable were not communicated clearly, and that created confusion and challenges throughout the implementation of the program (ACIP, 2002; Connolly and Milbank, 2002; Meckler, 2002). Later communications appeared to augment the confusion and created the perception (also discussed in Chapter 4) that the program was characterized by frequently shifting goals rather than by a clear purpose and effective implementation.

As the program progressed more slowly than expected, it became evident that the original goals and timeline would not be met. However, the 500,000 and 30-day figures had become de facto program goals, as the mass media seized on numerical figures as indicators of program progress both locally and nationally. In February 2003, many CDC officials cautioned the public and those involved in the program against focusing on numbers and acknowledged that CDC was moving away from the initial 30-day timeline, arguing that the variation in public health system structures across the country and in local needs and characteristics made it impossible and undesirable to require specific numbers and set a strict deadline (CDC, 2003d). In communication with members of the mass media in February 2003, DHHS and CDC personnel de-emphasized the focus on numbers of vaccinees and began to emphasize the importance of preparedness. One CDC spokesperson stated: "We're trying to do a better job of clarifying what the purpose of this program is, and the purpose of this program is to better prepare our country to respond to a bioterrorism event involving smallpox" (McGlinchey, 2003a). Despite that, CDC continued to urge rapid implementation of the smallpox vaccination program without guidance on how states could determine the pace and scope of their vaccination efforts (GAO, 2003).

Cardiac Adverse Events and Other Safety Concerns

In late March 2003, three vaccinees—two civilian women and one man in the military program—died from myocardial infarction (heart attack) within 5, 6, and 22 days of smallpox vaccination, respectively. All three had a history of heart disease or risk factors, including smoking and hypertension, so it was not immediately clear whether their deaths were related to vaccination. Later study showed that the deaths were consistent with what would have been expected in the population, and there was no evidence that smallpox vaccination created a higher-than-expected risk of heart attacks. But their deaths, combined with concern about a newly identified cardiac adverse event, had a substantial chilling effect on the willingness of volunteers to receive the vaccine.

A total of 1,000 people were vaccinated in the first 2 weeks of the program (different jurisdictions began at different times). After that, the number of vaccinees grew at a relatively steady rate of roughly 3,000–5,000 every week. That changed with the appearance of cardiac adverse events at the end of March 2003, when the program slowed down to fewer than 1,500 per week. By the end of April 2003, only a few hundred volunteers were being vaccinated every week (Henderson, 2003b). The number of weekly vaccinations continued to decline and never recovered, reaching a handful of vaccinees weekly, then monthly. Between April 30, 2004, and July 31, 2004, 25 people received smallpox vaccination, and during August 2004, 5 people were vaccinated (CDC, 2004a, 2004b, 2004c).

Cardiac Adverse Events

The myocardial infarction cases were only some of the cardiac adverse events associated with the civilian and military vaccination programs. Several cases of myocarditis and pericarditis (types of heart inflammation collectively labeled myo/pericarditis) were identified in the civilian program after smallpox vaccination, beginning in February 2003. Although they made a more subtle impression than fatal heart attacks, their association with vaccination was more worrisome. A report in the March 28, 2003, issue of *Morbidity and Mortality Weekly Report* listed seven cardiac adverse events in the civilian program: three myocardial infarctions, including the two fatal civilian cases noted above; two cases of angina; and two cases of myo/pericarditis (CDC, 2003f). By March 21, 2003, the military program had documented 10 cases of myo/pericarditis in addition to the heart attack noted above (CDC, 2003f; Connolly, 2003c). Recent and historical evidence supported an association between myo/pericarditis and smallpox vaccination (CDC, 2003k). The Department of Defense (DoD) identified a likely causal association between smallpox vaccination and myo/pericarditis (Halsell et al., 2003); the evidence of a causal association in the civilian population remained unclear (ACIP, 2003b).

Concern about cardiac complications associated with smallpox vaccine caused apprehension in people planning to be vaccinated and led many states to temporarily suspend vaccination and wait for CDC guidance (Connolly, 2003c; Kuhles and Ackman, 2003). The Advisory Committee on Immunization Practices (ACIP) and the ACIP Working Group on Smallpox Vaccination—created in February 2003 to monitor vaccination program communication, surveillance, and research activities (ACIP, 2003a)—held an emergency meeting on March 28, 2003, to make recommendations to CDC about medical screening of potential vaccinees and follow-up of persons with cardiovascular risk factors after vaccination (CDC, 2003h). The working group recommended the deferral of volunteers who had known cardiac disease, those who had three or more risk factors (for example, smoking, high blood pressure, and high blood cholesterol concentrations) for heart disease, and those over 50 years old (Neff, 2003a). ACIP accepted the first two recommendations but not the last, because of concerns that it would exclude a substantial proportion of potential civilian vaccinees likely to be older and previously vaccinated (and therefore considered less vulnerable to vaccine complications) (Neff, 2003b). ACIP also looked at historical evidence about myo/pericarditis, found largely in the context of military vaccination among young Finnish men (Helle et al., 1978; Kanjalainen et al., 1983). U.S. data from the 1960s were limited to pediatric vaccination, in which myo/pericarditis could have been missed (CDC, 2003h). Finally, ACIP recommended to CDC the following exclusion criteria: known underlying heart disease with or without symptoms and the presence of three or more of the known major cardiac risk factors (CDC, 2003a, 2003h). CDC accepted ACIP's recommendations and moved rapidly to revise the vaccination information package, screening materials, and informed consent form.

Myo/pericarditis, the cardiac complication not previously recognized among expected adverse events of smallpox vaccination, constituted a major safety finding and was later identified in the context of clinical trials of a second-generation smallpox vaccine. The pharmaceutical company Acambis in April 2004 temporarily suspended volunteer recruitment for the ACAM2000 clinical trials of cell-culture smallpox vaccine because of the occurrence of at least three cases of myo/pericarditis (Roos, 2004a). In

September 2004, the Food and Drug Administration lifted the clinical hold on enrollment in the ACAM2000 trials and concurred with Acambis that enrollment could be closed and analysis of the data could begin. Acambis undertook 12-month followup of affected study subjects.

Both DoD and CDC conducted followup of vaccinees with myo/pericarditis (Mootrey, 2003). Research on myo/pericarditis is needed, and efforts are already in progress. In July 2004, the National Institutes of Health provided funding for research on the effect of smallpox vaccine on cardiac cells in mice (Roos, 2004b).

Vaccination Program Safety Profile

In the weeks surrounding the beginning of the program, health care and public health organizations described their unease regarding specific safety issues related to the vaccination program. Although the program was voluntary, the potential of inadvertent transmission of vaccinia virus meant that adults and children who had neither consented to vaccination nor been screened for contraindications could become infected and face the risk of severe adverse events or even death (AAP, 2003). Some organizations also feared that the pace of the vaccination program could make it difficult to arrange staff schedules to provide time for leave or furlough in order to ensure patient safety (Burstein, 2002; Peterson, 2002; Schulman, 2002; Baker, 2003).

Reintroducing the smallpox vaccine in the absence of the disease required special attention to safety, including screening for contraindications and preventing the inadvertent transmission of vaccinia virus to contacts because the risk-benefit ratio was less clear in the absence of naturally occurring smallpox. CDC and its state and local counterparts worked to ensure safety at every step before, during, and after vaccination. CDC made every effort to develop effective and efficient screening methods and guidelines for pre-event smallpox vaccination clinics. In response to the present committee's recommendations, CDC developed an information sheet for contacts of vaccinees and modified the Pre-Event Vaccination System to document active surveillance of vaccine-related adverse events that required hospitalization or outpatient care, contraindications to vaccination among volunteers or their household contacts not identified before vaccination, and vaccinia-virus transmission to contacts (CDC, 2003e; IOM, 2003a). Volunteers were given multiple opportunities to learn about the vaccine and vaccination and to opt out if they determined that they were unable or unwilling to be vaccinated, and a thorough informed consent process was put into place.

The ACIP identified several contraindications to smallpox vaccination, and CDC included them in the screening process and in training and education materials. Prospective vaccinees would be excluded from vaccination for the following reasons: age (no one under 18 years old would be vaccinated in nonemergency situations), history of allergic reaction to vaccine or its components, breastfeeding, and moderate or acute illness. Prospective vaccinees would also be excluded if they or immediate household contacts had any of the following contraindications: pregnancy; disease, conditions, or treatments that cause immunosuppression or immune deficiency; and any acute, chronic, or exfoliative skin conditions, such as eczema and atopic dermatitis (CDC, 2003b). Furthermore, there are many people with compromised immune systems (because of HIV infection, immunosuppression for organ transplantation, or cancer therapy) for whom smallpox vaccine would hold a greater risk, and these conditions were included among the contraindications for smallpox vaccinations. Although there are many clinical data on reactions to smallpox vaccine, they predate contemporary immunosuppression. And very little information about fetal vaccinia and adverse events in inadvertently vaccinated pregnant women is available. After the vaccination of six civilians who later discovered that they were pregnant, ACIP established a pregnancy registry that would conduct follow-up of civilian and DoD pregnant women who were vaccinated (CDC, 2003g).

Concerns about program safety persisted. The present committee and the Association of State and Territorial Health Officials (ASTHO) recommended a pause between phases I and II to evaluate safety and ensure an adequate level of planning for expanded vaccination to a new population that required extensive communication and education for safety (for example, prevaccination screening and postvaccination site care). Phase III, intended to make the vaccine available to insistent members of the public, seemed even more problematic, in that it would pose public health threats, vast logistic challenges, and special and intensive communication requirements. Also, the final phase of the program would offer a potentially harmful vaccine in the context of an unknown risk, creating a philosophic conflict with health care and public health workers' injunction to "do no harm" (AAP, 2003; Libbey, 2002).

In February 2004, the program's safety profile reflected a small number of cases of inadvertent inoculation, indicating that vaccinees were probably effectively educated to prevent transmission. That and the fact that three of the four historically noted serious adverse events did not occur at all are also likely indicators of effective training and screening (see Table 3-1).

TABLE 3-1 Number of Reported Cases of Selected Adverse Events Associated with Smallpox Vaccination Among Civilians, by Type, United States, January 24-December 31, 2003

	Number of Cases[a]		
Adverse Events	Suspected	Probable	Confirmed
Eczema vaccinatum	—	—	—
Fetal vaccinia	—	—	—
Generalized vaccinia	2	—	1
Inadvertent inoculation, nonocular	11	—	9
Ocular vaccinia	1	—	2
Progressive vaccinia	—	—	—
Erythema multiforme major (Stevens-Johnson syndrome)	—	—	—
Myo/pericarditis	16	5	—
Postvaccinial encephalitis or encephalomyelitis	1	—	—
Pyogenic infection of vaccination site	—	—	—

SOURCE: CDC (2004d).

[a] "Adverse events that have been associated with smallpox vaccination are classified on the basis of evidence supporting the reported diagnoses. Cases verified by virologic testing are classified as confirmed. Cases are classified as probable if possible alternative etiologies are investigated and excluded and supportive information for the diagnosis is found. Cases are classified as suspected if they have clinical features compatible with the diagnosis, but either further investigation is required or investigation of the case did not provide supporting evidence for the diagnosis" (CDC, 2003m).

The War in Iraq

Military action in Iraq began on March 19, 2003. Both the events leading up to the war and the period after the declared end of major combat may have influenced public opinion and attitudes about and participation in the smallpox vaccination program. President Bush declared an end to major hostilities in Iraq in April 2003 (although military action continued).

As described in Chapter 2, the smallpox vaccination policy grew out of a series of discussions among top government officials about the possible existence of smallpox virus outside the two known repositories in Russia and the United States and about the threat of deliberate release of smallpox virus. The scope and content of intelligence considered in decision-making were not made known to the public until the publication of the Senate Intelligence Committee's Report on the U.S. Intelligence Community's Prewar Intelligence Assessments on Iraq (assuming that this evidence was used to make smallpox vaccination policy), which found the evidence of the presence of smallpox virus in Iraq to be weak (U.S. Senate Select Committee on Intelligence, 2004).

The rationale for the vaccination program was not formally linked with the possible and later impending war with Iraq, a nation suspected of possessing weapons of mass destruction (perhaps including smallpox virus, on the basis of information from the 1990s). However, the public comments of three public health officials (CDC Director Julie Gerberding, DHHS Secretary Tommy Thompson, and National Immunization Program Director Walter Orenstein) and two legislators (Senators Judd Gregg and Bill Frist) alluded to the war in a way that could be construed as suggestive of a link or suggested that the war served as an impetus for the increased number of vaccinees and rapid program implementation (Connolly, 2003a; Hallow, 2002; Manning and Sternberg, 2002; Rath and Turcotte, 2003; Reuters, 2003). Multiple mass media reports indicate that some public health and health care workers believed that the vaccination program was linked with the war, and public opinion about the vaccination program was split, not unlike public opinion about the war (Russell, 2003). Evidence from the mass media and from an ASTHO survey suggests that the perceived association between the war and the vaccination program was one of several reasons for suspicion and concern among prospective vaccinees, as well as a barrier to vaccination (ASTHO, 2003). Although government officials neither updated nor reiterated the smallpox threat assessment, mass media reports showed a downward shift in public perception about the level of risk of smallpox release and therefore a decreased motivation to receive the vaccine (Fiorill, 2003; Manning, 2003; McKenna, 2003; Yee, 2003). That shift in public perception may have contributed to the decline in the vaccination rate in April and May 2003.

The Compensation Plan

In April 2003, a compensation plan for people who experienced a smallpox vaccine injury was signed into law, largely addressing concerns about the adequacy of provisions available to protect people injured by smallpox vaccination and resolving some concerns about institutional liability in the event of inadvertent transmission of vaccinia.

Early in the implementation of the program, health care and public health organizations and labor unions expressed concern about the lack of adequate provisions for vaccine injury compensation and for some types of personal and institutional liability (GAO, 2003). Some states chose to wait until these issues were resolved to begin vaccination, and many prospective volunteers expressed confusion about what protections were available to them and reluctance to assume risks without adequate assurance of protection (MacLeod, 2003; Roos, 2003a). In January 2003, the American College of Emergency Physicians (ACEP), the American Hospital Association (AHA), and the American Nurses Association (ANA), and others found that the narrow definition of liability coverage provided under Section 304 of the Homeland Security Act seemed to provide protection to the vaccine manufacturer, the vaccinator, and the institution operating a vaccination clinic but left other institutions and people without coverage (such as hospitals that do not have vaccination clinics although their personnel may receive vaccination elsewhere and vaccinated personnel in a noncovered institution who may be liable for inadvertently infecting a patient). Furthermore, ACEP, AHA, and ANA were concerned about an incomplete and confusing patchwork of compensation solutions (for example, worker compensation not applicable to volunteers and differences among states) and the lack of a no-fault compensation mechanism for volunteers who experience complications and for people inadvertently infected by vaccinees. Although some states and institutions provided coverage under worker compensation or other mechanisms, available coverage was fragmentary at best. The American Public Health Association, the American College of Occupational and Environmental Medicine, the Service Employees International Union (SEIU), the Association of Federal, State, County, and Municipal Employees, and many others called for the development of comprehensive compensation mechanisms to protect people injured by smallpox vaccination (APHA, 2002; SEIU, 2002; August, 2003; Russell, 2003). SEIU and other health professionals' labor unions also called for a safer bifurcated needle (SEIU, 2002). The present committee urged CDC to clarify the status of compensation mechanisms as part of the informed consent process. As a result, CDC added information about compensation issues in the Vaccine Information Statement (Box 3-1).

On January 23, 2003, members of the Senate asked the White House to provide a plan for vaccine injury compensation (Daschle et al., 2003). Early proposals would provide coverage of vaccine injuries for those who would be vaccinated within 180 days of the program's initiation; this created concern about inappropriate pressure to receive the vaccine (Meckler, 2003b). The comprehensive compensation plan was proposed by DHHS in early March 2003, 6 weeks after the expected start of the vaccination program. The Senate Committee on Health, Education, Labor, and Pensions passed the smallpox compensation bill on April 2, 2003, and the Smallpox Emergency Personnel Protection Act of 2003 (SEPPA, PL 108-20) was signed into law by President Bush on April 30, 2003. The SEPPA

BOX 3-1
Compensation Plan Timeline

January 2003 – Members of the Senate ask the White House for smallpox vaccine injury compensation. Smallpox vaccination program begins.

March 6, 2003 – DHHS proposes a smallpox compensation plan.

April 2, 2003 – Senate Committee on Health, Education, Labor and Pensions passes smallpox compensation bill.

April 30, 2003 – President Bush signs into law the Smallpox Emergency Personnel Protection Act (SEPPA, PL 108-20) establishing a smallpox vaccine injury compensation program.

August 27, 2003 – SEPPA interim final rule: Smallpox Vaccine Injury Table published in Federal Register.

December 16, 2003 – SEPPA interim final rule: Administrative policies, procedures, and requirements guiding the program published in Federal Register.

SOURCES: Daschle et al. (2003); DHHS (2003d); Federal Register (2003a, 2003b).

interim final rule, with the smallpox vaccine injury table specifying the injuries, disabilities, conditions, and deaths that would be covered by the program (previously published in August 2003), was issued on December 16, 2003 (Federal Register, 2003b).

The General Accounting Office Report: An Early Assessment of Program Progress

On April 30, 2003, 3 months after the beginning of civilian vaccination, the General Accounting Office (GAO, now the Government Accountability Office) released its evaluation of the progress of the smallpox vaccination program.

GAO was asked to examine the implementation of the smallpox vaccination program and to describe program challenges. In an April 2003 report, GAO found that the program progressed more slowly than anticipated owing in part to a demanding program schedule that did not allow sufficient time for preparation either at CDC or state levels. GAO noted that CDC responded to questions about the lower-than-expected numbers of vaccinees by stating that even as few as 50,000 vaccinated people could mount an effective response (GAO, 2003). However, that number was not formally announced as the new target figure for the national pre-event vaccination program, and the report stated that CDC did not provide the evidence for the smaller number, nor did it outline what level of vaccination was necessary for smallpox preparedness (GAO, 2003; McGlinchey, 2003a).

As the smallpox vaccination program moved away from an emphasis on numbers to an emphasis on smallpox preparedness, public health agencies at the state and local levels reported that they lacked guidance about what preparedness meant and about how to assess whether they were prepared for a potential smallpox release (GAO, 2003; Selecky, 2003). The lack of clarity about program goals identified above remained a problem. The GAO report recommended that CDC provide guidance to its grantees for revising phase I vaccination targets and for expanding the program in the second phase.

Supplementary Funding for the Smallpox Vaccination Program

On May 5, 2003, DHHS notified the states that $100 million in supplemental funding would be made available to support smallpox vaccination efforts. The additional funding aimed to address state and local public health agency concerns about the costs imposed by the program. Although the overall effect of the funding has not been assessed, one local health official testified before a U.S. House of Representatives committee that the supplemental funding came too late for her public health agency, which had "cut other commitments" to implement the smallpox vaccination program (U.S. House of Representatives, 2004).

The timing of the smallpox vaccination program coincided with a period of intense budgetary crises in most state governments (NGA, 2003). Soon after the beginning of the program, ASTHO, the National Association of County and City Health Officials (NACCHO), and various state and local health officials, some of whom considered the program an unfunded mandate, provided program cost estimates that far exceeded CDC's estimate (Colacecchi and Jones, 2003; Libbey, 2003; Rosado, 2003). CDC's testimony before the Senate Committee on Health, Education, Labor, and Pensions on January 30, 2003, gave an estimated cost of vaccination of $10-15 per person, compared with the estimates of NACCHO and state and local health officials, which ranged from $100 to $400 per vaccinee (Colacecchi and Jones, 2003; Libbey, 2003). Although vaccination kits (vaccine, diluent, and needles) were provided to state and local public health agencies at no charge, public health agencies and their national representatives asserted that CDC's calculations did not include the activities and capabilities required to plan and implement smallpox vaccination clinics, including training, education, and communication (NACCHO, 2003a, 2003b). The National Association of Counties (NACo) and the National Governors Association (NGA) also expressed concern about the financial consequences of the smallpox vaccination program for the public health infrastructure and in the context of state and county budget deficits (NGA, 2003; Rosado, 2003). NGA, NACo, ASTHO, and NACCHO called for additional federal funding to prevent the diversion of funds from general bioterrorism preparedness and public health activities to smallpox-specific efforts and argued that funding would be especially needed to support the expansion of smallpox vaccination to a second phase (Hardy, 2002; Libbey, 2002, 2003; NGA, 2003). One estimate of the cost of phase II was $600 million to $1 billion (Kuhles and Ackman, 2003). The present committee and others called for an assessment of the full costs of the smallpox vaccination program (APHA, 2002; IOM, 2003b).

The April 2003 GAO report found that state and local health officials experienced substantial financial and workforce burdens on state and local public health agencies (GAO, 2003). ASTHO and NACCHO conducted additional study of the cost of the first phase of smallpox vaccination and found that it ranged from $79 to $1,784 per vaccination, and they estimated an average cost per vaccination of $265 and $204, respectively (NACCHO, 2003b).

The Monkeypox Outbreak

> In May and June 2003, a monkeypox outbreak was identified in Wisconsin; and cases were later found in Illinois, Indiana, Kansas, Missouri, and Ohio (CDC, 2003l). The disease, resembling smallpox, tested preparedness. Although familiarity with smallpox disease appeared to be an asset, at least one possibly systemic problem surfaced; CDC was not alerted about the outbreak for 13 days.

The monkeypox outbreak did not mark the first time during the course of the smallpox vaccination program that a naturally emerging infectious disease threat surfaced. In late 2002 and early 2003, a novel coronavirus emerged in China and spread rapidly to other nations along travel routes, causing widespread alarm and economic damage by crippling the tourism and travel industries from Hong Kong to Toronto (IOM, 2004). By summer 2003, when it seemed to recede, severe acute respiratory syndrome (SARS) had sickened about 8,000 people across Asia, Europe, and North America and caused the deaths of nearly 800. SARS placed enormous strains on many public health agencies in the United States. The emergence of SARS and later monkeypox during the course of the smallpox vaccination program was a reminder of the importance of public health preparedness for a wide array of potential problems (the "all-hazards" approach used by other agencies). Naturally occurring diseases, from West Nile virus to monkeypox to SARS, require capabilities, resources, training, education, and communication channels similar to those needed to respond to deliberate attack with bioweapons and could therefore serve as proxy events. The committee has discussed the usefulness of proxy events in its sixth report (see Appendix G) and has recommended that CDC support a system to ensure the continuing collection, synthesis, and sharing of lessons learned and best practices public health response to proxy events.

A child in Wisconsin was identified as having the first case of monkeypox in the United States during this outbreak. The child had contracted the disease from a sick pet prairie dog. The disease was ultimately traced to a Gambian giant rat and other exotic rodents that infected a number of prairie dogs. Humans were infected by contact with pets; most of the patients had confirmed exposure to infected rodents and no cases of solely human-to-human transmission were reported. By the end of the outbreak, 71 cases in the six states had been reported to CDC; 35 cases were laboratory-confirmed, and 36 were suspect and probable. On June 12, 2003, CDC made a recommendation, on the basis of expert opinion and limited evidence that people exposed to monkeypox be given smallpox vaccine (CDC, 2003j). Thirty people received smallpox vaccine to prevent transmission of monkeypox; 7 were vaccinated before exposure and 23 after exposure, and no severe adverse events were reported among vaccinees (CDC, 2003l).

Although there has been little systematic study of the monkeypox experience, the anecdotal reports of federal, state, and local public health agencies suggest that smallpox preparedness activities had a favorable effect on the response to the monkeypox outbreak (McGlinchey, 2003b). Clinicians were familiarized with poxvirus diseases, and communication linkages between the health care and public health communities (for example, for reporting and surveillance) were strengthened. Trained vaccinators were available to vaccinate affected people with smallpox vaccine, and vaccine supplies were available regionally. Unfortunately, a dysfunction in the system was identified when the initial cases of monkeypox were not reported to CDC for 13 days; local experts apparently tried to identify the pathogen by using only their local and state resources (CDC, 2003i; Mitchell, 2003). In a smallpox outbreak, such a delay could be expensive and deadly.

June 2003 ACIP Recommendation to End the Smallpox Vaccination Program

At the June 2003 ACIP meeting, the ACIP recommended that for safety reasons the federal government not expand smallpox vaccination beyond the health care and public health response team members still being vaccinated (ACIP, 2003b). (In May 2003, the present committee had called for a pause in the vaccination program to assess safety and to plan carefully before extending vaccination to more people.)

In June 2003, CDC reported that the number of vaccinees working in hospitals was small—only 40 percent of acute-care hospitals had at least one staff member vaccinated, and only 1 in 10 hospitals had two or more vaccinated staff members—a deficiency in numbers that could require a regional rather than a local response in some areas in the event of a smallpox-virus release (CDC, 2003a; Yee, 2003). The smallpox vaccination program did not come to an official stop in response to the ACIP recommendation, but the pace of vaccination continued to decline. By July 25, 2003, the total number of civilian vaccinees was 38,004—far short of the 500,000 that had been given as a program target and still short of the 50,000 that CDC had suggested in GAO's assessment (CDC, 2003c; GAO, 2003). A year later, on July 31, 2004, civilian vaccinations had reached a cumulative total of 39,579 (CDC, 2004c). Nearly 2 years after the beginning of the program, smallpox vaccination has all but come to a halt, with a mere handful of vaccinations each month.

In the months after the vaccination rate began to fall, CDC did not formally urge states and other jurisdictions to increase their vaccinees to specified numbers, and it did not take any steps to formally reiterate the need for the vaccine. A *Washington Post* article in July 2003 noted the recent silence on the part of White House and federal officials who made the decision to vaccinate and legislators who had been vocal supporters of the vaccination program (Connolly, 2003b). The same article quoted CDC Director Gerberding: " 'Can we stand up clinics across the country tomorrow to immunize our nation in 10 days? No,' she acknowledged. Still, we 'have made enormous progress.' "

In July 2004, DHHS adviser D.A. Henderson stated that the smallpox vaccination of first responders was no longer needed, because enough vaccine was available to vaccinate the nation, if needed, and many cities had improved their capability to respond to a potential smallpox attack (Calabresi and August, 2004; Malenic, 2004).

At the time this report was written, the program was languishing, and there was nearly complete silence on the part of the federal government about the status and future of this biopreparedness program; no official update of program progress or impact had been provided (see additional discussion in Chapter 4).

NOTEWORTHY FEATURES OF THE PROGRAM

Congressional Interest and Involvement

Members of Congress contributed to the smallpox vaccination program at various points in its evolution, from policy development to evaluation. Some policy-makers contributed to the early discussion of policy options. In the weeks and months before the smallpox vaccination program was announced, Senators Bill Frist and Judd Gregg and others publicly urged the government to consider making smallpox vaccine available to all Americans to facilitate individual choice (Frist, 2002; Gregg, 2002; McKenna, 2003). Several congressional committees and subcommittees held hearings on the subjects of smallpox vaccination and bioterrorism preparedness beginning soon after the September 11, 2001, attacks. Testimony before Congress as early as October 2001 (ASTHO, 2001) informed legislators about the need for a smallpox response plan, the need for additional resources, the need for a compensation mechanism for injuries associated with smallpox vaccination, and problems in the implementation of the program (NGA, 2003; U.S. House of Representatives, 2004). For example, at a July 2003 hearing of the Senate Committee on Health, Education, Labor and Pensions, members of the Senate expressed concerns about the slow progress of smallpox vaccination and questioned federal officials about possible causes, including delays in finalizing the table of vaccine-related injuries that could be compensated under the new federal compensation provisions (Heil, 2003). Congress also played an important role in moving the legislation to provide a comprehensive plan for compensation of people injured by smallpox vaccine (Rath and Turcotte, 2003).

Finally, members of Congress asked GAO to evaluate progress in the smallpox vaccination program; this led to the April 2003 report described above (GAO, 2003). In January 2004, a year after the beginning of smallpox vaccination, some members of Congress issued a report that critiqued the smallpox vaccination program and called for changes to ensure and strengthen smallpox preparedness (U.S. House of Representatives Select Committee, 2004).

The Relationship Between the Civilian and Military Vaccination Programs

The focus of this report is the implementation of CDC's civilian smallpox vaccination program. However, past committee reports and activities reflect its continuing interest in the parallel program implemented by DoD. The civilian and military programs are inherently related, and the committee believes that there is much to be learned from the two programs taken individually and together. DoD staff made presentations at the committee's meetings and responded to committee inquiries about the military program's progress, its administrative and educational efforts, and its safety system and related research.

The military vaccination program began immediately after the president's announcement on December 13, 2002, and has advanced at a steady and rapid pace, reaching and surpassing 600,000 vaccinees (DoD, 2004b). The smallpox vaccination program provided a unique opportunity for collaboration between CDC and DoD, and although the two programs involved very different circumstances and populations, there was much to be learned from both. The military population included a much higher percentage of young people never before vaccinated (and likely to be in very good health because of the nature of their job and their ages), whereas vaccination among the civilian population involved generally older people, most of whom had been vaccinated in the past. Also, the military program required vaccination for designated personnel, whereas the civilian program was voluntary. Unlike civilian vaccinees, who would pose a potential risk of inadvertent inoculation to spouses or household contacts, military personnel who were vaccinated were likely to live in settings and have duties that could expose a higher number of contacts to inoculation, not just spouses and intimate partners. For example, military activities and facilities are likely to require close physical interaction among personnel, several people may be required to use the same bedding consecutively, and laundry is processed in a communal fashion. Those factors had the potential to increase inadvertent exposure of nonvaccinated people to vaccination sites and secretions.

Both the military and civilian programs conducted follow-up of adverse events (CDC, 2003k), and the ACIP Working Group on Smallpox Vaccine Safety reviewed safety data generated by both programs. Although efforts were made to facilitate the flow of information between DoD and CDC, administrative difficulties and questions arose. For example, both CDC and DoD posted weekly updates of adverse events in their programs, but at times, information about adverse events in the military program was not communicated to the public or to the public health community in a timely fashion. Also, if there were inadvertent inoculation of civilian contacts of military vaccinees, it was not immediately clear which program—the civilian or the military—would include these cases in its adverse events surveillance.

Studies of reported adverse events (such as myocardial infarctions and myo/pericarditis) (CDC, 2003b) benefited from having the larger combined civilian and military vaccinees as potential study populations. For example, the data from the military supported the finding in the civilian population that cases of myo/pericarditis were associated with smallpox vaccination. However, it was also more difficult to identify adverse events specifically caused by the smallpox vaccine in the military population, because members of the military often received multiple concurrent vaccinations.

DoD has also made some important findings in its smallpox vaccination program. For example, in November 2003, two independent panels examined four deaths potentially related to DoD's vaccination program and found that one (the April 2003 death of a 22-year-old reservist) may have been triggered by several vaccinations she received, including smallpox vaccine (DoD, 2003, 2004a). In February 2004, DoD reported that an infant contracted tertiary vaccinia infection from breastfeeding (the mother was inadvertently inoculated by the father) (CDC, 2004e). In the August 25, 2004, Smallpox Vaccination Program Safety Summary, DoD reported that over 631,000 personnel had been vaccinated and that most adverse events had occurred at a rate lower than historical rates (DoD, 2004c).

Despite some early challenges, the collaboration between CDC and DoD gave the ACIP Working Group on Smallpox Vaccine Safety access to the substantial amount of data gathered by the much larger military program. The committee has previously expressed its hope that the Department of Defense Serum Repository and the Millennium Cohort Study will serve as resources for CDC as it follows up vaccinees and learns about the long-term sequelae of serious adverse events (IOM, 2003d).

PROGRAM CHALLENGES

A Push for Rapid Implementation Without Adequate Preparation

The committee has found that owing to the initial emphasis on rapid implementation of the smallpox vaccination program, CDC had little or no time to finalize or test many of the program components (such as the completeness or consistency of vaccine information and education materials) or to address identified barriers to implementation (IOM, 2003a, or refer to Appendix B in this report). That may explain many of the problems with the execution of the program, such as the financial and opportunity-cost problems reported by many state and local public health agencies, the lack of an adverse event compensation plan and the many delays in developing and implementing it with needed clarification on liability issues, unfinalized informed consent materials, and the lack of an appropriate and complete data system in the first 3 weeks of the program.

Although rapid program implementation would have been warranted in the face of an impending crisis, government's assurances that there was no imminent threat made the call for rapid implementation perplexing.

The Informed Consent Process

Like other aspects of smallpox vaccination program implementation, the informed consent process suffered from the program's rapid start and ambitious timeline. The early weeks of the program appeared to be caught up in a whirlwind of enormous effort on the part of CDC (GAO, 2003). CDC staff developed dozens of educational training materials, provided technical assistance and held regular conference calls with state public health agency leadership, and worked on communication plans. The crucial importance of the informed consent information and forms was recognized from the beginning, but additional time was needed to make corrections and improvements in the materials. That meant that some of the items were not final at the time vaccination began. The committee's concerns about the informed consent form were related to larger issues, such as the lack of adequate compensation provisions and the program's unique nature as a public health program established for national security reasons, that at a practical level implied a public health intervention with known risk and unknown benefits. For those reasons, the committee expressed concern in its first report to CDC that the informed consent form did not include an explanation of the state of compensation mechanisms for volunteers who would be injured by the vaccine (IOM, 2003a, or refer to Appendix B). The committee believed that there were ethical reasons for including clear language about compensation on the informed consent form, and it noted that there was a tension between the desire to maximize participation of appropriate candidates in the program and the imperative to minimize participation of those with contraindications and to create conditions that would allow those unwilling to receive the vaccine to feel comfortable in declining. CDC delayed for several weeks updating the informed consent and vaccination information materials with information about injury compensation to avoid deluging jurisdictions with yet another in a series of changes that seemed to cause dismay and logistical difficulties.

The Data System

An effective data system was needed before the program started. Unfortunately, the Pre-event Vaccination System (PVS) was not operational until 3 weeks after the vaccination program began. The haste of implementation did not allow CDC to ensure that the system met the needs of state public health agencies, nor did it allow time for the creation of an active adverse event surveillance system. Some states reported difficulties in using the PVS, including the fact that PVS relied on a readily available Internet connection, which some of the implementing entities lacked (Pezzino, 2003). The PVS was also needed to place rates of adverse events in context to facilitate accurate understanding, an appropriate alternative to having single cases get mass media attention. The committee discussed and made specific recommendations pertaining to CDC's data system in several of its earlier reports (IOM, 2003a, 2003b, 2003c) (see Appendixes B, C, and D). CDC later developed an active adverse events surveillance system.

The relatively slow progress of the program and the small numbers of vaccinees also complicated efforts to evaluate data for safety purposes (GAO, 2003). The committee is not aware of whether CDC has conducted a comprehensive assessment of the safety data system functioning, the completeness of the data gathered, and their relevance to the continuation of vaccination efforts.

Other Challenges

The smallpox vaccination program highlighted some of the challenges facing the health care delivery system and characterizing its relationship with public health. The program asked public health professionals and their health care colleagues to communicate and collaborate more intensively than usual. Mechanisms for communication (such as reporting by clinicians, and informing by public health authorities) between the health care and public health communities vary greatly (in both quantity and quality) across jurisdictions in all elements of concern to public health, including disease reporting in general (IOM, 2002a; Hirshon, 2003; Temte, 2003). The smallpox vaccination program and associated training and information activities required efforts that may have enhanced the channels available for communication. However, there was some concern in the clinician community that relying on the Internet as a main channel of communication posed a risk of bypassing clinicians who do not use the Internet or of getting lost in the midst of a barrage of other messages (Temte, 2003). Additional, redundant communication channels and extensive, regular training and education are needed to reach all clinicians and to facilitate the rapid movement of information between the health care and public health communities and among local, state, and national public health agencies.

The smallpox vaccination program also highlighted the fact that the health care system is under great strain. Many hospitals made considerable efforts to participate in the vaccination program and to conduct training and other preparedness activities, but the added burden brought into relief the other challenges facing them (such as overcrowding and staff shortages) and the health care system in general (Grady and Altman, 2003; HealthLeaders, 2003). Smallpox preparedness and the broad concerns of all-hazards preparedness served as a reminder that surge capacity may be a challenge for many communities in the event of a crisis—hospitals have limited beds available, there are staffing shortages, and there are large populations of uninsured people that will need prophylaxis or care in the event of a smallpox-virus release or other bioterrorist attack (Anderson, 2003). Furthermore, the first responder communities included in smallpox vaccination and other preparedness activities (because they have health and safety responsibilities and interact with the health care system) have other responsibilities, and additional interaction and dialogue are needed to ensure realistic expectations and smooth functioning of a multidisciplinary response to public health disasters, such as a smallpox-virus release.

FAVORABLE OUTCOMES

Despite the considerable challenges that arose in the course of the smallpox vaccination program, its implementation has provided opportunities for learning about smallpox vaccination and the conduct of biopreparedness programs and has led to some favorable outcomes. (The committee wrote on this subject at length in its fourth report, included here in Appendix E.)

Opportunities for Learning

Programmatically, CDC accomplished much in the implementation of the smallpox vaccination program, working under great time pressures to develop and enhance the range of capabilities needed to respond to a potential smallpox-virus release. CDC provided training in smallpox vaccination and smallpox disease to public health and medical personnel, developed communication plans and tools, and regularly interacted with state and local public health agencies, answering questions related to implementation and providing technical assistance.

Chapter 4 discusses two major lessons learned from the smallpox vaccination program, but the committee asserts that there are many lessons yet to be learned with respect to research and evaluation. There are many components of the smallpox vaccination program, both procedural issues and areas of scientific evidence, that could be mined for lessons that could be applied in future biopreparedness programs and in planning for other kinds of public health threats, such as pandemic influenza. For example, how did states select the people they initially considered to be potential smallpox vaccinees, and what has been learned about the composition and structure of response teams that might be useful in other types of public health emergencies? What has been learned from the compensation and liability quandary that would be useful in planning other biopreparedness activities? With regard to ethics, what can be learned from the evident tension between concern about the risks posed by the vaccine and altruism or between the imperative to have a voluntary program with truly informed consent and the need to implement a biopreparedness program to prepare the public health and health care workforce? What can be learned from the discussion about high-priority groups for vaccination and related complex decision-making processes? How well did the vaccine adverse events reporting systems (including active surveillance) work? CDC needs to complete, assess, and publish the results of its evaluative studies conducted during the program. Such findings are critical if the need arises to renew vaccination efforts, and they could be derived from a variety of studies described by CDC staff to the committee during open committee meetings. Important questions include these:

- What was the general rate of work-limiting or recreation-limiting activities due to symptoms or illnesses in the first month after vaccination?
- What are the current rates of serious adverse events related to smallpox vaccine in the civilian and military populations?
- What are current findings from the pregnancy registry, including pregnancy outcomes?

The committee urges that a concerted effort be made to document and publish all information from the program that could facilitate future programs at the intersection of public health and national security.

Other Favorable Outcomes

CDC's efforts and those of CDC's state and local partners facilitated the forging of multiple partnerships between state and local public health agencies and the health care and first responder communities (Gursky, 2003). Multiple presenters at the committee's meetings spoke of the partnerships among the health care and public health communities and between public health agencies and first responders (Anderson, 2003; Bresnitz, 2003; Fischler, 2003; Nikolai, 2003; Toomey, 2003).

The smallpox vaccination program provided coincidental preparation for the monkeypox event. A great deal of training about smallpox and, to a lesser extent, orthopoxviruses was implemented, and the health care community was more prepared to identify unusual rashes and probably more attuned to any symptoms out of the ordinary. That meant that when monkeypox appeared in the United States, there was a greater awareness and even readiness among health care providers. Because of the smallpox vaccination program, vaccine was readily available in all the states that had monkeypox cases, and trained and experienced personnel were available to screen, vaccinate, and follow up (Yee, 2003).

The smallpox vaccination program is also reported to have had a favorable effect on the state and local public health response to SARS, which emerged late in 2002 and continued through spring 2003 (Staiti et al., 2003). Although there is little empirical evidence to pinpoint or quantify improved performance, public health agencies have reported improved communication with their health care counterparts and an improved surveillance system (Judson, 2003; Selecky, 2003; Skivington, 2003; Witt, 2003).

Finally, the vaccination program provided opportunities to learn more about adverse vaccine effects in adults. Adverse events surveillance during implementation led to the identification of a new serious adverse event. Cases of myo/pericarditis were confirmed in the military program, and probable cases were identified in the civilian program, necessitating follow-up and future study.

The vaccination program served as a case study of biopreparedness with relevance for future similar endeavors. The committee has previously urged CDC to take full advantage of the data collected and experience gained in the course of implementing the program (IOM, 2003b, 2003d). Evaluation and research activities could be undertaken in areas ranging from the administrative to the scientific, from determining the overall cost of the smallpox vaccination program and specific components to assessing the opportunity cost to public health agencies and identifying long-term effects of vaccine-related adverse events.

CONCLUDING OBSERVATIONS

Implementation of the smallpox vaccination program began in January 2003 and is continuing. The rate of vaccination rose gradually for the first several weeks but then began a steep decline from which it never recovered—monthly vaccination numbers dropped to the single digits during summer 2004.

This chapter provides a summary of key milestones in the course of the program and other major events that occurred during implementation and may have affected or been affected by the program. The program experienced considerable implementation challenges. However, it also provided opportunities to gain experience with a broad multisector and interdisciplinary effort of biopreparedness and led to novel findings about potential complications from smallpox vaccine.

The committee hopes that CDC and its partners at the state and local levels will ensure that what has been accomplished and learned through the great investment of effort and resources is sustained and is integrated into the full spectrum of public health preparedness.

TABLE 3-2 Smallpox Vaccination Program Timeline

Date	Events (policy, program, and other developments)	IOM Committee Meeting or Report
September 2000	DHHS contracts with OraVax (now a part of Acambis, Inc.) for new smallpox vaccine to be delivered in 2004 (CIDRAP and IDSA, 2004).	
June 2001	ACIP recommendation on smallpox (vaccinia) vaccine: because of low risk of deliberate release and indeterminate risk to population, limit vaccination to laboratory or medical personnel working with non-highly-attenuated orthopox viruses (CDC, 2001). "Dark Winter," a war game for senior-level officials, is conducted by Center for Strategic and International Studies in partnership with Johns Hopkins Center for Civilian Biodefense Studies and ANSER Institute for Homeland Security. Exercise included a smallpox outbreak spreading to 25 states and 15 countries (ANSER Institute for Homeland Security, 2003).	
September 2001	Terrorist attacks in New York, Arlington (Virginia), and Pennsylvania. DHHS placed an order for 40 million doses of smallpox vaccine with Acambis (20-year contract for cell-culture vaccine) (IOM, 2002b).	
October 2001	Letters containing anthrax spores delivered through U.S. mail.	

TABLE 3-2 Continued

Date	Events (policy, program, and other developments)	IOM Committee Meeting or Report
November 2001	DHHS awards $428 million contract to Acambis/Baxter to produce smallpox vaccine (DHHS, 2001). NIH-funded researchers began to examine efficacy of diluted Dryvax smallpox vaccine (NIH, 2001).	
February 2002	CDC asks ACIP to review its recommendations on smallpox vaccination.	
April 2002	NIAID study finds that Dryvax smallpox vaccine may be diluted to expand supply (Frey et al., 2002; NIH, 2002). Dilutions of 1:5 and 1:10 resulted in take rates approximately as high as undiluted vaccine.	
June 2002	ACIP meets and drafts supplemental recommendations on smallpox vaccination (vaccinate up to 20,000 health care and public health workers) (ACIP, 2002). Public Health Security and Bioterrorism Preparedness and Response Act of 2002 signed into law (FDA, 2002).	
October 2002	ACIP meets again and updates recommendations on smallpox vaccination. ACIP also recommends offering vaccine to up to 500,000 health care and public health personnel (CDC, 2002a).	IOM Committee on Smallpox Vaccination Program Implementation convened at request of CDC
November 2002	President signs Homeland Security Act (White House, 2002a). Designated CDC staff members receive smallpox vaccination (epidemiologic investigation teams) (Associated Press, 2001). Mass media report that Bush administration intelligence review has concluded that four nations (Iraq, North Korea, Russia, and France) may possess covert and illegal stocks of smallpox virus (Gellman, 2002).	
December 2002	States submit to CDC smallpox response plans and smallpox pre-event vaccination plans (CDC, 2002c). CDC completes initial review of state smallpox vaccination plans President announces smallpox vaccination program.	First meeting of IOM Committee on Smallpox Vaccination Program Implementation

Continued

TABLE 3-2 Continued

Date	Events (policy, program, and other developments)	IOM Committee Meeting or Report
	HHS telebriefing on smallpox policy (White House, 2002b); initial goal: vaccinate 500,000 workers in 30 days.	
January 2003	Letter to White House issued by minority members of Senate calling for smallpox vaccine injury compensation. CDC begins shipping smallpox vaccine to states. Department of Homeland Security established. DHHS secretary authorizes civilian smallpox vaccinations. Civilian smallpox vaccination begins.	First report of IOM committee
February 2003	Media reports cite lack of a compensation plan as a barrier to smallpox vaccination (MacLeod, 2003; Meckler, 2003c). DHHS announces contracts to develop safer smallpox vaccines (DHHS, 2003b). DoD has vaccinated over 100,000 against smallpox. *Morbidity and Mortality Weekly Report (MMWR)* notifies of one case of angina 4 days after smallpox vaccination (CDC, 2003p). DoD reports first cases of myocarditis among personnel recently immunized with smallpox vaccine (CDC, 2003f).	Second meeting of IOM committee
March 2003	First civilian instances of myo/pericarditis identified, later classified as suspected and probable (CDC, 2003s). DHHS proposes smallpox vaccination compensation plan. Homeland security threat level changed to orange (high) (White House, 2003a). Surgeon general, CDC director, and others are vaccinated against smallpox (Kemper, 2003b). War with Iraq begins on March 19, 2003 (White House, 2003b). Maryland woman and Florida woman die from heart attack 5 and 22 days, respectively, after smallpox vaccination. Man dies from myocardial infarction 6 days after smallpox vaccination. ACIP recommends additional cardiac exclusion criteria for smallpox vaccination (CDC, 2003f; Kemper, 2003c). CDC issues Health Alert Network health advisory to avoid vaccinating people with	Second report of IOM committee

TABLE 3-2 Continued

Date	Events (policy, program, and other developments)	IOM Committee Meeting or Report
	cardiac risk factors and recommends temporary deferral for heart patients who volunteer for vaccination (CDC, 2003q). Multiple states temporarily postpone all smallpox vaccination clinics. CDC accepts ACIP's exclusion criteria and revises fact sheets, screening materials, and informed consent form.	
April 2003	More states suspend smallpox vaccination programs indefinitely, others for a limited length of time (Kemper, 2003c). Virginia defers initiation of smallpox vaccination. Media reports death of female reservist after receiving smallpox and anthrax vaccines (Mendieta, 2003; Roos, 2003c). GAO report *Smallpox Vaccination: Implementation of National Program Faces Challenges* finds that 6% of target population has been vaccinated by week 10 of program; data are insufficient to assess safety (GAO, 2003). On April 30, 2003, president signs into law Smallpox Emergency Personnel Protection Act of 2003, which establishes no-fault Smallpox Vaccine Injury Compensation Program (CDC, 2003r).	
May 2003	President declares end of major combat operations in Iraq (White House, 2003c). DHHS makes $100 million in supplemental funding available for the smallpox vaccination program (DHHS, 2003c). Monkeypox outbreak reported in several states including Wisconsin and Texas (CDC, 2003l). Media reports that in April and May, some states have begun offering smallpox vaccine to first responders (ABC 13 News, 2003; Murphy, 2003).	Third meeting of IOM committee Third report of IOM committee
June 2003	CDC Recommends smallpox vaccine to protect persons exposed to monkeypox (CDC, 2003j). ACIP recommends against expansion of smallpox vaccination program beyond "first phase" (ACIP, 2003c).	

Continued

TABLE 3-2 Continued

Date	Events (policy, program, and other developments)	IOM Committee Meeting or Report
August 2003	Oregon Health Sciences University researchers find that smallpox immunity may persist for decades, but there is disagreement about the meaning of the findings (Roos, 2003b).	Fourth report of IOM committee
October 2003	Ohio decides against offering smallpox vaccination to first responders (Shockman, 2003). *MMWR* reports that a review of death records shows that 1947 NYC smallpox vaccination campaign did not lead to increase in cardiac deaths (CDC, 2003o).	
November 2003	Two independent panels examine four deaths potentially related to DoD's smallpox vaccination program and found that one (April death of 22 year-old reservist) may have been triggered by vaccinations including vaccinia (DoD, 2003).	Fourth meeting of IOM committee
December 2003	Federal government issues interim final rule for Smallpox Emergency Personnel Protection Act of 2003 (SEPPA), plan for smallpox vaccine injury compensation. CDC updates smallpox case definitions.	Fifth report of the IOM committee
January 2004	HHS secretary's declaration regarding administration of smallpox countermeasures extended until and including January 23, 2005 (keeping SEPPA in place).	
February 2004	Military infant contracts vaccinia from breastfeeding (CIDRAP, 2004). DoD reports that 581,183 service members received smallpox shots from December 13, 2002, to February 11, 2004. Seventy-two vaccinees, or about 1 in 8,072, suffered myopericarditis, and there were 30 cases of vaccinia infection in contacts of vaccinees. Other complications included 36 cases of generalized vaccinia, most of which required only outpatient treatment, and one case of encephalitis (DoD, 2004d).	
March 2004		Fifth meeting of the IOM committee

TABLE 3-2 Continued

Date	Events (policy, program, and other developments)	IOM Committee Meeting or Report
April 2004	Acambis temporarily suspends volunteer recruitment for its clinical trials of cell-culture smallpox vaccine because of occurrence of at least three cases of myo/pericarditis in one trial (Roos, 2004a). DoD reports that 10 HIV-positive members of military who received smallpox vaccination did not experience adverse events (Tasker et al., 2004).	
May 2004	A review of New York City death certificates from 1946, 1947, and 1948 shows that the 1947 mass smallpox vaccination campaign in New York did not show an increase in cardiac deaths postvaccination (Thorpe et al., 2004).	
June 2004	DoD announces anthrax and smallpox vaccinations for all personnel deployed by Central Command and, for first time, select units in Pacific Command. Since December 2002, 625,000 troops have been vaccinated against smallpox (Malenic, 2004).	
July 2004	The Senate Select Committee on Intelligence issues report on US intelligence community's prewar intelligence assessments on Iraq; among other findings, report describes evidence on Iraq's possession of smallpox as weak (U.S. Senate Select Committee on Intelligence, 2004).	Sixth report of the IOM committee Sixth meeting of the IOM committee
September 2004	Aventis Pasteur vaccine produced in the 1950s shown to be effective, even in dilutions of 1:5 and 1:10 (Talbot et al., 2004).	
October 2004	Acambis and Bavarian Nordic A/S win $177 million U.S. government contract to produce safer smallpox vaccine (DHHS, 2004). CIA issues *Comprehensive Report of the Special Advisor to the Director of Central Intelligence on Iraq's WMD*. Report concludes that, although Iraq had capability to work with smallpox virus, there is "no direct evidence that Iraq either retained or acquired smallpox virus isolates or proceeded with any follow up smallpox related research" (CIA, 2004).	

REFERENCES

AAP (American Academy of Pediatrics). 2003. Testimony of Jon Abramson, Chair, Committee on Infectious Diseases of the American Academy of Pediatrics. Senate Health, Education, Labor, and Pensions Committee. Heading on the Smallpox Vaccination Plan: Challenges and Next Steps.

ABC 13 News. 2003. Virginia's First Responders Get Smallpox Vaccinations. *WSET/ABC 13 News.*

ACIP (Advisory Committee on Immunization Practices). 2002. Record of the Meeting of the Advisory Committee on Immunization Practices (Centers for Disease Control and Prevention, National Immunization Program). Atlanta, GA.

ACIP. 2003a. Record of the meeting of the Advisory Committee on Immunization Practices, February 26-27, 2003.

ACIP. 2003b. Record of the meeting of the Advisory Committee on Immunization Practices, June 18-19, 2003.

ACIP. 2003c. Advisory Committee on Immunization Practices (ACIP) Statement on Smallpox Preparedness and Vaccination. [Online] Available at http://www.bt.cdc.gov/agent/smallpox/vaccination/pdf/acipjun2003.pdf. Accessed July 17, 2003.

ANA (American Nurses Association). 2002. Statement to the IOM's Committee on Smallpox Vaccination Program Implementation.

Anderson R. 2003. Presentation Before the IOM Committee on Smallpox Vaccination Program Implementation. Transcript of Meeting Three on May 1, 2003, Washington, DC.

ANSER Institute for Homeland Security. 2003. Dark Winter. [Online] Available at http://www.homelandsecurity.org/darkwinter/index.cfm. Accessed September 14, 2004.

APHA (American Public Health Association). 2002. APHA Policy Statement on Smallpox Vaccination. [Online] Available at http://www.apha.org/legislative/policy/smallpox.pdf. Accessed June 17, 2003.

Associated Press. 2001, November 5. CDC Workers Get Smallpox Vaccination.

Associated Press. 2003, February 3. St. Vincent Won't Give Smallpox Vaccinations. *KARK.Com.*

ASTHO (Association of State and Territorial Health Officials). 2001. Testimony Before the Senate Committee on Appropriations, Subcommittee on Labor, Health and Human Services, and Education Appropriations, October 3, 2001. Bioterrorism Preparedness. [Online] Available at http://www.astho.org/templates/display_pub.php?u= JnB1Yl9pZD 0zMTQ=. Accessed December 12, 2004.

ASTHO. 2003. ASTHO Smallpox Preparedness Survey Results. [Online] Available at http://www.astho.org/pubs/spxsummaryb2.pdf. Accessed May 21, 2003.

August J (Assistant Director for Health and Safety, Department of Research and Collective Bargaining Services). 2003. Testimony for the American Federation of State, County and Municipal Employees (AFSCME). Senate Appropriations Committee: Labor, Health and Human Services and Education Subcommittee, January 29, 2003.

Baker M. 2003. Testimony on Behalf of the Service Employees International Union, AFL-CIO Before the U.S. Senate Committee on Health, Education, Labor, and Pensions on the Administration's Smallpox Vaccination Plan: Challenges and Next Steps. January 30, 2003. [Online] Available at www.SEIU.org.

Banks S, Hannan C. 2002. ASTHO Ensures State Health Officials Are Heard in Smallpox Debate. [Online] Available at http://astho.org/templates/displau_pub.php?pub_id=336. Accessed September 15, 2004.

Bavley A, Dvorak J. 2003, February 8. Safety Concerns Hinder Participation in Smallpox Vaccination Program. *Kansas City Star.*

Boston Herald. 2003, January 23. Editorial: Vaccine Dodgers Grow.

Bresnitz E. 2003. Presentation. Transcript from the IOM's Committee on Smallpox Vaccination Program Implementation Meeting Two on February 13, 2003, Washington, DC: 62-85.

Burstein J. 2002. Statement of the American College of Emergency Physicians. Transcript from the IOM's Committee on Smallpox Vaccination Program Implementation Meeting One on December 19, 2002, Washington, DC:267-271.

Calabresi M, August M. 2004, July 26. Was Smallpox Overhyped? (The Smallpox Scare: Was the Germ-Warfare Risk Overblown?). *TIME* 16.

CDC (Centers for Disease Control and Prevention). 2001. Vaccinia (smallpox) vaccine: recommendations of the Advisory Committee on Immunization Practices (ACIP), 2001. *Morbidity and Mortality Weekly Report* 50(RR-10):1-25.

CDC. 2002a. CDC Telebriefing Transcript: ACIP Smallpox Vaccine Meeting Briefing, October 17, 2002. [Online] Available at http://www.cdc.gov/od/oc/media/transcripts/t021017.htm. Accessed August 1, 2004.

CDC. 2002b. Supplemental Guidance for Planning and Implementing the National Smallpox Vaccination Program (NSVP).

CDC. 2002c. Press Release, December 12, 2002. CDC Initial Review of State Smallpox Vaccination Plans Complete. [Online] Available at http://www.cdc.gov/od/oc/media/pressrel/r021212.htm. Accessed August 1, 2004.

CDC. 2002d. CDC Telebriefing Transcript: HHS Teleconference on Smallpox Policy. [Online] Available at http://www.cdc.gov/od/oc/media/transcripts/t021214.htm. Accessed January 10, 2003.

CDC. 2003a. Interim Smallpox Fact Sheet: Smallpox Vaccine and Heart Problems. [Online] Available at http://www.bt.cdc.gov/agent/smallpox/vaccination/heartproblems.asp. Accessed January 15, 2001.

CDC. 2003b. Smallpox Fact Sheet—Information for Clinicians: Smallpox (Vaccinia) Vaccine Contraindications.

CDC. 2003c. Smallpox Vaccination Program Status by State, July 25, 2003.

CDC. 2003d. CDC Telebriefing Transcript: Smallpox Vaccine Adverse Events Monitoring and Response System. [Online] Available at http://www.cdc.gov/od/oc/media/transcripts/t030206.htm. Accessed March 11, 2003.

CDC. 2003e. Notice to readers: smallpox vaccine adverse events monitoring and response system for the first stage of the smallpox vaccination program. *Morbidity and Mortality Weekly Report* 52(05):88-89, 99.

CDC. 2003f. Cardiac adverse events following smallpox vaccination—United States, 2003. *Mortality and Morbidity Weekly Report* 52(12):248-250.

CDC. 2003g. Notice to readers: national smallpox vaccine in pregnancy registry. *Mortality and Morbidity Weekly Report* 52(12):256.

CDC. 2003h. Notice to readers: supplemental recommendations on adverse events following smallpox vaccine in the pre-event vaccination program: recommendations of the Advisory Committee on Immunization Practices. *Mortality and Morbidity Weekly Report* 52(13):282-284.

CDC. 2003i. CDC Telebriefing Transcript: Update: Monkeypox Investigation in the U.S.

CDC. 2003j. Updated Interim CDC Guidance for Use of Smallpox Vaccine, Cidofovir, and Vaccinia Immune Globulin (VIG) for Prevention and Treatment in the Setting of an Outbreak of Monkeypox Infections. CDC Guidelines and Resources. [Online] Available at http://www.cdc.gov/ncidod/monkeypox/treatmentguidelines.htm. Accessed December 15, 2004.

CDC. 2003k. Update: cardiac and other adverse events following civilian smallpox vaccination—United States, 2003. *Mortality and Morbidity Weekly Report* 52(27):639-642.

CDC. 2003l. Update: multistate outbreak of monkeypox—Illinois, Indiana, Kansas, Missouri, Ohio, and Wisconsin, 2003. *Mortality and Morbidity Weekly Report* 52(27):642-646.

CDC. 2003m. Update: adverse events following smallpox vaccination—United States, 2003. *Mortality and Morbidity Weekly Report* 52(13):278-282.

CDC. 2003n. Advisory Committee on Immunization Practices (ACIP) Statement on Smallpox Preparedness and Vaccination. [Online] Available at http://www.bt.cdc.gov/agent/smallpox/vaccination/pdf/acipjun2003.pdf. Accessed July 17, 2003.

CDC. 2003o. Cardiac deaths after a mass smallpox vaccination campaign—New York City, 1947. *Morbidity and Mortality Weekly Report* 25(39):933-936.

CDC. 2003p. Smallpox Vaccination Report Status and Adverse Events. [Online] Available at http://www.cdc.gov/od/oc/media/smpxrpt.htm. Accessed March 7, 2003.

CDC. 2003q. CDC Health Advisory (via Health Alert Network): Smallpox: People with Known Cardiac Disease Should Not Be Vaccinated. [Online] Available at http://www.phppo.cdc.gov/han/Documents/AlertDocs/OldAlerts/129.asp. Accessed January 26, 2005.

CDC. 2003r. Smallpox Emergency Personnel Protection Act of 2003: Benefits and Compensation for Smallpox Vaccine Injuries. [Online] Available at http://www.bt.cdc.gov/agent/smallpox/vaccination/bene-comp.asp. Accessed June 16, 2003.

CDC. 2003s. Smallpox vaccine adverse events among civilians—United States, March 4-10, 2003. *Mortality and Morbidity Weekly Report* 52(10):201-203.

CDC. 2004a. Smallpox Vaccination Program Status by State, April 30, 2004.

CDC. 2004b. Smallpox Vaccination Program Status by State, August 31, 2004.

CDC. 2004c. Smallpox Vaccination Program Status by State, July 31, 2004.

CDC. 2004d. Update: adverse events following civilian smallpox vaccination—United States, 2003. *Mortality and Morbidity Weekly Report* 53(05):106-107.

CDC. 2004e. Secondary and tertiary transfer of vaccinia virus among U.S. military personnel—United States and worldwide, 2002-2004. *Morbidity and Mortality Weekly Report* 53(05):103-105.

CIA (Central Intelligence Agency). 2004. Comprehensive Report of the Special Advisor to the Director of Central Intelligence on Iraq's WMD. [Online] Available at http://www.cia.gov/cia/reports/iraq_wmd_2004/. Accessed January 26, 2005.

CIDRAP (Center for Infectious Disease Research and Policy). 2004, February 12. Contact Vaccinia in Soldier's Baby Linked to Breast-feeding. *CIDRAP News*.

CIDRAP and IDSA (Infectious Diseases Society of America). 2004. Smallpox: Current, Comprehensive Information on Pathogenesis, Microbiology, Epidemiology, Diagnosis, Treatment, and Prophylaxis. [Online] Available at http://www.cidrap.umn.edu/cidrap/content/bt/smallpox/biofacts/smllpx-summary.html. Accessed August 23, 2004.

Colacecchi J, Jones M. 2003. Testimony Before the Senate Appropriations Committee: Senate Labor, Health and Human Services and Education Appropriations Subcommittee, January 29, 2003. State Smallpox Pre-event Phase 1 Vaccination Program Estimated Costs. [Online] Available at http://appropriations.senate.gov/releases/record.cfm?id=190233. Accessed January 21, 2005.

Connolly C. 2003a, February 24. Bush Smallpox Inoculation Plan Near Standstill; Medical Professionals Cite Possible Side Effects, Uncertainty of Threat. *Washington Post*, A6.

Connolly C. 2003b, July 17. Focus on Smallpox Threat Revived. *Washington Post*, A3.

Connolly C. 2003c, March 29. 2 States Halt Smallpox Shots: Pentagon Reports First Post-Inoculation Fatal Heart Attack. *Washington Post*.

Connolly C, Milbank D. 2002, December 14. U.S. Revives Smallpox Shot. Bush Says He Will Receive Vaccine with Military, Emergency Workers. *Washington Post*, A1.

Daschle T, and 21 members of Senate (Democrat). 2003, January 22. Letter to President George W. Bush.

DHHS (Department of Health and Human Services). 2001, November 28. News Release: HHS Awards $428 Million Contract to Produce Smallpox Vaccine. Acambis/Baxter Will Produce 155 Million Doses by End of 2002.

DHHS. 2003a, January 24. News Release: HHS Secretary Authorizes Smallpox Vaccination Program. [Online] Available at www.hhs.gov/news/press/2003pres/20030124e.html. Accessed January 25, 2003.

DHHS. 2003b, February 25. News Release: HHS Announces Contracts to Develop Safer Smallpox Vaccines.

DHHS. 2003c, May 5. News Release: Secretary Thompson to Release $100 Million to Assist States with Smallpox Vaccination Programs.

DHHS. 2003d, March 5. News Release: HHS Proposes Smallpox Vaccination Compensation Plan. [Online] Available at http://www.hhs.gov/news/press/2003pres/20030305.html. Accessed March 7, 2003.

DHHS. 2004, October 7. News Release: HHS Awards $232 Million in Biodefense Contracts for Vaccine Development.

DoD (Department of Defense). 2003. Panels Issue Reports on Vaccine Adverse Event Cases: Vaccination Possibly Related to Soldier's Illness and Death. Press release, November 19, 2003.

DoD. 2004a. Vaccination Possible Cause of Soldier's Illness and Death. [Online] Available at http://www.vaccines.mil/documents/337safetypanelQA.pdf.

DoD. 2004b, June 30. News Release: Anthrax, Smallpox Protection Policies Updated. News Release No. 624-04. [Online] Available at http://www.defenselink.mil/releases/2004/nr20040630-0955.html. Accessed January 30, 2005.

DoD. 2004c. DoD Smallpox Vaccination Program Safety Summary. [Online] Available at http://www.smallpox.army.mil/event/SPSafetySum.asp.

DoD. 2004d. Smallpox Vaccination Program Summary: DoD Smallpox Vaccination Program as of February 11, 2004.

Everett W, Coffin S, Zaoutis T, Halpern S, Kim J, Strom B. 2002. Smallpox Willingness: A National Study of Emergency Department Personnel. Presented to the IOM Committee on Smallpox Vaccination Program Implementation on December 19, 2002.

FDA (Food and Drug Administration). 2002. The Bioterrorism Act of 2002. [Online] Available at http://www.fda.gov/oc/bioterrorism/bioact.html. Accessed January 26, 2005.

Federal Register. 2003a. Smallpox Vaccine Injury Compensation Program: Administrative Implementation. August 27, 2003, Washington, DC, 51492-51499. [Online] Available at http://www.gpoaccess.gov/fr/index.html.

Federal Register. 2003b. Smallpox Vaccine Injury Compensation Program: Administrative Implementation. December 16, 2003, Washington, DC, 70080-70106. [Online] Available at http://www.gpoaccess.gov/fr/index.html.

Fiorill J. 2003, October 24. U.S. Smallpox Official Acknowledges Vaccination "Targets Were Not Achieved". *Global Security Newswire.*

Fischler D. 2003. Presentation Before the IOM Committee on Smallpox Vaccination Program Implementation. Transcript of Meeting Four on November 6, 2003, Washington, DC.

Frey SE, Newman F, Cruz J, Shelton WB, Tennant JM, Polach T, Rothman AL, Kennedy JS, Wolff M, Belshe RB, Ennis FA. 2002. Dose-related effects of smallpox vaccine. *New England Journal of Medicine* 346(17):1275-1280.

Frist B. 2002, August 9. Op-Ed: Deciding Who Is Protected Against Smallpox. *New York Times.*

GAO (General Accounting Office). 2003. Smallpox Vaccination: Implementation of National Program Faces Challenges. Washington, DC: General Accounting Office, GAO-03-578.

Gellman B. 2002, November 5. Findings Spur New Smallpox Concerns. *Albany (NY) Times Union*.

Grady D, Altman L. 2003, March 25. Experts See Gains and Gaps in Planning for Terror Attack. *New York Times*.

Gregg J. 2002, October 6. Commentary: Let the Public Choose on Smallpox Vaccine. *Washington Post*.

Gursky E. 2003. Progress and Peril: Bioterrorism Preparedness Dollars and Public Health. Century Foundation. [Online] Available at http://www.tcf.org/Publications/Homeland Security/Gursky_Progress_Peril.pdf. Accessed January 30, 2005.

Hallow R. 2002, November 24. Governors Seek Access to Smallpox Vaccine. *Washington Times*, A4.

Halsell JS, Riddle JR, Atwood JE, Gardner P, Shope R, Poland GA, Gray GC, Ostroff S, Eckart RE, Hospenthal DR, Gibson RL, Grabenstein JD, Arness MK, Tornberg DN. 2003. Myopericarditis following smallpox vaccination among vaccinia-naive U.S. military personnel. *Journal of the American Medical Association* 289(24):3283-3289.

Hardy G. 2002. Statement of the Association of State and Territorial Health Officials. Presentation Before the IOM Committee on Smallpox Vaccination Program Implementation. Transcript of Meeting One on December 19, 2002, Washington, DC.

HealthLeaders. 2003. Smallpox Scare: Hospitals May Incur Costs, Downtime from Vaccinations. Green Sheet, February 2003. [Online] Available at http://www.healthleaders.com/magazine/2003/feb/greensheet.php. Accessed July 7, 2004.

Heil E. 2003, July 24. Panel Questions HHS on Low Smallpox Vaccinations. *GovExec.com*. [Online] Available at http://www.govexec.com/dailyfed/0703/072409cd2.htm. Accessed September 29, 2003.

Helle EP, Koskenvuo K, Heikkila J, Pikkarainen J, Weckstrom P. 1978. Myocardial complications of immunisations. *Annals of Clinical Research* 10(5):280-287.

Henderson J. 2003a. National Smallpox Vaccination Program Update. Presentation Before the IOM Committee on Smallpox Vaccination Program Implementation on May 1, 2003.

Henderson J. 2003b. Update on National Smallpox Preparedness: Smallpox Preparedness Indicators. Presentation Before the IOM Committee on Smallpox Vaccination Program Implementation on November 6, 2003.

Hirshon J. 2003. Presentation to the IOM Committee on Smallpox Vaccination Program Implementation. Transcript of Meeting Four on November 6, 2003, Washington, DC.

IOM (Institute of Medicine). 2002a. The Future of the Public's Health in the 21st Century. Washington, DC: The National Academies Press.

IOM. 2002b. Scientific and Policy Considerations in Developing Smallpox Vaccination Options: A Workshop Report. Washington, DC: The National Academies Press.

IOM. 2003a. Review of the Centers for Disease Control and Prevention's Smallpox Vaccination Program Implementation: Letter Report #1. Washington, DC: The National Academies Press.

IOM. 2003b. Review of the Centers for Disease Control and Prevention's Smallpox Vaccination Program Implementation: Letter Report #2. Washington, DC: The National Academies Press.

IOM. 2003c. Review of the Centers for Disease Control and Prevention's Smallpox Vaccination Program Implementation: Letter Report #3. Washington, DC: The National Academies Press.

IOM. 2003d. Review of the Centers for Disease Control and Prevention's Smallpox Vaccination Program Implementation: Letter Report #4. Washington, DC: The National Academies Press.

IOM. 2004. Learning from SARS: Preparing for the Next Disease Outbreak. Washington, DC: The National Academies Press.

Judson F. 2003. Presentation Before the IOM Committee on Smallpox Vaccination Program Implementation. Transcript of Meeting Three on May 1, 2003, Washington, DC.

Karjalainen J, Heikkila J, Nieminen MS, Jalanko H, Kleemola M, Lapinleimu K, Sahi T. 1983. Etiology of mild acute infectious myocarditis. Relation to clinical features. *Acta Medica Scandinavica* 213:65-73.

Kemper V. 2003a, January 17. States Lag at Start of Smallpox Program. *Los Angeles Times.*

Kemper V. 2003b, March 14. Few Volunteer for Smallpox Vaccination. *Los Angeles Times.*

Kemper V. 2003c, March 29. Guardsman Dies After Receiving Smallpox Vaccine; California Suspends All Inoculations and Wants New Federal Guidelines for Adverse Reactions. *Los Angeles Times.*

Kuhles D, Ackman D. 2003. The federal smallpox vaccination program: where do we go from here? *Health Affairs* (Web Exclusive) W3:503-510.

Libbey P. 2002. Presentation Before the IOM Committee on Smallpox Vaccination Program Implementation. Transcript of Meeting One on December 19, 2002, Washington, DC.

Libbey P. 2003. Testimony on Behalf of NACCHO (National Association of County and City Health Officials) Before the Subcommittee on Labor, Health, and Human Services, Education and Related Agencies, Committee on Appropriations, U.S. Senate. Hearing on Smallpox Vaccination, January 29, 2003.

MacLeod M. 2003, February 2. State Puts Smallpox Program on Hold Until Feds Resolve Liability Issue. *Macomb Daily* [Michigan].

Malenic M. 2004. U.S. to Expand Military Vaccinations. *Global Security Newswire.*

Manning A. 2003, April 22. Second Round of Smallpox Vaccinations Begins. *USA Today.*

Manning A, Sternberg S. 2002, October 7. Officials Ponder Timing, Sequence of Immunizations. *USA Today.*

Marchione M. 2003, February 7. Health Workers Enlist in Smallpox Fight; State Giving Hospitals Time to Educate Workers About Risk of Shot. *Milwaukee Journal Sentinel,* 15A.

McCullough M. 2003, February 7. Americans Aren't Rolling Up Their Sleeves for Smallpox Inoculation. *The Salt Lake Tribune.*

McGlinchey D. 2003a, February 26. CDC Says It Never Aimed for 500,000 Smallpox Vaccinations. *Global Security Newswire.*

McGlinchey D. 2003b, June 12. Monkeypox Outbreak Tests Bioterrorism Response System. *Global Security Newswire.*

McKenna M. 2003, February 15. No Vaccination for Nation's Fear; Unease Hinders Smallpox Program. *Atlanta Journal-Constitution.*

McNeil D. 2003, February 7. Many Balking at Vaccination for Smallpox. *New York Times.*

Mendieta A. 2003. A Young Soldier from the South Suburbs Died of a Mysterious Illness Before She Could Fulfill Her Dream of Serving Her Country on the Front Lines. *Chicago Sun-Times,* 6.

Meckler L. 2002, October 5. US Divided on Smallpox Policy. *Associated Press.*

Meckler L. 2003a, February 22. Smallpox Vaccinations Off to Slow Start. *Associated Press.*

Meckler L. 2003b, April 2. Lawmakers Split on Smallpox Compensation. *Associated Press.*

Meckler L. 2003c, February 5. Concerns About Compensation for People Injured by the Smallpox Vaccine Are Hampering Inoculation Program. *Associated Press.*

Mitchell S. 2003, June 12. Monkeypox Shows Gap in Bioterror Readiness. *United Press International.*

Mootrey G. 2003. Presentation Before the IOM Committee on Smallpox Vaccination Program Implementation. Transcript of Meeting Three on May 1, 2003, Washington, DC.

Murphy W. 2003, April 14. FDNY Sets Terms for Smallpox Vaccinees. *Newsday.*

NACCHO (National Association of County and City Health Officials). 2003a. Impact of Smallpox Vaccination Program on Local Public Health Services. Research Brief No. 9.

NACCHO. 2003b. Costs of Smallpox Vaccination Program: Summary of Preliminary Data. Research Brief No. 10.

Neff J. 2003a. Advisory Committee on Immunization Practices Smallpox Vaccine Safety Working Group: Summary of Vaccination Program Safety Monitoring, April 2003.

Neff J. 2003b. Presentation Before the IOM Committee on Smallpox Vaccination Program Implementation. Transcript of Meeting Three on May 1, 2003, Washington, DC.

New York Times. 2002, December 22. Editorial: Ducking Smallpox Vaccinations.

NGA (National Governors Association). 2003. Statement of the National Governors Association for the Senate Labor, Health and Human Services and Education Appropriations Subcommittee on Smallpox Vaccination Funding. Senate Appropriations Commitee: Senate Labor, Health and Human Services and Education Appropriations Subcommittee.

NIH (National Institutes of Health). 2001. Fact Sheet: Study Seeks to Determine Effectiveness of Diluted Smallpox Vaccine. [Online] Available at http://www.vrc.nih.gov/factsheets/btsmallpox.htm. Accessed January 26, 2005.

NIH. 2002. Press Release: NIAID Study Results Support Diluting Smallpox Vaccine Stockpile to Stretch Supply. [Online] Available at http://www.nih.gov/news/pr/mar2002/hhs-28.htm. Accessed January 26, 2005.

Nikolai K. 2003. Presentation Before the IOM Committee on Smallpox Vaccination Program Implementation. Transcript of Meeting Three on May 1, 2003, Washington, DC.

Ornstein C, Bonilla D. 2003, February 6. Smallpox Plan Divides Hospitals: Fifteen in the County Refuse Vaccinations for Employees. Nine Accept; Most Are Undecided. *Los Angeles Times.*

Ornstein C, Richardson L. 2003, February 8. U.S. Far Behind Schedule for Smallpox Vaccinations. *Los Angeles Times.*

Pasternack N. 2003, February 5. State to Give Vaccine: First Shots Will Be for Health Workers. *Olympia (WA) Olympian.*

Peterson C. 2002. Presentation Before the IOM Committee on Smallpox Vaccination Program Implementation. Transcript of Meeting One on December 18, 2002, Washington, DC.

Pezzino G. 2003. Presentation Before the IOM Committee on Smallpox Vaccination Program Implementation. Transcript of Meeting Three on May 1, 2003, Washington, DC.

Rath E, Turcotte J. 2003, March 6. Press Release: Senator Gregg to Move Smallpox Compensation Legislation Through Senate. Office of Judd Gregg, U.S. Senator for New Hampshire.

Reuters. 2003, March 27. Experts Urge Caution in US Smallpox Plan.

Roos R. 2003a, February 5. Many Doses of Smallpox Vaccine Shipped, But Few Shots Given so Far. *CIDRAP News.*

Roos R. 2003b, August 21. D.A. Henderson Critiques Report on Duration of Smallpox Immunity. *CIDRAP News.*

Roos R. 2003c, November 19. Vaccines Might Have Contributed to Death of Army Reservist. *CIDRAP News.*

Roos R. 2004a, April 13. Myopericarditis Cases Complicate Acambis Smallpox Vaccine Trials. *CIDRAP News.*

Roos R. 2004b, June 16. Pilot Study to Probe Cardiac Effects of Smallpox Vaccine. *CIDRAP News.*

Rosado E. 2003. Fact Sheet: Smallpox. National Association of Counties.

Russell S. 2003, January 18. Smallpox Vaccine Plan Starts Tuesday, Despite Concerns; Some Health Workers May Opt Out Over Risks, Compensation Issues. *San Francisco Chronicle.*

Schulman R. 2002. Presentation Before the IOM Committee on Smallpox Vaccination Program Implementation. Transcript of Meeting One on December 18, 2002, Washington, DC.

SEIU (Service Employees International Union). 2002. As Bush Plan for Mass Smallpox Stirs Controversy, Nation's Largest Health Care Organization Says Hospital Workers, Patients Will Face Unnecessary Risk. [Online] Available at http://www.seiu.org/media/press_releases/press.cfm?ID=1096. Accessed January 8, 2003.

Selecky M. 2003. Presentation Before the IOM Committee on Smallpox Vaccination Program Implementation. Transcript of Meeting Three on May 1, 2003, Washington, DC.

Shockman L. 2003, March 28. Nationwide Smallpox Protection Program for Health Workers Is Shy of Goal. *Toledo [Ohio] Blade.*

Skivington S. 2003. Presentation Before the IOM Committee on Smallpox Vaccination Program Implementation. Transcript of Meeting Three on May 1, 2003, Washington, DC.

Staiti A, Katz A, Hoadley J. 2003. Has Bioterrorism Preparedness Improved Public Health? Center for Studying Health System Change Issue Brief No. 65.

Talbot T, Stapleton J, Bready R, Winokur P, Bernstein D, Germanson T, Yoder S, Rock M, Crowe J, Edwards K. 2004. Vaccination success rate and reaction profile with diluted and undiluted smallpox vaccine: a randomized controlled trial. *Journal of the American Medical Association* 292(10):1205-1212.

Tasker S, Schnepf G, Lim M, Caraviello H, Armstrong A, Bavaro M, Agan B, Delmar J, Aronson N, Wallace M, Grabenstein J. 2004. Unintended smallpox vaccination of HIV-1 infected. *Clinical Infectious Diseases* 38(9):1320-1322.

Temte J. 2003. Presentation Before the IOM Committee on Smallpox Vaccination Program Implementation. Transcript of Meeting Four on November 6, 2003, Washington, DC.

Thorpe L, Schwartz S, Manning S, Marx M, Frieden T. Mass smallpox vaccination and cardiac deaths, New York City, 1947. *Emerging Infectious Diseases* 10(5):917-920.

Toomey K. 2003. Presentation Before the IOM Committee on Smallpox Vaccination Program Implementation. Transcript of Meeting Two on February 13, 2003, Washington, DC.

U.S. House of Representatives. 2004. U.S. Representative Thomas M. Davis (R-VA) Holds Hearing on Health System Preparedness. House Government Reform Committee.

U.S. House of Representatives Select Committee on Homeland Security (Democratic Members). 2004. A Biodefense Failure: the Smallpox Vaccination Program One Year Later.

U.S. Senate Select Committee on Intelligence. 2004. Report on the U.S. Intelligence Community's Prewar Intelligence Assessments on Iraq. [Online] Available at http://intelligence.senate.gov/iraqreport2.pdf. Accessed July 8, 2004.

Washington Times. 2003, January 23. Editorial: Smallpox refuseniks.

Washington Post. 2002, December 19. Editorial: Doctors' Orders.

White House. 2002a. President Bush Signs Homeland Security Act. Remarks by the President at the Signing of H.R. 5005 the Homeland Security Act of 2002. [Online] Available at http://www.whitehouse.gov/news/releases/2002/11/20021125-6.html. Accessed January 26, 2005.

White House. 2002b. President Delivers Remarks on Smallpox. [Online] Available at http://www.whitehouse.gov/news/releases/2002/12/20021213-7.html. Accessed January 8, 2003.

White House. 2003a. National Threat Level Raised. Statement by Homeland Security Secretary Tom Ridge. [Online] Available at http://www.whitehouse.gov/news/releases/2003/03/20030317-8.html. Accessed January 26, 2005.

White House. 2003b. President Bush Addresses the Nation. [Online] Available at http://www.whitehouse.gov/news/releases/2003/03/20030319-17.html. Accessed January 26, 2005.

White House. 2003c. President Bush Announces Major Combat Operations in Iraq Have Ended. Remarks by the President from the USS Abraham Lincoln at Sea off the Coast of San Diego, California. [Online] Available at http://www.whitehouse.gov/news/releases/2003/05/iraq/20030501-15.html. Accessed January 26, 2005.

Witt D. 2003. Presentation Before the IOM Committee on Smallpox Vaccination Program Implementation. Transcript of Meeting Three on May 1, 2003, Washington, DC.

Yee D. 2003, June 19. CDC: Not Enough Health Workers Have Smallpox Shots. *Associated Press.*

Yih W, Lieu T, Rego V, O'Brien M, Shay D, Yokoe D, Platt R. 2003. Attitudes of healthcare workers in U.S. hospitals regarding smallpox vaccination. *BMC Public Health* 3:20.

4

Lessons Learned from the Smallpox Vaccination Program

As the committee observed in its first report, the smallpox vaccination program is not a typical public health program, but rather a biopreparedness program predicated on national security considerations (IOM, 2003a). Bioterrorism preparedness is a recent addition to the scope of work of public health agencies, and it presents opportunities and challenges (such as new types of information restrictions and new domains of uncertainty) as public health agencies learn to work with national security and defense entities on matters of shared concern.

The smallpox vaccination program is a case study in blending public health and national security interests to prepare for an event of low likelihood and high consequence—bioterrorism in the form of a smallpox virus release. The program will not be the last of its kind as long as terrorism, specifically bioterrorism, continues to be a threat. Therefore, discerning broad lessons to be learned from the smallpox vaccination program is important for ensuring the success of similar future programs. The present chapter highlights the committee's major findings about the program and provides a conclusion and a recommendation based on those findings.

ABSENCE OF EXPLICIT SCIENTIFIC AND PUBLIC HEALTH RATIONALE FOR THE PROGRAM

In 2002, most public health officials and health care workers who participated in surveys or in several forums discussing smallpox vaccination expressed support for a limited pre-event smallpox vaccination effort and willingness to be vaccinated if they were designated as members of smallpox response teams (Banks and Hannan, 2002; Everett et al., 2002; IOM, 2002; Yih et al., 2003). Yet the high degree of support for limited smallpox vaccination to prepare the nation to respond to attack did not generate a substantial turnout of volunteer vaccinees; by the end of 2004, fewer than 40,000 people had been vaccinated, far short of original estimates of turnout. The committee found several possible and related reasons for that incongruity.

First, the scientific and public health rationale that led to the smallpox vaccination policy was never fully explained to key constituencies—traditional partners in the development and implementation of public health strategies, including state and local public health agencies—that provided input to the process but whose advice and perspectives were not reflected in the final policy. Although the committee recognizes that the terrorist attacks of 2001 were a dramatic and persuasive reminder of the importance of biopreparedness, it was never made clear to the public health and health care communities why smallpox was selected as a primary target for biopreparedness, how pre-event smallpox vaccination was identified as a core strategy, and why vaccination was urgent.

Second, the scientific and public health rationale that led to the structure of the smallpox vaccination program (in its final form, characterized by the phases and numbers discussed elsewhere in this report) was never fully explained. The ultimate policy called for a much higher number of vaccinees than the original, cautious estimate provided to the government by the Advisory Committee on Immunization Practices (ACIP), and the rationale for offering the vaccine to 500,000 initially, then to up to 10 million, and finally to insistent members of the public was not made clear to important constituencies. Instead, confusing and contradictory information was presented to the public and the public health community about the policy and program.

Third, the limited amount of information that was provided to explain the rationale for the policy and for the structure of the program was neither updated nor reiterated during the course of the program despite strong signals that updating or reiteration was needed.

Fourth, program implementation was characterized by a lack of review of the program's course and reassessment of starting assumptions. Despite calls for a pause to assess program progress and safety, the program continued. As its pace waned, there was no apparent attempt to reassess or review program implementation and its trajectory.

Finally, and most centrally, the ability of the Centers for Disease Control and Prevention (CDC) to speak authoritatively as the nation's public health leader, on the basis of the best available scientific reasoning, was severely constrained, presumably by the top levels of the executive branch.

Because the smallpox vaccination program involved both public health and national security considerations, it is understood that the latter could involve classified information and thus limit what could be made available to the public. However, the apparent, unexplained constraints on CDC led to an environment in which the public health and health care communities and their leaders did not receive all the information needed to make institutional and individual decisions regarding smallpox vaccination (Selecky, 2003; Smith, 2003). There is little to suggest that the scientific and public health reasoning that typically characterizes the development of public health policies was a priority in this case. The expert input of public health leaders and other relevant constituencies was not reflected in the final structure of the smallpox vaccination policy. Agencies and organizations expected to be important partners in implementing the program expressed concerns and questions about it, and those concerns ultimately affected the program's outcomes. Key constituencies remained skeptical about the need for the program, and their lack of buy-in led to poor participation in the vaccination program. At the institutional level, this is illustrated by the request of the Association of State and Territorial Health Officials (ASTHO) for an explanation of the rationale for the program (Selecky, 2003) several months after the beginning of vaccination. Among individual public health and health care workers, receiving what they perceived as insufficient information left them unable to accept smallpox vaccination.

Lack of Scientific and Public Health Rationale for the Existence of the Vaccination Program

In 2003, in *Health Affairs*, Kuhles and Ackman wrote:

> The key message we received from potential vaccinees was that civilians are unlikely to voluntarily assume personal risk without good reason. Before performing an invasive procedure, physicians are required to undertake an informed-consent process with the patient, which spells out the indications, alternatives, and risks. The government owes its health care, public health, and first-responder communities the same consideration, particularly as it relates to the indications for vaccination, which thus far has been lacking.

Surveys of public health and health care workers (ASTHO, 2003; Everett et al., 2002; Yih et al., 2003), interviews (Kuhles and Ackman, 2003; Markowitz and Rosner, 2004), and newspaper articles (*Associated Press*, 2003; Bavley and Dvorak, 2003; Connolly, 2003a; Denogean, 2003; McCullough, 2003; McNeil, 2003; Ornstein and Bonilla, 2003; Wheeler, 2003) have shown that personal decision-making about smallpox vaccination was shaped by perceptions about known and considerable vaccine risk and unknown vaccine benefit in the absence of disease. The question of vaccine benefit was linked with the rationale for the vaccination program. On the basis of mass media coverage of program progress and a variety of additional sources, including presentations to the present Institute of Medicine (IOM) committee, it appears that despite the expressed sense of personal commitment (May et al., 2003) to protecting the public's health, both individuals and institutions found the information available for decision-making inadequate in quantity and quality and ultimately not sufficiently conducive to an affirmative decision regarding vaccination.

Communication about the smallpox vaccination policy and the decisions that led to it was incomplete and vague, particularly information quantifying or explaining the available evidence about the threat of smallpox and information about the epidemiologic and public health reasoning regarding whom and when to vaccinate. Although sensitive, classified information may have been involved, it does not appear that the complete facts needed for decision-making and buy-in at the state and local levels were shared with constituencies, and failure to do that had a detrimental effect on the program's progress and, more important, may have compromised the relationship of trust between CDC and the public health community.

The president's announcement stated multiple times that the government had no information that a smallpox virus release was imminent (White House, 2002). Information provided by the Department of Health and Human Services (DHHS) and CDC largely reiterated the president's statements and shed no additional light on the evidence that led to the decision to begin pre-event smallpox vaccination (U.S. Department of State, 2002). At least some of the information appeared to be many years old, dating back to the fall of the Soviet Union (Gellman, 2002), and it was never made clear to the public what accumulation of evidence made smallpox vaccination an urgent priority. The president's announcement that the threat was not imminent, although not zero, restated what had been the case for at least a decade. Undoubtedly, the events of September and October 2001 were important in shaping how old information was being viewed (White House, 2002).

A complete risk-benefit analysis in the face of extreme ambiguity seemed impossible, and both institutional and personal decisions regarding vaccination were complicated by the lack of information. The factual information available to institutions and individuals considering participation in the voluntary vaccination program consisted primarily of the following:

- The president's statement about the threat assessment.
- The statements of other federal officials (including the director of CDC) about the threat assessment.
- The recent occurrence of domestic terrorism and bioterrorism.

- The immediacy of war with a nation that the administration asserted had weapons of mass destruction, including biologic weapons.
- Historical evidence about the vaccine.
- Historical evidence about the disease.
- The provisions of Section 304 of the Homeland Security Act.

The resulting sense of uncertainty proved to be problematic. As one clinician stated, the perceived lack of evidence regarding a possible smallpox virus release was a deterrent to vaccination. "It is not enough for someone—whether it is the president or the secretary of state—to say, 'I'm worried about this; trust me'. . . . We need more than that today as a profession and as a society," he observed (Connolly, 2003a). In a presentation to this committee, the president of a large health and hospital system stated (Anderson, 2003) that he did not believe he had the evidence to support the vaccination of "even the core 100 [vaccinees]. It was our concern that there was evidence that we didn't have, that we weren't being given, or it wasn't being shared, that something was more serious here than we thought. Maybe there was a weaponized product, that somebody had broken through, and that we weren't being told about." The hospital epidemiologist of a university health system stated (Edmond, 2003) that "we didn't want the decision to vaccinate to be one that was ideological. We wanted it to be an evidence-based decision." On the basis of the information available to it, the leadership of that university health system developed an institutional policy to undertake only planning for postevent vaccination and to implement smallpox vaccination only in any of three scenarios: if a smallpox case occurred anywhere in the world, if information were provided by the federal or state government about a serious smallpox risk, or if smallpox stocks were found outside the two approved repositories. Representatives of a large health plan also listed among problems with the program the perception that the case for smallpox vaccination was "never sufficiently compelling" and that the uncertainty surrounding the policy and program created distress and skepticism among staff (Skivington and Witt, 2003). Finally, interviews conducted with health officials and other public health experts in the early months of the program's implementation indicated that some did not believe that a convincing case had been made to justify the pre-event vaccination program (Kuhles and Ackman, 2003; Markowitz and Rosner, 2004).

The Input of Key Constituencies

The committee's knowledge of the circumstances surrounding the development of the policy is derived primarily from official CDC and DHHS transcripts of press conferences, testimony before Congress, presentations at IOM committee meetings, and, to a lesser extent, mass media reports (when multiple reports corroborating an event were available). During the development of the smallpox vaccination policy, there was communication among CDC, DHHS, the Office (later the Department) of Homeland Security, and the White House (Cohen and Enserink, 2002). Multiple constituencies (including various entities in the health care, public health, and first responder communities) provided written and oral input to CDC and to Congress (for example, at CDC-organized forums across the nation) in the months before the policy was developed and during its implementation. For example, during summer 2002, CDC engaged its state and local partners (such as representatives of ASTHO and the Council of State and Territorial Epidemiologists) in numerous discussions and provided multiple opportunities for comment about the policy options being considered (ASTHO, 2002; CDC, 2002a; IOM, 2002). In June 2002, ASTHO held a conference call and then conducted a survey to determine its members' views on strategies for smallpox preparedness. The survey found that a majority of state health officials were opposed to pre-event vaccination of the general public, but most supported pre-event vaccination of designated response teams (Banks and Hannan, 2002). Consensus reached at the June 2002 ACIP meeting reflected a similar opposition to pre-event vaccination of the general public and support for vaccination of specific groups of responders (CDC, 2002b). The ultimate policy decision on vaccinating members of the general public and on vaccinating health care workers differed from the consensus of key constituencies, and it is unclear to what extent their expertise and input were considered.

The collaborative nature of public health in the United States, described in the IOM report *The Future of the Public's Health in the 21st Century*, makes partnership and communication essential to any program's success. Within that process, the credibility of information and decisions from the national level sets the stage for all later decisions and actions by state and local health departments and their partners. Not knowing what evidence was considered and not receiving information about it from CDC—as evidenced by the fact that key partners, such as ASTHO, requested clarification (to the committee's knowledge never provided) of the rationale behind the policy and the structure of the program—may have affected the public health community's trust in CDC, as is evident in the expressed perceptions and concerns of many in the public health and health care communities (ASTHO, 2003; Pendley, 2003; Markowitz and Rosner, 2004). A recent CDC analysis of the swine influenza vaccination program of 1976 noted the importance of ensuring the credibility of decisions made by CDC (DHHS, 2004). The Neustadt and Fineberg analysis (1983) of the swine flu program also concluded that the program demonstrated an "insensitivity to the long-term credibility of institutions."

The final vaccination policy differed considerably from the recommendations of public health leaders and other important constituencies, and those groups were left with questions about the rationale for the vaccination program. That contrasts with the implementation of more typical public health programs and with the principles of public health practice. First, the ethos of public health attaches great importance to the empowerment and participation of a broad constituency in decision-making; a high degree of openness and collaboration also is consistent with the democratic principle of public accountability (Gostin, 1995). Second, effective policymaking requires identifying potential obstacles, and those are likely to be known or anticipated by key constituencies. The implementation of the vaccination program reveals missed opportunities at the level of policymaking to identify or adequately address potential obstacles to implementation (discussed in Chapter 3). For example, in addition to unease about compensation and liability issues, state and local public health agencies expressed concern that implementing a vaccination program of massive proportions, beyond the initial 500,000 vaccinees, would have safety implications and enormous resource requirements (Connolly, 2002; Hardy 2002; Libbey, 2003a, 2003b; Rosado, 2003).

That the policy was not consistent with the recommendations of key constituencies and its rationale was not clearly and adequately explained to them may also have led to difficulties in balancing competing priorities. For example, the vaccination program's single-agent focus and great resource requirements burdened the public health system to the detriment of other public health activities, including the routine activities of public health and preparedness for other kinds of emergencies. Smallpox efforts were all-consuming for many local public health agencies, especially smaller health departments. Despite the bioterrorism grants that had been made available to states, state and local public health officials expressed frustration at the program's vast underestimation of its direct and opportunity costs and argued that the vaccination program necessitated a diversion from bioterrorism plans that they had already developed in anticipation of funding (ASTHO, 2003; Cook, 2003; GAO, 2003; Kuhles and Ackman, 2003; Markowitz and Rosner, 2004; NACCHO, 2003a, 2003b; Staiti et al., 2003; U.S. House of Representatives, 2004). Of local public health agencies surveyed by the National Association of County and City Health Officials (NACCHO) in March 2003, 79 percent reported that smallpox activities adversely affected their other bioterrorism preparedness efforts (NACCHO, 2003a). County health officials also reported on opportunity costs of diverting staff to smallpox activities and on delaying or deferring other public health programs (Kuhles and Ackman, 2003; Madlock, 2003; Nikolai, 2003; NACCHO, 2003b; Markowitz and Rosner, 2004; U.S. House of Representatives, 2004). As one county public health agency struggled with a tuberculosis outbreak, its efforts were complicated by the fact that its resources were greatly strained by a combination of budget cuts and the demands of the smallpox vaccination program. Other local health departments reported diverting staff from their regular activities, delays in childhood immunizations, cancelled family planning clinics, cuts in tobacco control and maternal and child health services, and other changes or cuts in services routinely provided by public health agencies (Connolly, 2003b; Cook, 2003; Hughes, 2003; Staiti et al., 2003).

Planning for the smallpox vaccination program appears not to have included sufficient analysis of the potential effect of vaccination activities on the provision of essential public health services and on other preparedness efforts or analysis of the added costs of implementing such a large vaccination program (GAO, 2003; IOM, 2003b, 2003c). It remains unclear to what extent the supplementary funding provided by DHHS in May 2003 ameliorated the fiscal challenges experienced by some jurisdictions.

Lack of Scientific and Public Health Rationale for the Structure of the Vaccination Program

The rationale for the program's structure also was not fully explained. As discussed in Chapter 3, ACIP's June 2002 recommendation to CDC and DHHS called for the vaccination of up to 20,000 people: public health personnel who would serve on smallpox public health investigation teams and health care personnel staffing designated "smallpox hospitals" (CDC, 2002b). John Modlin, ACIP chair, acknowledged the group's unease with the unknown risk of smallpox virus release, but he believed that its recommendation to DHHS and CDC was made carefully. "The committee has been told that the risk is low but not zero. We obviously can't put a number on that but we . . . assume that it's low, and I think the decision that we made . . . balanced that low or very low risk with . . . the known risk from the vaccine" (CDC, 2002c). In October 2002, after the mass media had reported on the various figures being considered by the administration, one of which was 500,000 vaccinees, ACIP revised its recommendation in recognition that hospitals would probably resist being designated as smallpox hospitals and, more important, that smallpox-stricken persons would go to the nearest emergency department rather than to a designated location (Altman, 2002; Brown, 2002; CDC, 2002b; Cohen and Enserink, 2002). ACIP's revised vaccination target was 500,000. The ACIP chair acknowledged that that was a "back-of-the-envelope" calculation based on the assumption that if the nation's roughly 5,100 acute-care hospitals each vaccinated roughly 100 people, the total would be about a half-million vaccinated health care workers. That may explain in part how the target for the first phase of the program was derived, although to some the 500,000 figure seemed oddly coincidental with the estimate first suggested by White House officials, and there was some initial concern that ACIP was pressured to modify its earlier recommendation (Brown, 2002; Cohen and Enserink, 2002) (see also discussion in Chapter 2).

The rationale for the second and third phases of the program, vaccinating 10 million responders and insistent members of the general public, respectively, which surpassed and even diverged from ACIP recommendations and from the advice of constituencies such as the American Public Health Association, the American Academy of Family Physicians, the Emergency Nurses Association, and others that called for limited vaccination (AAFP, 2002; APHA, 2002; ENA, 2002; IDSA, 2002; May et al., 2003), was never shared with those who would implement the program or who would volunteer to be vaccinated. There was no apparent public health reasoning behind the decision to offer vaccine to the public. In fact, the present committee stated in its fourth report to CDC that "offering vaccination to members of the general public is contrary to the basic precepts of public health ethics, which focus on a fair and reasonable balance of risks and benefits among individuals and for the population as a whole" (IOM, 2003b; see Appendix E). The nation's public health and health care communities expected an explanation of the public health reasoning behind the policy that would include an epidemiologic justification for offering vaccination to the three types of vaccinees identified, evidence that vaccinating response teams before a smallpox virus release would ensure a better and faster response to an attack, evidence that vaccinating other types of responders (such as firefighters and police) would substantially improve response effectiveness, and evidence that implementing specific pre-event vaccination activities would be an optimal use of resources as part of bioterrorism preparedness efforts. The committee is unaware of evidence showing whether and how the advantages and disadvantages of various pre-event vaccination options were carefully weighed and compared or evidence that decisions were made accordingly.

Confusing and Contradictory Information About the Policy and the Program

The contradictory and confusing information provided during the implementation of the smallpox vaccination program may have constituted another barrier to implementation of the program and may have undermined CDC's credibility further. For example, the announcement of the policy and later explanations assured Americans that there was no imminent risk of smallpox virus release (U.S. Department of State, 2002; White House, 2002). Nevertheless, the federal government repeatedly called for rapid implementation of the vaccination program. CDC's initial guidance to the states called for implementing vaccination within 30 days (CDC, 2002d). After the program began, representatives of the public health community remarked on the challenging timeline and called for slower implementation (Hardy, 2002; Libbey, 2003a, 2003b). Although the initial 30-day timeline was later changed and CDC acknowledged that flexibility would be needed because of administrative difficulties and variation among states, CDC continued to call for rapid implementation without specifying the reason (CDC, 2003a, 2003c; Ornstein and Bonilla, 2003; Russell, 2003). CDC's emphasis on safety *and* speed seemed contradictory and generated confusion and an atmosphere of near-crisis in which public health agencies at all levels felt compelled to undertake smallpox vaccination activities about which they had doubts (ASTHO, 2003; Connolly, 2003b; Cook, 2003; McKenna, 2003; NACCHO, 2003a; Pezzino, 2003). In addition, owing to the remarkable speed with which the program was implemented, a number of administrative and procedural components were not ready for implementation, as discussed in greater detail in Chapter 3. Although impending crisis would have justified a rapid response, that was not the case that was made. Instead, the rush to vaccinate as many personnel as possible as rapidly as possible gave rise to concerns about the wisdom of exposing people to an unsafe vaccine in the absence of a known threat of disease.

As described in Chapter 3, the present IOM committee and ASTHO urged CDC to pause after the first phase of vaccination to assess program safety and to plan for the next phase, and ACIP recommended terminating the program because of the occurrence of cardiac adverse events and their unknown long-term safety ramifications (CDC, 2003d; IOM, 2003d; Meckler, 2003a). The present committee repeated its call for a pause in the vaccination program in another report in which that was the primary recommendation (IOM, 2003b); however, despite its acknowledgment of the importance of safety, CDC stated that it expected the program to progress seamlessly from one phase to the next, at least in part to maintain momentum (Henderson, 2003; McGlinchey, 2003a). It is not clear whether CDC discussed the merits and costs of a pause in the vaccination program with its state and local counterparts. In the end, multiple state and local programs paused or stalled simply for lack of volunteer vaccinees.

Lack of Updating or Reiteration of the Rationale

The juxtaposition of impending war with the uncertainty surrounding the rationale for the vaccination policy and the lack of information pertaining to the smallpox threat assessment may have contributed to the program's slow progress. In January and February 2003, simultaneously with the implementation of smallpox vaccination, the administration was demonstrating to the nation and international allies that a war in Iraq was necessary to prevent the use of weapons of mass destruction. That clearly contentious matter was debated in Congress, in the mass media, and elsewhere. An attack on Iraq was argued on security, economic, foreign relations, military, and other grounds.

Although the federal government did not explicitly link the war with Iraq and the vaccination program and at times even denied that the rationale for the program was related to the rationale for the war, several officials (DHHS Secretary Thompson, CDC Director Gerberding, and CDC National Immunization Program Director Walt Orenstein) and legislators (Senators Bill Frist and Judd Gregg) made statements that could be interpreted as suggesting that the war was a factor in the decisions made about the smallpox vaccination policy and program or as asserting the importance of vaccination in view of developments related to the war and the possibility of a bioterrorrist attack (Frist, 2002; Gregg, 2002; Hallow, 2002; Manning and Sternberg, 2002; Pear, 2003; Rath and Turcotte, 2003; Tanner, 2003; *Washington Post*, 2002). Whether formally linked with the war or not, by its timing the smallpox vaccination policy was caught up in the larger debate with its emotional and polarizing consequences. Similarly, there was debate in some quarters about the efficacy and necessity of the vaccination program. According to the April 2003 General Accounting Office (GAO, now the Government Accountability Office) report, and to local health officials, hospital administrators, and others who were interviewed by the media or who addressed this committee, many people concluded that the risk of a smallpox attack was associated with the contentious war with Iraq (Anderson, 2003; Judson, 2003; Kuhles and Ackman, 2003; Krupnick, 2003; Manning, 2003; McKenna, 2003; McNeil, 2003). As the weeks passed, major combat in Iraq ended; the homeland security threat level, which had been increased before the war, was lowered; and the smallpox threat did not materialize. In September 2003, the U.S.-led Iraq Survey Group reported that it did not find weapons of mass destruction in Iraq; in particular, the group found no evidence of smallpox (Linzer, 2003; CIA, 2004; UN Security Council, 2004). Unfortunately, the smallpox threat assessment was neither updated nor reiterated, and that left many prospective volunteers in the public health and health care communities to draw their own conclusions about the threat status and may have further eroded their trust, given what they were (or were not) hearing from their federal-level partners. Those factors may have contributed to a waning sense of urgency; combined with concerns about cardiac adverse events, they go far to explain the declining rate of vaccination.

At the May 2003 meeting of the present IOM committee, ASTHO summarized what the nation's health officials considered requirements for advancing smallpox preparedness, including a definition of the full scope of smallpox preparedness, a national consensus on who should be asked to consider voluntary vaccination (before an event) and why, a clear articulation of the best available intelligence information regarding the nation's potential risk of smallpox, and a clear statement of all known benefits and risks associated with smallpox vaccination (Selecky, 2003). Even months into the vaccination program, public health officials were actively seeking more information about the threat of smallpox virus release and the rationale for smallpox vaccination.

The Senate Select Committee on Intelligence *Report on the U.S. Intelligence Community's Prewar Intelligence Assessments on Iraq* (2004) and the report of the special adviser to the director of central intelligence on Iraq's weapons of mass destruction found much of the evidence on the existence of weapons of mass destruction in Iraq to be weak, including the evidence on smallpox (CIA, 2004). The significance of those reports is not that the evidence that may have been used to make the vaccination policy had been brought into question but rather that the evidence and the extent of uncertainty about it were not communicated to relevant constituencies as part of a discussion of the scientific and public health rationale for the vaccination program. Policies and programs are sometimes found to have been based on flawed information and are accordingly changed or terminated. Public health decisions are sometimes made in the face of great uncertainty, but the uncertainty is generally openly discussed. The Senate and Central Intelligence Agency reports give rise to questions about why a sense of uncertainty about the probability of smallpox virus release was not more openly conveyed, with more information about the rationale for the policy, and why the threat assessment was not clarified, changed, or confirmed as the sense of urgency in the program diminished and the rate of vaccination dropped. Although DHHS and CDC officials expressed concern about the loss of momentum in the pre-event smallpox vaccination program and the apparent complacency among health care and public health workers, there was neither a formal reiteration of the threat assessment nor a formal reassessment of whether and how the program should continue (Fiorill, 2003; Meckler, 2003b). If the decision to vaccinate was based on some type of evidence, how could the decision remain unchanged when the evidence apparently changed? Again, the absence of a science-based and public health-based public explanation to either continue or end the program may have constituted a threat to trust.

Lack of Review of the Program's Course and Lack of Reassessment of Starting Assumptions

In its report on another controversial vaccination program, the swine influenza program of 1976, GAO (1977) recommended that "when decisions must be based on very limited scientific data, HEW [the Department of Health, Education, and Welfare, predecessor of DHHS] should establish key points at which the program should be formally evaluated." Another analysis of the swine influenza program (Neustadt and Fineberg, 1978) recommended "a comprehensive definition and review of assumptions everyone can see and weigh before decision and remember after. The review thus should be public." The multiple assumptions and decisions involved in the swine influenza vaccination policy were never clarified before or during the program, and the program lacked designated points for stopping to assess program progress and safety and to plan for the future.

In the case of the smallpox vaccination program, the transition between the first and second phases of the vaccination campaign seemed to offer an appropriate point for stopping to evaluate assumptions, assess safety, and plan for what would be needed for a new population of vaccinees. The executive director of the American Public Health Association underscored the need to reassess assumptions before progressing to a new population of vaccinees (McKenna, 2003). As noted, in May 2003, the present committee called for a pause in the vaccination program before the second phase (IOM, 2003d). In June 2003, ACIP recommended that CDC not proceed with smallpox vaccination beyond the initial group of health care and public health response team members (CDC, 2003d). ACIP cited the cardiac adverse events: the fatal myocardial infarctions that prompted the development of cardiac exclusion criteria and the military and probable civilian cases of heart inflammation (myo/pericarditis) that came to be considered serious adverse events related to vaccination. Subsequent to ACIP's or IOM's calls to stop or pause, CDC Director Gerberding reiterated the agency's commitment to proceeding with smallpox vaccination (CDC, 2003e). Although CDC's rapid and appropriate response to the cardiac adverse events may provide partial evidence of the effectiveness of the adverse event active surveillance system and demonstrate the emphasis on safety, this IOM committee remained concerned that without a programmatic pause, states would have no opportunity to benefit from a national-level evaluation and perspective on the smallpox vaccination program. Given the much higher numbers of vaccinees expected in the second phase of vaccination, the potential for complications and other challenges seemed greater and therefore justified careful evaluation of phase I and planning for phase II, especially the communication, training, and education needs.

CDC's Role in Providing Scientific and Public Health Reasoning for Policy

Even in ordinary circumstances, policy-making in the federal government is a complex and somewhat amorphous process. Conflicting values and priorities and multiple sources of evidence and data are involved (Gostin, 1995). The process that led to the smallpox vaccination policy may have been similar to the development of other public health policies, except for its unusual marriage of public health and national security. Although many principles that guide other public health programs appeared to apply, the nature of the problem to be addressed by the policy made it likely that most decisions would, in time, be scrutinized and criticized. The decision to take preventive action in circumstances in which preparation itself poses a risk or cost (as in the case of smallpox vaccine) would be criticized if the threatened event did not occur. Without a doubt, a decision to do nothing would be criticized if the threat did materialize. The smallpox vaccination program occurred in an environment of great uncertainty, so it required a clear explanation of its scientific and public health rationale and required every reasonable effort to ensure transparency and effective, regular communication among public health agencies at the federal, state, and local levels.

The presentations of multiple public health and health care leaders at the committee's meetings, substantial coverage by the mass media, surveys and briefs from ASTHO and NACCHO, findings of the 2003 GAO report, a summary of interviews with public health workers (Markowitz and Rosner, 2004), and ultimately the slow and halting progress of the vaccination program itself provided the committee with ample evidence that many in the public health and health care communities were skeptical or confused about the rationale for the program. The committee asserts that the reaction of the public health community in particular to the program (for example, deferring or refusing participation) indicates that the trust of public health agencies, officials, and workers in CDC as the nation's public health leader was compromised. As National Institute of Allergy and Infectious Diseases Director Anthony Fauci stated (2002),

> because people of good intentions disagree on government policy regarding smallpox vaccination in the context of a bioterrorist threat, the general public must understand the decision-making process as well as the rationale behind decisions that may affect their health and their lives. The need to be forthcoming is of particular importance, given the terrible trauma caused by the unforeseen events of September 11, 2001, as well as the anxiety associated with the continued threat of bioterrorist attacks. Because the population feels powerless, it must rely heavily on the deliberations and decisions of government leaders.

Explaining the decision-making process behind the smallpox vaccination policy to the public was important for both ethical and practical reasons (to inform and to reassure). Yet the federal government provided little public communication during program implementation. For the people expected to implement and participate in the program, explaining the decision-making process seemed crucial for the preparedness program's very existence, to safeguard the trust between CDC and its public health partners, and to secure the agreement and participation of public health agencies, health care organizations, professional associations, and other constituencies.

CDC has long been a leader in protecting the public's health by playing many roles, including supporting state and local health departments, supporting and evaluating the nation's immunizations programs, and performing the epidemiology and laboratory functions of communicable disease control. CDC's leadership role and the centrality of scientific evidence to its mission (CDC, 2004) are apparent in the agency's relationships with public health agencies and in CDC's performance in response to major crises, such as the SARS outbreak of 2003. The committee asserts that CDC's leadership role depends in part on the agency's ability to function as the definitive voice of science-based public health; its decisions and recommendations must always be seen as emerging logically from the best available scientific and public health reasoning. Many in the public health community did not perceive that to be the case during the smallpox vaccination program. Indeed, the national security context may have complicated CDC's ability to provide and communicate scientific and public health reasoning in the development of smallpox vaccination policy; CDC leadership may have been unable to disclose some of the underlying data, or such information may not have been made available to CDC itself.

The committee recognizes that public health policy decisions are not made solely on the basis of conclusive scientific data although science is accorded an extremely high value. The circumstances surrounding the smallpox vaccination policy at the interface between public health and national security interests were conducive to decision-making with little or no attention to public health and scientific imperatives. Those circumstances made CDC's role as the voice of science-based public health even more critical, yet CDC appeared unable to communicate in its typically transparent and clear manner. Furthermore, the implementation of the smallpox vaccination program was characterized by targets that were established and changed, phases that were established and eliminated, and recommendations that were sought—from ACIP and from the present IOM committee—and then not followed (Brown, 2002; CDC, 2002b, 2003b; McGlinchey, 2003a). Although it is not surprising that the program changed and its goals shifted, little or no explanation was given of the reasoning behind the decisions. In the short term of the program's implementation, the unanswered questions and concerns that overshadowed the program contributed to problems and delays. In the long term, those issues may have created barriers to strengthening preparedness and may have impaired reliance on CDC as the nation's definitive public health leader and one of the best sources of science-based, timely, and accurate public health information.

Based on the lessons learned from the smallpox vaccination program, the committee concludes that a policy strategy and a mechanism are needed to balance the need for scientific evidence and public health analysis with the imperatives of national security, ensuring in the process that the authoritative voice of CDC, the nation's public health leader, will be preserved.

OUTCOME UNKNOWN: HAS SMALLPOX PREPAREDNESS BEEN ENHANCED?

The smallpox vaccination program did not progress according to expectations, and its overall contribution to smallpox and public health preparedness is unclear (GAO, 2003; Gursky, 2003; U.S. House of Representatives Select Committee, 2004). The perception that the vaccination program's focus was on numbers of vaccinees rather than on smallpox preparedness was apparently created and perpetuated by a failure to communicate effectively about goals and objectives and about program progress and challenges.

Focus on Numbers Rather than Preparedness

The initial distinction between pre-event vaccination plans and post-event plans may have caused some confusion because vaccination of response teams is an activity that could be simply included among smallpox post-event plans as the only type of vaccination activity that occurs in advance of a smallpox virus release. The CDC director's statement in November 2003 that the agency never had a vaccination program but had a preparedness program (a comment described by the mass media as a denial of the program's existence) amounted to a distinction that had not been adequately communicated to the public or to the media (McGlinchey, 2003b; National Press Club, 2003). The vaccination effort was officially titled "the National Smallpox Vaccination Program" (CDC, 2002d), and it was meant to be one component of preparedness: vaccination of workers who would help to shorten the response time in the event of a smallpox virus release. However, the way in which the program was portrayed made its focal point "How do we get to these numbers?" rather than "What do we have to do to protect the country from this potential threat?" Ideally, vaccination would have been described as one activity in a comprehensive smallpox preparedness program. The ineffective communication on that important point might have misrepresented the program's goals, adversely shaped the opinion of many in the public health and health care communities, and created confusion in the mass media.

Within several weeks of the beginning of the vaccination program across the nation, the mass media reported a halting start (slow in comparison with the pace suggested by the initial 30-day timeline) as prospective vaccinees weighed substantial unknowns against what they knew about potential vaccine complications and in the absence of an adequate compensation plan (Bavley and Dvorak, 2003; GAO, 2003; Kemper, 2003; McCullough, 2003; Ornstein and Bonilla, 2003). The vaccination rate dropped steeply in April and May 2003 in the wake of cardiac adverse events and the announced end of major combat in Iraq. As DHHS and CDC officials were questioned about the number of vaccinees necessary for preparedness, the figure of 50,000 was offered although no additional guidance was made available to advise states on the numbers they would need to "effectively investigate an outbreak, care for patients, and vaccinate members of the public", especially given the variation among states and the difference between the number achieved and initial estimates (GAO, 2003). The value and legitimacy of the vaccination program were further questioned in news reports that documented shifting goals and CDC's often uneasy communication on the matter, for example, a change in the DHHS-CDC position on the numbers of vaccinees, denial that there had been a change in the program's focus, and the claim that preparedness, not numbers of vaccinees, had been the focus all along (Roos, 2003; Shockman, 2003). Public health officials even expressed some concern that they might have inadvertently created an exaggerated perception of the risk posed by the vaccine by being exceedingly cautious in informing prospective vaccinees about possible complications (Connolly, 2003a).

In a program already beset by ambiguity and unanswered questions, numbers seemed to constitute one concrete element, but the lack of an explanation of the scientific evidence and public health reasoning that went into shaping the smallpox vaccination program left the numbers—and the expectations of key actors, the mass media, and the public—ungrounded in factual information. Because preparedness was not defined from the beginning and the concept of broad preparedness was not reiterated and reinforced during the course of the program, numbers, however inexact, became a proxy for preparedness. The lack of clarification of the relationship between vaccination and preparedness allowed vaccination to obscure and even supersede comprehensive preparedness in rhetoric and in practice. Little or no explanation or evidence was provided to explain whether preparedness was related to vaccination; whether vaccination was required for preparedness and, if so, what number of vaccinees; and what constitutes preparedness. In fact, some of the early communication from CDC implied that preparedness required vaccination and that rapid vaccination was essential for preparedness (CDC, 2003a). Not until several weeks into the program did CDC state that "preparedness is not numbers," echoing statements made by ASTHO and by the present IOM committee (Cook, 2003; IOM, 2003d; Kuhles and Ackman, 2003; NACCHO, 2003a; Selecky, 2003). Months into the program, when CDC attempted to reorient program focus toward the full scope of preparedness, the efforts were perceived as an attempt to divert attention from a troubled program (McGlinchey, 2003b). The pattern of confusing vaccination numbers with preparedness continued. In 2004, the DHHS secretary responded to a question about the status of smallpox vaccination, stating that "we would like to be able to keep increasing that vaccination number, so that every state is ready" and perhaps reinforcing the perception that numbers were a correlate of readiness (DHS, 2004).

Despite the late effort to differentiate preparedness and vaccination, the committee has determined that many people and institutions were able to distinguish between the two. For example, public health agencies worked on training staff, developing communication plans, and other preparedness activities while hospital administrators who decided not to receive or implement vaccination at the time continued to work on planning, training, education, and other elements of preparedness (Edmond, 2003; Selecky, 2003; Toomey, 2003).

There are other challenges to the claim that preparedness was the program goal from the beginning. If preparedness, not numbers, was the program's focus, the frenetic pace of vaccination imposed at the beginning of the program was not needed. If the program had all along been about preparedness and not about numbers of vaccinees, CDC could have decided to delay the program because of concerns about compensation, the states could have been encouraged to proceed with their planning, training and education, and related preparedness efforts while deferring vaccination until compensation and other issues were resolved. The federal government's single-minded and intense focus on vaccination and vaccination targets also imposed great burdens on public health agencies that may have affected not just the routine work of the agencies (the Ten Essential Public Health Services) but their ability to develop comprehensive smallpox preparedness in the context of bioterrorism preparedness.

Is the Nation More Prepared Against Smallpox?

It is unclear whether smallpox preparedness has been strengthened. Government officials have said that preparedness has been improved, but the committee is not aware of the evidence that such readiness has been reached. That type of evidence, properly communicated, is critical to reassure the public that local, state, and federal public health agencies have the equipment, staff, and other resources to mount an effective response to an attack that uses smallpox virus. Smallpox preparedness also has broader implications for other types of preparedness. For example, the capacity to implement mass vaccination requires many of the plans and resources that are needed to implement mass distribution of other types of countermeasures, from iodine tablets to anthrax prophylaxis.

At the committee's November 2003 meeting, the director of CDC's Office of Terrorism Preparedness and Emergency Response (OTPER), Joseph Henderson, presented the agency's efforts to define and measure public health preparedness, including smallpox preparedness. CDC had developed 4 preparedness goals, 22 objectives, and 127 indicators, 10 of which specifically addressed smallpox preparedness. CDC intended the indicators to serve as a way to "scorecard" preparedness nationally and state by state and as a way to evaluate compliance with grant guidance (Henderson, 2003). This IOM committee was asked to review the smallpox preparedness indicators (in the context of the larger bioterrorism indicators project) and to advise CDC on their appropriateness and on ways to determine when an indicator had been met. The committee devoted its fifth report, included here as Appendix F, to a review of the indicators and included an assessment of relevant constituencies (state and local public health agencies, health care professionals, health care institutions, and first responders), whose input was solicited at the November 2003 meeting. In that report, the committee stated that preparedness for public health emergencies (including a potential smallpox event) should be part of overall continuous quality improvement of the public health system (IOM, 2003e).

CDC appears to have continued its work on the performance indicators; but at the time the present report was being written, no indicators or other assessment tool had been implemented. In May 2004, at the meeting of the DHHS secretary's Council on Public Health Preparedness, a CDC official stated that efforts to develop assessment tools were continuing and summarized CDC's Evidence-Based Performance Goals for Public Health Disaster Preparedness—42 performance goals and 47 measures (Knutson, 2004). In July 2004, at the CDC–American Medical Association First National Congress on Public Health Readiness, the director of CDC's OTPER noted that CDC's Evidence-Based Performance Goals for Public Health Disaster Preparedness—more recently, consisting of 35 performance goals and 45 measures—would be available for review on August 31, 2004 (Schable, 2004).

The committee is unaware of the current status of the performance goals and measures. On the basis of available information, the committee has concluded that the nation's smallpox preparedness has not yet been formally, systematically, and comprehensively evaluated. Therefore, if the smallpox vaccination effort was in fact part of a larger preparedness program, it is unclear whether the effort succeeded in strengthening preparedness. An early program objective was to build the capacity of every state to vaccinate its entire population within 10 days of a smallpox virus release. Although an ASTHO survey has found that most states believe they are prepared to complete mass vaccination within 10 days and the DHHS secretary has stated that most states "could vaccinate every person . . . within 10 days, and that's our goal" (DHS, 2004), there are no data to confirm that states and the nation as a whole would be able to accomplish that. Furthermore, defining preparedness is still a necessity because it is unclear what information has been used to determine that 10 days was an appropriate target. The window of opportunity for smallpox prophylaxis is believed to be 3-4 days after exposure (CIDRAP and IDSA, 2004). If so, aiming to vaccinate all within 10 rather than 3 days would probably be insufficient for the prevention of next-generation cases if exposure were widespread—and certainly insufficient to avert public concern about whether everyone can obtain protection if needed.

After nearly 2 years of great effort, considerable expenditures, and the smallpox vaccination of nearly 40,000 people, the nation remains with insufficient evidence that it is prepared to respond to a smallpox virus release. In fact, the delay evidenced in the response to the monkeypox outbreak (CDC was informed of the outbreak 13 days after its start), which could be considered a proxy for a bioterrorist attack, indicates that considerable gaps in preparedness remain (Mitchell, 2003).

The committee recommends that, in collaboration with its state and local partners and in the context of broad bioterrorism preparedness, CDC define smallpox preparedness; set goals that reflect the best available scientific and public health reasoning; conduct regular, comprehensive assessments of preparedness at the national level and by state; and communicate to the public about the status of preparedness efforts.

This will inform and reassure Americans about the public health system's ability to protect their health and will help jurisdictions continuously improve and learn from the process of preparing for public health emergencies, including smallpox virus release.

CONCLUDING OBSERVATIONS

Trust is a unifying theme among the committee's findings. The committee asserts that a relationship of trust between CDC and the public health and health care communities is a critical requirement in the implementation of biopreparedness programs. When a policy has the potential to greatly affect the public's health, an explanation of the evidence base and rationale that led to the policy becomes necessary to justify and mobilize public health action. The rationale of the smallpox vaccination program was never adequately explained to key constituencies and communication with CDC was constrained by unknown factors. As a result, the public health and health care communities seemed unable to trust the government and CDC fully when they called for smallpox vaccination in large numbers and at a rapid pace. The pace of vaccination ultimately declined, and the number of vaccinees reached fell far short of initial expectations. CDC's credibility has been recognized to be an important asset.

The role of CDC as the nation's public health leader—providing scientific and public health reasoning to inform the process of policy-making and to explain the rationale for policy to key constituencies—must be safeguarded. The reality and perception of CDC's independence to communicate openly and transparently came into question during the implementation of the smallpox vaccination program. It is essential to preserve the public health and health care communities' trust in CDC's leadership; therefore, when reasons of national security limit CDC's ability to perform its role, that fact should be made explicit and public.

The trust of the general public in government and government's ability to protect the public's health also is a critical requirement for responding to bioterrorism (and other public health threats). Communication experts (Covello and Sandman, 2001; Sandman, 2002) and a recent survey (Lasker, 2004) have shown that people's trust in the government must be handled with great care, but it is an essential requirement for effective communication; people are less likely to panic and more likely to participate constructively during an emergency if they believe they can trust government agencies to provide accurate and timely information.

The public's confidence in the public health system's capacity to protect people in a bioterrorism event efficiently and effectively depends on evidence and reassurance that CDC and the nation's public health agencies are prepared. Although considerable resources and effort have been invested in the smallpox vaccination program, it remains unclear whether the nation is more prepared than it was before to respond to an attack with smallpox virus; preparedness has not been defined, clear goals have not been set, and there has been no comprehensive and systematic assessment of smallpox preparedness. Such an assessment is necessary to demonstrate that the nation is prepared and to communicate that to the public.

Since the eighteenth century, American governments at all levels have determined that public health is an appropriate concern. The history of the agencies established shows regular debates about the array of activities to be expected and the degree to which decision makers and the public agree with the rationale that prompts action. Decisions about regulation of drinking water, protection of the food chain, immunization of children, and many other matters reflect those concerns. Without a regular exchange of trustworthy information and clarity of rationale, the ability of the public health community to act decisively when needed is compromised. The committee believes that it is crucial for the highest level of the executive branch of the federal government to examine the consequences of the unclear rationale for the smallpox vaccination policy and for CDC itself to undertake a careful and transparent analysis of the problems encountered by the smallpox vaccination program, from problems with implementation to the lack of known outcomes. Only such an effort, in collaboration with public health partners at the state and local levels, can lay the foundation for a preparedness program that can build on the trust so central to a public health community and can reassure the public that the nation's public health system is prepared to protect their health.

REFERENCES

AAFP (American Academy of Family Physicians). 2002. Panel calls for limited smallpox vaccination. *FP Report* 8(8).

Altman L. 2002, August 25. Health Workers Await Official Smallpox Policy. *New York Times*.

Anderson R. 2003. Presentation Before the IOM Committee on Smallpox Vaccination Program Implementation. Transcript of Meeting Three on May 1, 2003, Washington, DC.

APHA (American Public Health Association). 2002. News Release: APHA Calls for Measured, Deliberate Approach to Smallpox Vaccinations. [Online] Available at http://www.apha.org/news/press/2002/smallpoxresponse.htm. Accessed December 13, 2002.

Associated Press. 2003, February 1. State Begins Smallpox Inoculations. *Billings [Montana] Gazette*.

ASTHO (Association of State and Territorial Health Officials). 2002. 2002 Infectious Diseases Committee Annual Report—September. [Online] Available at http://www.astho.org/?template=_infectious_disease_committee.html.

ASTHO. 2003. ASTHO Smallpox Preparedness Survey Results (April 25, 2003). [Online] Available at http://www.astho.org/pubs/spxsummaryb2.pdf. Accessed July 7, 2003.

Banks S, Hannan C. 2002. ASTHO Ensures State Health Officials Are Heard in Smallpox Debate. [Online] Available at http://astho.org/templates/displau_pub.php?pub_id=336.

Bavley A, Dvorak J. 2003, February 8. Safety Concerns Hinder Participation in Smallpox Vaccination Program. *Kansas City Star*.

Brown D. 2002, October 17. Panel Alters Advice on Smallpox Shots: Wider Use for Health Workers Backed. *Washington Post*, A3.

CDC (Centers for Disease Control and Prevention). 2002a, May 30. Media Advisory: Smallpox Public Forums. [Online] Available at www.cdc.gov/od/oc/media/pressrel/a020530.htm. Accessed January 31, 2005.

CDC. 2002b. Centers for Disease Control and Prevention, National Immunization Program Record of the Meeting of the Advisory Committee on Immunization Practices, June 19-20, 2002, Atlanta, GA.

CDC. 2002c. CDC Telebriefing Transcript, June 20, 2002: Smallpox Vaccine. [Online] Available at http://www.cdc.gov/od/oc/media/transcripts/t020620.htm. Accessed January 31, 2005.

CDC. 2002d. Supplemental Guidance for Planning and Implementing the National Smallpox Vaccination Program (NSVP), November 22, 2002. [Online] Available at http://www.bt.cdc.gov/agent/smallpox/vaccination/pdf/supplemental-guidance-nsvp.pdf.

CDC. 2003a. CDC Telebriefing Transcript, January 17, 2003: CDC Smallpox Vaccination Update. [Online] Available at http://www.cdc.gov/od/oc/media/transcripts/t030117.htm. Accessed August 6, 2004.

CDC. 2003b. CDC Telebriefing Transcript: Update on Monkeypox and Severe Acute Respiratory Syndrome (SARS) Investigations. [Online] Available at http://www.cdc.gov/od/oc/media/transcripts/t030619.htm. Accessed July 5, 2003.

CDC. 2003c. CDC Telebriefing Transcript: Smallpox Vaccine Adverse Events Monitoring and Response System. [Online]. Available at http://www.cdc.gov/od/oc/media/transcripts/t030206.htm. Accessed March 11, 2003.

CDC. 2003d. Advisory Committee on Immunization Practices (ACIP) Statement on Smallpox Preparedness and Vaccination. [Online]. Available at http://www.bt.cdc.gov/agent/smallpox/vaccination/pdf/acipjun2003.pdf. Accessed July 17, 2003.

CDC. 2003e. CDC Telebriefing Transcript: Safer, Healthier Summer. [Online] Available at http://www.cdc.gov/od/oc/media/transcripts/t030626.htm. Accessed July 1, 2003.

CDC. 2004. About CDC. [Online] Available at http://www.cdc.gov/aboutcdc.htm. Accessed December 17, 2004.

CIA (Central Intelligence Agency). 2004. Comprehensive Report of the Special Advisor to the Director of Central Intelligence on Iraq's WMD. [Online] Available at http://www.cia.gov/cia/reports/iraq_wmd_2004/.

CIDRAP (Center for Infectious Disease Research and Policy) and IDSA (Infectious Diseases Society of America). 2004. Smallpox: Current, Comprehensive Information on Pathogenesis, Microbiology, Diagnosis, Treatment, and Prophylaxis. [Online] Available at http://www.cidrap.umn.edu/cidrap/content/bt/smallpox/biofacts/smllpx-summary.html.

Cohen J, Enserink M. 2002. Rough-and-tumble behind Bush's smallpox policy. *Science* 298:2312-2316.

Connolly C. 2002, December 24. Smallpox Plan May Force Other Health Cuts. *Washington Post,* A1.

Connolly C. 2003a, February 24. Bush Smallpox Inoculation Near Standstill; Medical Professionals Cite Possible Side Effects, Uncertainty of Threat. *Washington Post*, A6.

Connolly C. 2003b, March 10. Smallpox Campaign Taxing Health Resources. *Washington Post,* A4.

Cook R. 2003, April 5. Smallpox Planning Detracts from Core Public Health, Officials Say. *Associated Press.*

Covello V, Sandman P. 2001. Risk Communication: Evolution and Revolution. Baltimore, MD: Johns Hopkins University Press, pp. 164-178.

Denogean AT. 2003, February 3. Health Officials Weigh Smallpox Vaccinations Pros, Cons. *Tucson [Arizona] Citizen.* Local News.

DHHS (Department of Health and Human Services). 2004. Appendix 11: Lessons Learned from 1976 Swine Influenza Program—Draft. In *Draft Pandemic Influenza Preparedness and Response Plan.* [Online] Available at http://www.hhs.gov/nvpo/pandemicplan/annex11.swineflu.pdf. Accessed August 30, 2004.

DHS (Department of Homeland Security). 2004. Press Conference, January 29, 2004: Bio-Surveillance Program Initiative Remarks by Secretary of Homeland Security Tom Ridge and Secretary of Health and Human Services Secretary Tommy Thompson.

Edmond M. 2003. Presentation Before the IOM Committee on Smallpox Vaccination Program Implementation. Transcript of Meeting Three on May 1, 2003, Washington, DC.

ENA (Emergency Nurses Association). 2002. Letter to President George W. Bush. December 12, 2002. [Online] Available at http://www.ena.org/news/news/SmallpoxLetter.htm. Accessed December 16, 2002.

Everett W, Coffin S, Zaoutis T, Halpern S, Kim J, Strom B. 2002. Smallpox Willingness: A National Study of Emergency Department Personnel. Presentation Before the IOM Committee on Smallpox Vaccination Program Implementation on December 19, 2002.

Fauci AS. 2002. Smallpox vaccination policy—the need for dialogue. *New England Journal of Medicine* 346(17):1319-1320.

Fiorill J. 2003, October 24. US Smallpox Official Acknowledges Vaccination "Targets Were Not Achieved". *Global Security Newswire.*

Frist B. 2002, August 9. Deciding Who Is Protected Against Smallpox. *New York Times.*

GAO (General Accounting Office). 1977. The Swine Flu Program: An Unprecedented Venture in Preventive Medicine. Washington, DC: HRD-77-115.

GAO. 2003. Smallpox Vaccination: Implementation of National Program Faces Challenges. Washington, DC: General Accounting Office, GAO-03-578.

Gellman B. 2002, November 5. Findings Spur New Smallpox Concerns. *Albany (NY) Times Union.*

Gostin L. 1995. The Formulation of Policy by the Three Branches of Government. In *IOM, Society's Choices: Social and Ethical Decision-Making.* Washington, DC: National Academy Press.

Gregg J. 2002, October 6. Let the Public Choose on Smallpox Vaccine. *Washington Post.*

Gursky E. 2003. Progress and Peril: Bioterrorism Preparedness Dollars and Public Health. Century Foundation. [Online] Available at http://www.tcf.org/Publications/Homeland Security/Gursky_Progress_Peril.pdf. Accessed January 30, 2005.

Hallow R. 2002, November 24. Governors Seek Access to Smallpox Vaccine. *Washington Times,* A4.

Hardy G. 2002. Statement of the Association of State and Territorial Health Officials. Presentation Before the IOM Committee on Smallpox Vaccination Program Implementation, Meeting One on December 19, 2002, Washington, DC.

Henderson J. 2003. Presentation Before the IOM's Committee on Smallpox Vaccination Program Implementation. Transcript of Meeting Three on May 1, 2003, Washington, DC.

Hughes C. 2003, September 28. Public Health Programs Feared Lost in New Battle. *Albany (NY) Times Union.*

IDSA (Infectious Diseases Society of America). 2002. Letter to President George W. Bush. December 3, 2002. [Online] Available at http://www.idsociety.org.

IOM (Institute of Medicine). 2002. Scientific and Policy Considerations in Developing Smallpox Vaccination Options: A Workshop Report. Washington, DC: The National Academies Press

IOM. 2003a. Review of the Centers for Disease Control and Prevention's Smallpox Vaccination Program Implementation: Letter Report #1. Washington, DC: The National Academies Press.

IOM. 2003b. Review of the Centers for Disease Control and Prevention's Smallpox Vaccination Program Implementation: Letter Report #4. Washington, DC: The National Academies Press.

IOM. 2003c. Review of the Centers for Disease Control and Prevention's Smallpox Vaccination Program Implementation: Letter Report #2. Washington, DC: National Academies Press.

IOM. 2003d. Review of the Centers for Disease Control and Prevention's Smallpox Vaccination Program Implementation: Letter Report #3. Washington, DC: The National Academies Press.

IOM. 2003e. Review of the Centers for Disease Control and Prevention's Smallpox Vaccination Program Implementation: Letter Report #5. Washington, DC: The National Academies Press.

Judson F. 2003. Presentation Before the IOM Committee on Smallpox Vaccination Program Implementation. Transcript of Meeting Three on May 1, 2003, Washington, DC.

Kemper V. 2003, February 6. Smallpox Vaccine Hits a Snag: Compensation. *Los Angeles Times*, 18.

Knutson D. 2004. State and Local Terrorism Preparedness and Emergency Response: Status Update, Presentation to the Secretary's Council on Public Health Preparedness, May 4, 2004.

Krupnick M. 2003, January 24. CNA Calls Smallpox Program "Political." Nursing Union Official Says Bush's Plan Carries More Risks Than Benefits. *Contra Costa Times,* A1.

Kuhles D, Ackman D. 2003. The federal smallpox vaccination program: where do we go from here? *Health Affairs* (Web Exclusive) W3:503-510.

Lasker R. 2004. Redefining Readiness: Terrorism Planning Through the Eyes of the Public. New York: New York Academy of Medicine, Center for the Advancement of Collaborative Strategies in Health.

Libbey P. 2003a. Statement of Patrick M. Libbey, Executive Director National Association of County and City Health Officials. Presentation Before the Secretary's Council on Public Health Preparedness, January 14, 2003. [Online] Available at http://www.naccho.org/advocacydoc650.cfm. Accessed January 31, 2005.

Libbey P. 2003b. Testimony of Patrick M. Libbey, Executive Director, National Association of County and City Health Officials Before the Senate Appropriations Committee: Senate Labor, Health and Human Services and Education Appropriations Subcommittee.

Linzer D. 2003, September 18. No Evidence Iraq Stockpiled Smallpox. *Associated Press.*

Madlock Y. 2003. Presentation Before the IOM Committee on Smallpox Vaccination Program Implementation. Transcript of Meeting Three on May 1, 2003, Washington, DC.

Manning A. 2003, April 22. Second Round of Smallpox Vaccinations Begins. *USA Today.*

Manning A, Sternberg S. 2002, October 7. Officials Ponder Timing, Sequence of Immunizations. *USA Today.*

Markowitz G, Rosner D. 2004. Smallpox Campaign and Population Health Programs Emergency Preparedness, Bioterrorism, and the States: The First Two Years After September 11. New York: Milbank Memorial Fund.

May T, Aulisio MP, Silverman RD. 2003. The Smallpox Vaccination of Health Care Workers: Professional Obligations and Defense Against Bioterrorism. *Hastings Center Report* September-October 2003.

McCullough M. 2003, February 7. Americans Aren't Rolling Up Their Sleeves for Smallpox Inoculation. *The Salt Lake Tribune.*

McGlinchey D. 2003a, February 26. CDC Says It Never Aimed for 500,000 Smallpox Vaccinations. *Global Security Newswire.*

McGlinchey D. 2003b, November 19. CDC Director Denies Existence of Smallpox Immunization Program. *GovExec.Com.*

McKenna M. 2003, February 15. No Vaccination for Nation's Fear; Unease Hinders Smallpox Program. *Atlanta Journal-Constitution.*

McNeil D. 2003, February 7. Many Balking at Vaccination for Smallpox. *New York Times.*

Meckler L. 2003a, February 22. Smallpox Vaccinations Off to Slow Start. *Associated Press.*

Meckler L. 2003b, July 17. CDC: Smallpox May Still Be a Threat. *Associated Press.*

Mitchell S. 2003, June 12. Monkeypox Shows Gap in Bioterror Readiness. *United Press International.*

NACCHO (National Association of County and City Health Officials). 2003a. Impact of Smallpox Vaccination Program on Local Public Health Services. Research Brief No. 9.

NACCHO. 2003b. Costs of Smallpox Vaccination Program: Summary of Preliminary Data. Research Brief No. 10.

National Press Club. 2003. National Press Club Luncheon with Dr. Julie Gerberding, Centers for Disease Control and Prevention, November 14, 2003.

Neustadt R, Fineberg H. 1983. The Epidemic That Never Was: Policy-making and the Swine Flu Affair. New York: Vintage Books.

Neustadt RE, Fineberg HF. 1978. The Swine Flu Affair: Decision-making on a Slippery Disease. U.S. Department of Health, Education, and Welfare.

Nikolai K. 2003. Presentation Before the IOM Committee on Smallpox Vaccination Program Implementation. Transcript of Meeting Three on May 1, 2003, Washington, DC.

Ornstein C, Bonilla D. 2003, February 6. Fifteen in the County Refuse Vaccinations for Employees. Nine Accept; Most Are Undecided. *Los Angeles Times*.

Pear R. 2003, March 7. Threats and Responses: Biological Defense Officials Seek Smallpox Compensation Fund. *New York Times*, A15.

Pendley L. 2003. Commentary: Smallpox Vaccinations Prompt Questions. *Santa Fe New Mexican*, A7.

Pezzino G. 2003. Presentation Before the IOM Committee on Smallpox Vaccination Program Implementation. Transcript of Meeting Three on May 1, 2003, Washington, DC.

Rath E, Turcotte J. 2003. Press Release, March 6, 2003: Senator Gregg to Move Smallpox Compensation Legislation Through Senate. Office of Judd Gregg, U.S. Senator for New Hampshire.

Roos R. 2003, May 14. In Funding Guidelines, HHS Urges States to Press on with Smallpox Efforts. *CIDRAP News*.

Rosado E. 2003. Fact Sheet: Smallpox. National Association of Counties. [Online] Available at http://www.naco.org/ContentManagement/ContentDisplay.cfm?ContentID=7042. Accessed January 31, 2005.

Russell S. 2003, January 18. Smallpox Vaccine Plan Starts Tuesday, Despite Concerns; Some Health Workers May Opt Out Over Risks, Compensation Issues. *San Francisco Chronicle*.

Sandman PM. 2002. Smallpox Vaccination: Some Risk Communication Linchpins. [Online] Available at http://www.spsandman.com/col/smallpox.htm. Accessed January 31, 2003.

Schable C. 2004. Readiness: Where Are We? Where Do We Need to Be? Presentation to the CDC-AMA First National Congress on Public Health Readiness, July 22, 2004. [Online] Available at http://www.ama-assn.org/ama/noindex/category/11053.html. Accessed January 31, 2005.

Selecky M. 2003. Presentation Before the IOM Committee on Smallpox Vaccination Program Implementation. Transcript of Meeting Three on May 1, 2003, Washington, DC.

Shockman L. 2003, March 28. Nationwide Smallpox Protection Program for Health Workers Is Shy of Goal. *Toledo [Ohio] Blade*.

Skivington S, Witt D. 2003. Kaiser Permanente Smallpox Vaccination Implementation Overview. Slide presentation before the IOM Committee on Smallpox Vaccination Program Implementation, May 1, 2003.

Smith S. 2003. Smallpox vaccination: national security & individual risk. *Virtual Mentor (American Medical Association Ethics Resource Center)* 5(2).

Staiti A, Katz A, Hoadley J. 2003. Has Bioterrorism Preparedness Improved Public Health? Center for Studying Health System Change, Issue Brief: Findings from HSC No. 65.

Tanner L. 2003. CDC Encourages Health Workers at Conference to Get Smallpox Shots. *Associated Press*.

Toomey K. 2003. Presentation Before the IOM Committee on Smallpox Vaccination Program Implementation. Transcript of Meeting Two on February 13, 2003, Washington, DC.

UN (United Nations) Security Council. 2004. Nineteenth Quarterly Report on the Activities of the United Nations Monitoring, Verification and Inspection Commission in Accordance with Paragraph 12 of Security Council Resolution 1284 (1999). Geneva: United Nations, S/2004/924. [Online] Available at http://www.un.org/Depts/unmovic/new/documents/quarterly_reports/s-2004-924.pdf. Accessed February 14, 2005.

U.S. Department of State. 2002. White House Press Briefing (Officials Detail Smallpox Vaccination Plans; Will Consider Vaccination Requests from Allies and Friends.). U.S. Department of State, Office of International Information Programs.

U.S. House of Representatives. 2004. U.S. Representative Thomas M. Davis (R-VA) Holds Hearing on Health System Preparedness. House Government Reform Committee. Available from Federal Document Clearing House, Inc, via Lexis-Nexis.

U.S. House of Representatives Select Committee on Homeland Security (Democratic Members). 2004. A Biodefense Failure: The Smallpox Vaccination Program One Year Later. [Online] Available at http://www.house.gov/hsc/democrats/pdf/press/040129_A BiodefenseFailureOneYearLater. pdf. Accessed February 2004.

U.S. Senate Select Committee on Intelligence. 2004. Report on the U.S. Intelligence Community's Prewar Intelligence Assessments on Iraq. [Online] Available at http:// intelligence.senate.gov/iraqreport2.pdf.

Washington Post. 2002. Voluntary Smallpox Vaccination Urged. Offer to General Population Represents a Shift in Policy. *Washington Post,* A1.

Wheeler T. 2003, February 6. Medical Workers Leery of Smallpox Vaccine. *Beacon Journal [Ohio]*.

White House. 2002. President Delivers Remarks on Smallpox. [Online]. Available at http:// www.whitehouse.gov/news/releases/2002/12/20021213-7.html. Accessed January 8, 2003.

Yih W, Lieu T, Rego V, O'Brien M, Shay D, Yokoe D, Platt R. 2003. Attitudes of healthcare workers in U.S. hospitals regarding smallpox vaccination. *BMC Public Health* 3(20):20.

Appendixes

A

Recommendations from Letter Reports #1-6

RECOMMENDATIONS FROM LETTER REPORT #1

Issues of Timing

The committee recommends that the Centers for Disease Control and Prevention (CDC) develop and communicate the criteria (e.g., types and rates of adverse reactions) that would trigger a reconsideration of the current systems in place to protect vaccinees and their contacts (e.g., the October 2002 Advisory Committee on Immunization Practices [ACIP] recommendations on contraindications, screening, care of the vaccination site, and administrative leave).

To most effectively evaluate the progress and outcomes of the first phase, the committee recommends that CDC utilize the variation in implementation by hospitals and health departments (e.g., differences in granting administrative leave, types of bandages used, different site care instructions, degree of patient contact, adverse reaction investigation) to obtain safety data, and to analyze these data before embarking on subsequent phases of the vaccination program.

Compensation for Adverse Reactions to the Smallpox Vaccine

The committee recommends that CDC and its state and local public health partners immediately work to clarify each state's worker's compensation program's position on coverage for smallpox vaccine–related injuries and illnesses for workers covered under their programs.

The committee recommends that CDC and the Department of Health and Human Services support all efforts, some of which might be administratively or legislatively bold and creative, to bring this issue of compensation for smallpox vaccine adverse reactions—including those reactions that occur despite non-negligent manufacture and administration of the vaccine—to speedy resolution.

Workforce Issues Resulting from Vaccination

The committee recommends that during phase I, CDC assess the effects of the current situation regarding administrative leave, disseminate the analysis widely, and before phase II begins, decide whether the ACIP recommendation needs to be reassessed. Any evidence of transmission of vaccinia virus to a patient from an immunized health care worker should lead to an active case investigation or to an immediate reassessment of policy.

Opportunity Costs

The committee recommends that CDC work with their public health partners to document as well as possible the true costs of the smallpox program.

Informed Consent Process

The committee recommends that all consent documents include a statement that the risks of the smallpox vaccine, while very low, are predictably higher than the risks associated with most other vaccines, but that the benefit is presently unknown—possibly very low (absent exposure to smallpox) or very high (in the event of exposure).

The committee further recommends that informed consent forms include explicit notification of the availability, or lack thereof, of compensation for adverse reactions.

Comprehension of Screening Materials

Understanding that different populations may interpret the educational and screening materials somewhat differently, the committee recommends that CDC pretest the educational and screening materials in populations with different educational, socioeconomic, and cultural backgrounds before these materials are used for the first phase of the pre-event smallpox vaccination program, if this is possible given the time frame. If not, then material should be evaluated after phase I, and modified before phase II.

Educating Household Contacts

The committee recommends that CDC develop specific educational materials for household contacts of potential vaccinees.

The committee recommends that the materials also include instructions about how household members can avoid accidental infection with vaccinia, should the household member choose not to disclose the contraindication to the vaccinee.

The committee recommends that CDC consider using the blood-donation opt-out and informed consent processes as models for the pre-event smallpox vaccination program.

Reasons for Declining Vaccine

The committee recommends that CDC collect data on the reasons why potential vaccinees choose not to be vaccinated.

Using the Pre-Event Vaccination System (PVS) to Collect Data on Adverse Reactions

The committee strongly recommends that active surveillance for adverse reactions be employed, rather than relying exclusively on the passive surveillance systems that already exist (e.g., VAERS). The committee recommends that CDC use the Pre-Event Vaccination System (PVS) as the primary data collection system for adverse reactions.

The committee recommends a follow-up on a subset of individuals in PVS rather than a telephone survey of vaccine recipients. The follow-up survey could be used to gather information on long-term effects from the vaccine, as well as information on cases of accidental vaccinia infection in household members of vaccinees, rather than focusing on obtaining data on common adverse reactions.

Evaluation of Risk Factors for Known Adverse Reactions

The committee strongly recommends analysis of the phase I PVS data as a series of nested case-control studies, with results available before moving on to phase II of the vaccination program.

Establishment of a Data Safety and Monitoring Board (DSMB)

If CDC is unable to assure this independent functioning of the DSMB, the committee recommends that the proposed organizational arrangement be reconsidered.

CDC Safety System Guidance to States

The committee recommends CDC evaluate each state's capacity for managing adverse reactions before indicating that a state is ready to begin vaccinations.

Focus Areas of Training and Education

The committee recommends that CDC expand the scope of their training and education regarding the identification, treatment, and reporting of serious adverse reactions to all clinicians.

The committee recommends that the first communication clinicians should receive is basic information about the details of the pre-event smallpox vaccination program.

Communication Planning

The committee recommends that CDC's communication efforts about smallpox vaccination clearly separate public health issues from national security matters. The latter are best addressed by representatives of the administration more directly involved in such matters, and not by representatives of scientific agencies. Therefore, the responsibility of CDC is to deliver clear, consistent, and science-based public health communications.

The committee recommends that CDC identify a single "voice" for the national vaccination program, a credible individual with a strong scientific background and an experienced communicator who can serve as the key CDC spokesperson. Additionally, the agency should develop several back-up sources for the media who can offer the same level of informed comment and thoughtful observation as the program's primary "voice."

The committee recommends that more attention be given to developing a variety of materials and channels to inform and educate the public about the immunization program before vaccinations begin.

RECOMMENDATIONS FROM LETTER REPORT #2

A Focus on Preparedness

The committee recommends that CDC work with states to decide what more is needed to achieve smallpox preparedness, if anything. Further, given the routine turnover in personnel, each state should evaluate what it needs to maintain this preparedness.

A Need for Evaluation

The committee recommends that CDC comprehensively evaluate the program and its outcomes in order to improve its implementation and to protect the vaccinees and the public.

Communication

The committee recommends CDC revisit and communicate to the public the program's objectives in view of state-level realities, and provide a preliminary perspective on the national and state success in reaching those objectives. The CDC should continue to support, as well as build on the experience of state and local health departments who are developing their communication strategies about state and local program implementation.

The committee recommends that CDC and its state and local partners develop communications strategies that:

- Provide adequate quality and quantity of information.
- Are timely.
- Reassure the public that efforts are in progress to protect them in the event of a smallpox attack.

The committee recommends CDC develop and offer journalists training materials and opportunities specifically designed for the media, explaining the program's clinical components, providing the best available scientific evidence, and dedicating staff experts to provide technical support to media representatives.

Training and Education

The committee recommends that all print materials addressed to a diverse audience (e.g., the public) should be easily read and understood by all members of that audience. Also, all communication materials in other languages should be culturally appropriate.

The committee recommends that educational and training materials be tested for ease of comprehension with samples representing a cross-section of the sex, race, ethnicity, and level of education.

Data to Assess Vaccine and Program Safety

The committee recommends that a data field be added to PVS to indicate which version of the Pre-Vaccination Information Packet was provided to the vaccinee, in order to document what information was given to the vaccinee prior to consent.

The committee recommends that CDC consider adding a data field to HSVMS to indicate whether a serious adverse event occurred or whether a VAERS report was filed (understanding that more complete information about circumstances surrounding the adverse event will be entered into VAERS and the Active Surveillance System).

The committee recommends that CDC work to ensure that a qualified health professional monitors, conducts a "take" reading, and provides a regular vaccination site inspection for each vaccinee in the program and enters the relevant data into the appropriate smallpox vaccination program data system.

The committee recommends that whenever the ACIP working group issues findings/recommendations to the ACIP and through it to the director of CDC, it carefully consider concurrent release to the public and do so if it would be in the interest of transparency and maintaining the public's trust in the program.

The committee recommends that CDC be very clear about what types of adverse events will be reported to the public and when.

The committee recommends that the vaccination report webpage use categories that correspond to the categories presented in the MMWR adverse event reports.

The committee recommends that CDC report on a regular basis how effective screening practices have been at identifying contraindications (e.g., pregnancy, HIV status, eczema or atopic dermatitis) prior to vaccination.

The committee recommends that CDC work with the Department of Defense (DoD) to decide how adverse events that involve both the civilian and military populations will be reported.

Compensation

The committee recommends that CDC gather data on the reasons why potential vaccinees are declining vaccination and document the extent to which lack of compensation is identified as a barrier, among other possible barriers (e.g., uncertainty surrounding risk of smallpox, fear of transmitting virus to contacts, extent to which local programs are encouraging vaccination).

The committee recommends that the compensation language be easy to read and understandable to a wide range of audiences.

The committee recommends that potential vaccinees be reminded of the current compensation situation before they formally give their consent to be vaccinated.

Funding

The committee recommends that this inquiry be broad in scope and include not only cost to local and state health departments, but also the financial impact on the provision of other essential public health services, the costs incurred by participating hospitals, and estimates of costs of expanding the vaccination program to additional health care and public health workers and emergency first responders.

RECOMMENDATION FROM LETTER REPORT #3

The committee recommends CDC facilitate the efforts of states that wish to pause to evaluate the process and outcomes of their vaccination efforts to date, and plan for next steps before deciding whether and when to begin vaccination of new personnel. CDC should provide states with a target date for when CDC expects to have completed its revision of materials, data systems (adding new occupational categories, etc.), and guidelines. States that have identified a need for more vaccinated volunteers to carry out specific smallpox response functions will then be able to set their own timeline for vaccinating these new groups.

RECOMMENDATIONS FROM LETTER REPORT #4

A Standard for Smallpox Preparedness

The committee recommends that CDC provide guidance to assist state public health agencies (and their partners,[1] as appropriate) in establishing a baseline level or a minimum standard of preparedness for a smallpox attack, after which, each state could individually assess its priorities and further expand its preparedness against smallpox and other threats to the public's health as needed.

Preparing Key Responders

The committee recommends that CDC support the establishment of state and/or local, and if appropriate, national, voluntary registries of individuals who have undergone vaccination to be mobilized, trained, and assigned as needed in the event of a smallpox attack. Such registries would include all willing vaccinated personnel not associated with a response team, ranging from retired or relocated health care or public health workers to military reservists and former military personnel.

Using Scenarios to Test Preparedness

The committee recommends that CDC facilitate the development of a range of scenarios for potential smallpox attack(s), including one or more multi-threat scenarios, and urge states to use these to expand and continuously improve their plans to respond to a wide range of possibilities.

Vaccination of Members of the General Public Who Insist on Receiving Smallpox Vaccine

The committee recommends that CDC proceed with a deliberate and stepwise approach toward meeting the president's policy of offering vaccine to members of the general public who insist on receiving it by:

[1]State partners may include, but not be limited to, emergency management agencies, law enforcement, fire and emergency medical services, hospital and other health care associations.

- Conducting brief quantitative surveys to determine public interest and desire for smallpox vaccine. These surveys should include public and private health agencies as well as the general public, in order to understand the potential scope of public interest.
- Determining the budgetary and other requirements that would meet the demand noted.
- Identifying, monitoring, and referring people to existing or planned smallpox vaccine clinical research trials or other well-structured clinical arrangements that meet the basic requirements of medical and public health ethics, including assurances for safety of vaccinees and their contacts, acceptable balance between risk and benefit, and acceptable distribution of scarce public health resources to meet all preparedness as well as other public health goals. The committee encourages CDC to consider utilizing a pilot program or some other means of evaluating the initial experiences with this effort.

Communicating About and Coordinating the Response to Adverse Events

To help ensure that the adverse event reporting and follow-up procedures work as seamlessly as possible, the committee recommends that CDC coordinate better with their state partners and provide feedback to local partners who reported the adverse event.

Streamlining Data Collection

The committee recommends that CDC pursue ways to streamline the data systems that are used in the smallpox vaccination program, improving user-friendliness and integrating the multiple systems to avoid duplicate data entry, especially considering that any future expansion of the vaccination program would require a larger number and greater diversity of data system users, some of whom may be using these systems for the first time.

Utility of the Active Surveillance System

Because the civilian smallpox vaccination program is a true partnership between CDC, states, and local jurisdictions, the committee recommends that CDC continue and expand their communication with states and local jurisdictions about the imperativeness of their participation in the Active Surveillance System, stressing that the safety of the vaccination program cannot be guaranteed without their full participation and cooperation.

Pregnancy Screening

Considering that the rate of inadvertent exposure to smallpox vaccine during pregnancy is lower than expected and it is impossible to detect all pregnancies at the time of vaccination, the committee does not recommend extra pregnancy screening efforts at this time.

Evaluation and Safety Studies

The committee recommends that CDC begin developing a structured, prioritized research agenda that can aid decision-making as the smallpox preparedness program moves forward.

The committee recommends that in the short term, studies of the serious adverse events should receive the highest priority. For safety-related questions, in the longer term, studies examining long-term outcomes for those who experienced both serious and mild adverse events and studies of how mild adverse events contributed to lost work or social function should be a high priority. For system-related questions, in the longer- term, studies of cost and opportunity costs should be a high priority.

RECOMMENDATIONS FROM LETTER REPORT #5

If CDC intends to use scenarios as a planning tool, the committee recommends that the scenarios represent a range of possible situations, be used to help guide state and local planning activities, and facilitate state and local assessment of their level of preparedness.

The committee recommends that a flexible, incremental, science-based decision-making and management structure for smallpox response that includes all levels of government be developed and communicated to state and local agencies so that the consequences of a smallpox outbreak can be managed effectively.

The committee recommends that CDC consider conducting the preparedness assessments on a multi-year basis.

The committee recommends that CDC address its immediate need of measuring cooperative agreement compliance with a concise and simple set of indicators, and then use this set of indicators as the foundation of a longer, deliberative, national process to develop measures that address the full range and appropriate balance of preparedness activities.

The committee recommends that federal agencies and CDC, specifically, be held accountable for their unique federal responsibilities in an emergency response and assessed on their progress in facilitating national public health emergency preparedness.

The committee recommends that CDC consider utilizing the 10 Essential Public Health Services as a framework for the readiness indicators.

The committee recommends that CDC collaborate with Health Resources and Services Administration (HRSA) to integrate the preparedness indicators into one document, in order to help the health care and public health communities work hand-in-hand to plan, implement plans, and evaluate their readiness to respond to threats (including, but not limited to, a smallpox attack) and to avoid requiring duplicate reporting from states.

RECOMMENDATIONS FROM LETTER REPORT #6

The committee recommends that all federal entities concerned with bioterrorism preparedness (e.g., CDC, HRSA, and ODP) should more actively coordinate guidance and funding activities. Federal agencies should also work together to develop mechanisms that facilitate coordination and collaboration among their grantees at the state and local levels. Federal efforts should include the clarification of primary responsibility and authority in bioterrorism events, to ensure that CDC can fulfill its unique role as the nation's public health agency.

The committee recommends that CDC should collaborate with all of its partners to strengthen preparedness by applying research findings and experience in public health emergency response, bioterrorism preparedness, and disaster management. In order to strengthen the evidence base for public health preparedness, CDC should:

- Strengthen the link between public health research and practice;
- participate in and promote interdisciplinary research about preparedness;
- support a system to assure the ongoing collection, synthesis, and sharing of lessons learned and best practices from public health preparedness exercises and public health response to proxy events; and
- in coordination with the appropriate federal-level partners, such as AHRQ, evaluate the effectiveness, design, and opportunity costs of preparedness strategies, such as exercises.

The committee recommends that CDC should use the Evidence-Based Performance Goals for Public Health Disaster Preparedness to develop standards against which CDC, states, and localities may regularly measure their performance in exercises and in response to proxy events. Public health agency performance in exercises and proxy events should be used to identify gaps in preparedness and to improve planning, communication, and coordination at the agency and interagency levels, as part of a process of continuous quality improvement in preparedness planning and response. Preparedness drills and exercises should not be evaluated individually, but their cumulative and long-term impact on preparedness, such as generalizability to other potential hazards, must be considered in the evaluation process.

B

Review of the Centers for Disease Control and Prevention's Smallpox Vaccination Program Implementation, Letter Report #1

January 16, 2003
Dr. Julie Gerberding
Director
Centers for Disease Control and Prevention
1600 Clifton Road, NE
Atlanta, GA 30333

Dear Dr. Gerberding:

The Centers for Disease Control and Prevention (CDC) asked the Institute of Medicine (IOM) to convene an expert committee to advise it and its public health colleagues on the implementation of a pre-event smallpox vaccination program. The IOM agreed to provide this advice through a series of timely reports. We are pleased to communicate to CDC observations, conclusions, and recommendations from the first meeting of the committee of volunteer experts who have agreed to serve the IOM in this effort. The committee's areas of expertise include internal medicine, infectious diseases (including smallpox), dermatology, pediatrics, nursing, epidemiology, public health law and ethics, public health practice, emergency medicine, and pharmacology.

CDC charged the IOM committee with providing guidance on how to best implement the president's policy regarding pre-event smallpox vaccination, addressing the following eight areas:

- the informed consent process;
- contraindications screening;
- the system in place to assess the safety profile of the smallpox vaccine;
- guidance for the treatment of vaccine complications;
- professional training programs CDC is developing;
- the communications efforts;
- guidance CDC offers to states in developing their implementation plans; and
- overall progress at achieving the goals of the program.

Given the rapid pace of planning for the smallpox vaccination program, the committee realizes that while it has been working on this report, CDC has been moving ahead, and at the time of the report's release, it is possible that CDC has already accomplished some of the components the committee is recommending.

In addition to CDC's partners, many in the general public will be interested in this communication. Moreover, all reports of IOM committees are released to the public. We thus provide some background information directed at readers less familiar with the issue. This letter is divided into general statements about implementing the recently announced pre-event smallpox vaccination program, followed by targeted recommendations on the specific components of the committee's charge.

Our intent is to help CDC and its partners across the country implement President Bush's pre-event smallpox vaccination policy as safely as possible. We begin by offering our professional admiration for the hard work of CDC staff and their public health partners in our states and territories, major metropolitan areas, counties, and local communities who have been working under conditions of many uncertainties to prepare for this program. We hope we can help make these efforts even more successful.

BACKGROUND INFORMATION AND COMMITTEE PROCESS

On September 30, 2002, the Centers for Disease Control and Prevention (CDC) entered into a contract with the Institute of Medicine (IOM) of the National Academies to provide targeted advice on the implementation of a "pre-event" or precautionary smallpox vaccination program. An independent, nongovernmental, nonprofit organization operating under the 1863 congressional charter to the National Academy of Sciences, the IOM has provided advice on matters of health and medicine for over 30 years. The IOM often tackles issues of importance to CDC's public health mission, including matters of vaccine financing, supply, development, and—

perhaps most relevant to this project—safety. The IOM operates by convening ad hoc committees of the nation's experts, invoking policies and procedures developed over many years to ensure the advice is free from sponsor or other interested-party influence, unbiased with respect to the questions at hand, and based on evidence.

The last case of smallpox in the United States occurred in 1949. General vaccination against smallpox—accomplished with cutaneous administration of a closely related virus, vaccinia virus—ceased in the United States in 1972, when the threat of smallpox disease disappeared due to eradication efforts, which were declared complete by the World Health Organization on May 8, 1980. Only two official stocks of smallpox (variola) virus remained—under the auspices of the governments of the United States and the Soviet Union. It has often been rumored and suggested that some of the virus possessed by the Soviet Union could have been given illegally to people attempting to use the virus as a biological weapon, though factual evidence to support this concern has not been made public. The events of September and October 2001 increased U.S. concerns about all types of possible terrorism, including the potential for biological terrorism. Thus, attention turned to considerations of initiating vaccination against smallpox. CDC has been concurrently developing "post-event" vaccination plans (mass vaccinations after a smallpox release) and—the focus of this committee—"pre-event" plans (precautionary vaccination of smallpox response teams, first responders, and the general public).

On December 13, 2002, President Bush announced his policy on pre-event vaccination against smallpox (White House, 2002). Vaccination of select military personnel, including the president in his role as Commander-in-Chief, began immediately thereafter. At the time of this writing, voluntary vaccination of state-based teams of public health disease investigators and of hospital-based teams of health care workers (who would respond to the first case of smallpox, should it ever appear) is scheduled to begin in late January 2003. The president has asked that this round of vaccinations be completed as quickly as possible and that a broader vaccination effort commence thereafter. As currently understood, the subsequent vaccinations will encompass the voluntary vaccination of all health care workers and those commonly defined as first responders, such as firefighters, police, and emergency medical personnel. Vaccination of the general public is specifically not recommended, but the president also announced the intent to provide vaccinations to those members of the public who request the intervention. The IOM's Committee on Smallpox Vaccination Program Implementation met for the first time December 18-20, 2002, to begin addressing their charge, stated most succinctly as providing advice on how best to implement the policy as announced by President Bush.

The committee has not been asked to, and will not, comment on the president's policy decision to recommend voluntary smallpox vaccination to health care, public health, and emergency personnel under a precautionary program, and to allow but not recommend access to the vaccine by people not included within those groups. The extensive expertise the committee brings to this issue will focus on program implementation.

The committee realizes that this is an atypical vaccination campaign, and that it is neither a research study nor an ideal public health program. Rather, it is a public health component of bioterrorism preparedness. The committee was constituted to help CDC and its partners at state and local health departments, hospitals, health clinics, and private medical offices throughout the country implement a program with inherent serious risks and with publicly unknown and unstated benefits, and to do so rapidly, within a timeline that has not been explicitly outlined. Thus, the committee has chosen to address to the best of its ability at this time questions specifically posed to it by CDC and, when evidence or time does not permit a reasoned answer, to pose questions that, if answered, might allow for better and more evidence-based advice. Due to the time pressures inherent in this vaccination campaign, this report presents the committee's recommendations on the first set of vaccinations described in the President's policy announcement. Subsequent reports will provide recommendations relevant to further vaccination efforts, hopefully informed by experience gained from the initial effort.

For practical reasons, the committee uses the term "phase I" to describe the planned vaccination of 500,000 public health and health care workers who volunteer to be part of smallpox response teams, and "phase II" to refer to the subsequent vaccination of 10 million health care and public health workers and other emergency responders. However, it is unclear what the rounds of vaccination are being called by CDC ("phases" seems most frequently used) and clarification also is needed about the target population for later vaccination efforts.

Much of the evidence on which the committee bases its conclusions derives from two sources—the historical medical literature on the effects of smallpox vaccine (vaccinia virus), and presentations from and material prepared by CDC at the time of the first committee meeting (noting that the committee has not received updated drafts of materials, such as consent forms). In addition, these sources are supplemented by material presented to the committee by interested partners in the vaccination program and anecdotal information about state, local, and hospital-level response around the country available in recent print media. A list of all materials reviewed by the committee is available to the general public through the National Academies' Public Access and Records Office (http://www4.nationalacademies.org/onpi/paro.nsf; phone: (202) 334-3543; e-mail: publicac@nas.edu). Before addressing the specific items in its charge, the committee summarizes its key messages and then addresses some general considerations.

SUMMARY OF KEY MESSAGES

The committee urges CDC to:

1. Highlight the unique nature of the smallpox vaccination program as a public health component of a national bioterrorism preparedness policy, focusing on the delivery of clear, consistent, science-based information.
2. Proceed cautiously, allowing continuous opportunity for adequate and thoughtful deliberation, analysis, and evaluation. Embark on phase II only after adequate evaluation of phase I has occurred.
3. Use a wide range of methods for proactive communication, training, and education, and customize it to reach diverse audiences, including potential vaccinees, all health care providers, and the general public.
4. Designate one credible, trusted scientist as key national spokesperson for the campaign, and sharpen and expand communication plans and strategies to ensure rapid, transparent, and sustained contact with the media throughout implementation.

GENERAL CONSIDERATIONS

National Security Concerns and the Unknown Balance of Risks and Benefits

The smallpox vaccination program has been competently planned by public health authorities, and decades of experience in vaccination programs and in clinical medicine have been brought to bear on this process. The planning of public health interventions, particularly immunization programs, includes cautioned and deliberate consideration of the risks of the intervention compared to its benefit. The benefit of this public health program is the likelihood that the vaccine will prevent morbidity and mortality from smallpox viral infection, if smallpox reappears. Nevertheless, there is evidence that the risks of the intervention are significant (Neff et al., 1967; Lane et al., 1969, 1970—citation used by CDC to explain adverse reaction rates); the smallpox vaccine may be the least safe vaccine ever used on a wide scale.

Although the vaccine to be used in the first two phases of the program is the same calf lymph–derived vaccine stored since the 1970s, the host characteristics on a population level have changed significantly. First, a high proportion of the population has not been immunized against smallpox, and there is evidence that primary vaccinees are more likely to experience serious adverse reactions compared to those being revaccinated (Lane et al., 1969). The vaccine also carries significant risks for some members of the population—those with various types of immune suppression, such as HIV infection or due to cancer chemotherapy, those with certain diseases such as eczema and atopic dermatitis, and close personal contacts of vaccinees who have such contraindications. The U.S. population has many more people at high risk for serious adverse reactions now compared to the 1960s, when most data concerning the safety profile of the vaccine were collected. Furthermore, it is assumed that with rigorous efforts at screening those at risk and with intensive efforts at educating vaccinees about caring for the vaccination site, accidental inoculation of high-risk contacts of vaccinees can be minimized. However, the actual risks will only be known after the vaccination program is operative.

The benefit of the vaccine also is unknown at this time. There is no reason to believe that the efficacy of the vaccine at preventing smallpox infection has changed, both in its protection of individual vaccinees and the additional protection it offers to others by blocking smallpox transmission to the unvaccinated, although there is no way to ascertain whether the vaccine would be effective against bioengineered smallpox. However, the assumed benefit of the vaccine includes an estimate of the risk of encountering smallpox virus; this estimate was derived by the President and his advisors with a view to national security issues, facts and considerations not communicated to the committee.

Based on the administration's statement that the risk of a smallpox attack is indeterminate (not zero but currently assumed to be very low) (White House, 2002), the benefit of the vaccination program to the public also is not zero but is assumed to be very low. The benefit to any individual might indeed be zero if the individual never encounters the smallpox virus. However, in the event of exposure to smallpox virus, the benefit to individuals may be very high. Given this profile of high vaccination risk and likely very low to zero benefit, the administration's policy to offer vaccination to public health, medical, and emergency workers must be implemented in a most prudent and cautious manner.

In general, public health interventions are undertaken with recognition of some benefit to some individuals, no effect on others, and the possibility of some risk to a small percentage of the population (e.g., folic acid supplementation of the food supply), with expectation of overall benefit to the population receiving the intervention. This precautionary program is a public health component of national bioterrorism preparedness, and those who assume the vaccine's risks may have a small likelihood of individually benefiting from it.

In this context, it is imperative to highlight the voluntary nature of this vaccination campaign and the paramount importance of safety, to protect the volunteers assuming this risk. The sense of urgency required by national security considerations should be kept in balance with the President's stated goal of safety. Therefore, learning from experience, making midcourse corrections on every aspect of the program, and maintaining constant and consistent communications with the public are integral to developing the safest program possible. Like all Americans, the committee hopes that the risk of smallpox disease reappearing approaches zero and that an abundance of caution can prevail. Therefore, information on the progress and outcomes of implementation—including but not limited to safety concerns and the experience of states and local communities—needs to be shared, analyzed, and discussed at every step before proceeding further. If the risk of smallpox disease (and thus the benefit of the vaccine) is truly very low, deliberation is key to ensuring the safest program possible.

Issues of Timing

The pre-event smallpox vaccination program is a complicated and enormous task. Given the presidential directive for rapid implementation, the states, major metropolitan areas, and territories charged with developing plans for implementing the first phase of the program had very little time to respond to the guidance CDC issued for developing a program. At the time of the committee's December 2002 meeting and in subsequent media accounts, several states expressed concern that the original ambitious time frame was not realistic (Young, 2003). Concurrently, CDC revealed that it would relax the 30-day timeline for the first phase of vaccination, but without providing specifics about the changed timeline (CDC, 2002a; Orenstein, 2002; Strikas, 2002). At the time of writing this report, the committee had not received written confirmation of this change.

The committee hopes that local health department and hospital readiness will dictate the launch date for phase I in each state or community, and duration of each state vaccination program. Furthermore, sufficient time should be allowed between the two phases to ensure adequate assessment and plan revision by CDC and its partners at the state and local levels.

Although advising deliberate and careful planning and implementation, the committee recognizes that the unique context of this program may change at any time, as new information about the nature and extent of threats to the public's health may become available to public health authorities. For example, the confirmation of a suspected smallpox case would immediately signal a change in policy and mandate the rapid implementation of vaccination plans.

As phase I, and ultimately, phase II are completed, it is advisable that CDC evaluate the long-term sustainability of the vaccinated smallpox response teams. There will be some turnover among the first vaccinated cohort of response team members, and CDC would need to determine how it can ensure that public health and health care smallpox response teams maintain an adequate number of vaccinated members with the necessary expertise for each team. The commencement of phase II vaccinations may help eliminate the concern over the immediate sustainability of response teams vaccinated during phase I, but the need for new rounds of vaccinations for newly designated members of response teams should be considered once phase I and phase II vaccinations have been completed.

An important task for CDC and its medical and public health partners will be to develop an agreed-upon set of questions that must be answered satisfactorily throughout phase I and before phase II can begin. The questions, borrowed from analyses of the Swine Flu program of the late 1970s (GAO, 1977), are "What evidence on which things, when and why, would make us change the course we now propose, and to what?" (Neustadt and Fineberg, 1978).

Should a deliberation about the fundamental nature of the policy not be possible, at a minimum **the committee recommends that CDC develop and communicate the criteria (e.g., types and rates of adverse reactions) that would trigger a reconsideration of the current systems in place to protect vaccinees and their contacts (e.g., the October 2002 Advisory Committee on Immunization Practices [ACIP] recommendations on contraindications, screening, care of the vaccination site, and administrative leave).** For example, CDC might wish to consider from how many vaccinees it will require data and at what rate of specific serious adverse reactions (in vaccinees or their contacts) CDC would consider the program riskier than currently expected and the contraindication screening less adequate than needed (or safer than currently expected).

Hospitals and health departments will implement the first phase of the pre-event vaccination program in slightly different ways, depending upon the circumstances and needs of their communities. Much could be learned from this differential administration of the program. Since this program is a very unusual public health intervention, it will be important to gather data on which practices and techniques are most effective in different types of settings. **To most effectively evaluate the progress and outcomes of the first phase, the committee recommends that CDC utilize the variation in implementation by hospitals and health departments (e.g., differences in granting administrative leave, types of bandages used, different site care instructions, degree of patient contact, adverse reaction investigation) to obtain safety data and to analyze these data before embarking on subsequent phases of the vaccination program.**

Clarity

The committee urges that CDC and the Department of Health and Human Services (DHHS) proceed in their public discussions and program guidance with attention to clarity, focusing on issues such as timelines and terminology.

First, there has been confusion on the part of the committee, and likely others as indicated by media reports on the subject (Altman and O'Connor, 2003; Young, 2003), about the characteristics of program phases, the numbers of people estimated to be vaccinated, when vaccinations will begin, and the estimated duration of each phase. Specific wording should be chosen (e.g., waves, phases, stages), clearly defined, and then used consistently in all communications from CDC and DHHS. In addition, all communications should be clear about whether particular guidance refers to pre-event (precautionary) smallpox vaccination or to post-event (response and control) vaccination. This is particularly important for any discussion of contraindications, which are very different under the situation of post-exposure vaccination. In this regard, the pre-event program must be explained as part of a general program of public health preparedness for bioterrorism and other threats to the public's health.

It is clear to the committee and other interested parties that the stated policy of the president is an absolutely voluntary vaccination program for hospitals that may choose whether to have a smallpox response team and for public health and health care workers who may volunteer to be members of a response team, but this matter bears continual emphasis in communications and planning.

Finally, some administration and other policy statements about the early part of vaccination implementation have described the group to be vaccinated as "first responders" or "response teams." The committee believes there is a need to more clearly explain in policy and planning materials that in the event of a smallpox release, the first responders (i.e., those who are likely to first encounter or identify smallpox) will be public health and health care teams. Fire, police, and emergency personnel commonly described as first responders may have a role to play in mass vaccination, in addition to law enforcement's role in investigating the criminal aspects of a smallpox virus release.

Compensation for Adverse Reactions to the Smallpox Vaccine

Although not a specific "line-item" within its contractual charge, the committee interprets general issues of compensation for adverse reactions as integral to its stated charge to assess the overall progress at achieving the goals of the program. [The committee will use the term "adverse reactions" to describe both the common (i.e., local and systemic reactions) and serious adverse reactions (e.g., generalized vaccinia, serious cases of accidental inoculation, eczema vaccinatum, progressive vaccinia, vaccinia keratitis, and encephalitis). There may be some suspected adverse reactions that are not yet recognized as being causally associated with the vaccine. If these suspected adverse reactions are determined to be causally associated with the smallpox vaccine, then compensation should address these reactions as well.] It does so because it believes that the currently stated plans for compensation for adverse reactions could seriously affect achievement of the stated goal of the program—to increase the nation's bioterrorism preparedness. A number of hospitals have said that they will not participate in the pre-event vaccination program until these issues are resolved (McKenna, 2002; Price, 2002). The committee believes that resolution of the adverse reaction compensation issues is important for the informed consent process, clearly a part of the committee's charge. Concerns about lifelong disability resulting from the vaccine (particularly neurological disability from postvaccinal encephalitis) also may arise, and the committee encourages consideration of how to address disability issues. Implications of the pre-event vaccination program for issues related to health insurance, disability insurance, and life insurance also should be considered.

The committee notes that the Homeland Security Act of 2002 (Public Law No. 107-296) provides a federal mechanism to compensate vaccinees who are injured due to negligent manufacture or administration of the smallpox vaccine (but does not cover adverse reactions that occur despite non-negligent manufacture and administration). This has encouraged manufacturers and vaccine administration sites to participate in the pre-event vaccination program, as it reduces their liability exposure for adverse reactions. The Homeland Security Act does not, however, provide reimbursement to vaccinees for costs associated with participating in the program when there are no instances of negligence. These costs may include administrative leave (with possible loss of salary) in order to avoid accidental infection of vulnerable patients in their workplace; lost income due to time away from work while recuperating from adverse reactions that occur despite non-negligent manufacture and administration of the vaccine, particularly for nonsalaried workers; and unreimbursed medical expenses associated with treating adverse reactions that occur despite non-negligent manufacture and administration of the vaccine. In addition, the committee notes with concern that there may be some people, such as patients and family members, who are infected accidentally by contact with a vaccinee, despite efforts to care for the vaccination site appropriately. Recognizing this, contacts should be considered part of the population that is vulnerable to adverse reactions and, thus, losses from the vaccine. This is not unlike the policy of vaccine-associated paralytic polio in contacts of people who received the oral polio vaccine in the National Vaccine Injury Compensation Program. Without reimbursement for these losses, the committee fears that some, perhaps many, public health and health care workers will decline vaccination, thus undermining the effectiveness of the program's implementation.

Some of these adverse reactions may be covered by state worker's compensation programs. However, there is much uncertainty surrounding the types of vaccine adverse reactions and circumstances leading to those vaccine adverse reactions that would be coverable under each state's worker's compensation law. Public health and health care workers who are considering vaccination need accurate information about the rights and protections that are available to them under their state's worker's compensation law. **The committee recommends that CDC and its state and local public health partners immediately work to clarify each state's worker's compensation program's position on coverage for smallpox vaccine–related injuries and illnesses for workers covered under their programs.**

At the time of the issuance of this report, the implications of the Homeland Security Act were not fully understood by many of the state and local public health and health care partners in the smallpox vaccination program. This led to confusion and concern that individuals who have volunteered to be part of the nation's defense against bioterrorism—the public health and health care workers who participate in precautionary vaccination and their family members who are at risk of accidental inoculation—are inadequately protected financially from liability, compared to the much smaller group of public health and health care workers who agree to administer the vaccine (AHA, 2002; McDonough, 2003).

The committee heard during discussion that these concerns have been raised with DHHS and other administration officials (SEIU, 2002). These concerns may change as more is learned about the adverse reaction rates during phase I of the vaccination program. The committee also understands that the 108th Congress might address these issues. The committee urges timely attention and communication about the progress of these deliberations. Without this, concerns about the financial burden for caring for the adverse reactions of the smallpox vaccine (and the sobering consideration that some small but real number of vaccinees or their contacts could die or suffer permanent disability subsequent to vaccination) could greatly decrease the number of people who volunteer for smallpox vaccination. This could seriously affect the program's achievement of its overall goals of increasing U.S. terrorism preparedness. **The committee recommends that CDC and DHHS support all efforts, some of which might be administratively or legislatively bold and creative, to bring this issue of compensation for smallpox vaccine adverse reactions—including those reactions that oc-**

cur despite non-negligent manufacture and administration of the vaccine—to speedy resolution.

Workforce Issues Resulting from Vaccination

Recognizing that this first phase of smallpox vaccination will only involve public health and health care response teams, the committee encourages CDC to consider some additional issues that may affect the willingness of health care workers to participate in the pre-event smallpox vaccination program.

As phase I vaccinations begin, hospital patients could be adversely affected by the absence of health care workers from patient care duties because of adverse reactions or possible administrative leave (Altman, 2002). Most hospitals are not staffed with sufficient redundancy to absorb such staff losses safely (AHA, 2002). Depending upon the size of response teams at individual hospitals, staggering vaccinations may be a prudent step for ensuring the safety of not only the vaccinees, but also the patients. This may extend the period originally anticipated for the first phase of vaccinations. However, this will help ensure that hospitals proceed with vaccinations only as quickly as safety will allow.

It should be noted that in the Department of Defense's initial experience vaccinating approximately 170 military personnel, there were no cases of secondary infections in contacts (Vogel, 2003). However, the committee notes that the controlled conditions of the military setting cannot always be replicated in a civilian setting.

The same concerns regarding absence of workers from hospitals during the period of phase I vaccinations also applies to state and local public health departments. Considering that the median size of a local public health department in the United States is 14 staff (NACCHO, 2001), having even a small number of staff unable to perform their duties for a few days because of adverse reactions to the vaccine could have a detrimental effect on the ability of the local public health departments to keep their standard public health programs operating sufficiently. These concerns become of even greater importance to public health departments that have even fewer staff. In terms of timing of smallpox response team vaccinations, the committee agrees with the Advisory Committee on Immunization Practices (ACIP) recommendation that hospitals and health departments stagger vaccinations within individual institutions if this is deemed desirable by the individual programs (CDC, 2002e). The committee recognizes that staggering vaccinations might prove incompatible in some instances with the necessity of minimizing vaccine wastage.

In addition to concerns about potential absenteeism and its effects on hospital functioning and patient care, there are questions about the possible need for or usefulness of administrative leave as a way to support health care worker decision-making and perhaps to ensure patient safety. When ACIP met in October 2002, members discussed the issue of administrative leave for health care workers who would receive the vaccine in the pre-event vaccination program. In their recommendation, they stated, "With respect to administrative leave for health care workers, the ACIP does not believe that health care workers need to be placed on leave because they received a smallpox vaccination. Administrative leave is not required routinely for newly vaccinated healthcare workers unless they are physically unable to work due to systemic signs and symptoms of illness, extensive skin lesions which cannot be adequately covered, or if they do not adhere to the recommended infection control precautions. It is important to realize that the very close contact required for transmission of vaccinia to household contacts is unlikely to occur in the healthcare setting" (CDC, 2002e).

The issue of administrative leave is complicated. CDC has no authority to resolve the issue of costs for administrative leave; it can only provide guidance based on ACIP recommendations as stated above. Nevertheless, the committee is sympathetic to the concerns of workers who might not participate in the program without adequate accommodation, but also to the financial and staffing problems that hospitals or health departments would have in offering administrative or other paid leave. Ideally, any individual or institution that wished to use an administrative or other paid leave policy would be able to do so. However, this may not be feasible to resolve for phase I of the program, given the short period until vaccinations begin and the reportedly short duration of phase I. **Therefore, the committee recommends that during phase I, CDC assess the effects of the current situation regarding administrative leave, disseminate the analysis widely, and before phase II begins, decide whether the ACIP recommendation needs to be reassessed. Any evidence of transmission of vaccinia virus to a patient from an immunized health care worker should lead to an active case investigation or to an immediate reassessment of policy.** In order to provide an appropriate evidence base for such a reassessment, CDC might wish to:

- Develop preliminary standards of care for the types and extent of contact recently vaccinated health care workers should have with patients, taking into account that hospitals care for different spectra of patients with respect to age, disease types, and disease severity;
- Survey and analyze the effect of the vaccine on absenteeism; and
- Analyze how the cost of offering administrative leave with pay compares with the cost of not offering administrative leave with pay (e.g., accidental inoculations in patients, medical errors due to health care workers not functioning at the proper level due to adverse reactions), using data from hospitals and health departments that decide on their own to offer administrative leave with pay.

Opportunity Costs

The committee is concerned and heard concerns from CDC's state and local partners that the smallpox vaccination program will incur great costs that are hard to document (AHA, 2002; ANA, 2002; Burstein, 2002; Connolly, 2002a, 2002b; Hardy, 2002; NACCHO, 2002; Altman and O'Connor, 2003; *Associated Press*, 2003; Mitchell, 2003; Richmond, 2003)—these costs include items such as:

- fewer resources (e.g., time, staffing, money, public service announcements, etc.) for public health programs than planned, due to the needs of the smallpox program, which could delay the development of plans for dealing with a smallpox release;
- hospitals' costs to enhance bioterrorism preparedness and response capabilities, often with limited financial assistance from the federal, state, or local governments;
- negative effects on the public's perceptions of inoculations in general due to misunderstanding of the special characteristics of the smallpox vaccine; and
- medical errors that occur because of short-staffing due to absenteeism subsequent to vaccine-related illness (Nakamura and Weiss, 2002).

The committee recommends that CDC work with their public health partners to document as well as possible the true costs of the smallpox program. The committee has no specific recommendations at this time on how to do this, but a concerted effort to assess these costs is important and could help in shaping the smallpox immunization program as it expands.

SPECIFIC CONSIDERATIONS

Informed Consent Process

As noted above, the committee believes that it should be recognized that the pre-event smallpox vaccination program is not a typical public health program, but rather, a matter of national public health preparedness against a national security threat. Given the difficulty in characterizing or quantifying the actual threat, the benefit to vaccinees is unknown, and this reality should be recognized and communicated to potential vaccinees to enable an informed decision regarding vaccination. Health care workers who are volunteering to be a part of smallpox response teams are making a decision for the public good, as well as for personal protection. Some data, as well as reports from media sources, indicate that the potential personal benefit (i.e., protection) is an important factor in health care worker decisions to receive the vaccine (Everett et al., 2002). A further consideration in ensuring truly informed consent is the administration's responsibility to communicate promptly changes in the threat assessment to all health care workers considering vaccination, as well as the general public.

With regard to the consent documents and all other communications, the committee urges continued attention to the tensions inherent in ensuring appropriate participation in the program. That is, there is a tension between maximizing participation of those appropriate for and consenting to vaccination—those with appropriate medical and public health responsibilities who are at risk for infection (should it appear) and without true contraindications themselves or in close personal contacts—and minimizing participation by those at high risk for adverse reactions (or in contact with those at high risk for adverse reactions), or those who for whatever reasons do not wish to be vaccinated.

The committee has two specific concerns about the informed consent aspects of this program. President Bush stressed in his announcement of December 13, 2002, that this is a voluntary program for public health and health care workers (White House, 2002). The committee is pleased with the emphasis on the voluntary nature of the program but stresses that consent is not a simple matter. It is easy to imagine situations whereby a potential vaccinee will not feel free to decline vaccination. A potential vaccinee might not wish to disclose fears about the risk of the vaccine, particularly in regard to one's own or a personal contact's HIV or pregnancy status, or even the fear of treating a smallpox victim. While in large hospitals or public health departments, other vaccinees might be available to volunteer for service, in small hospitals, a potential vaccinee might be the only worker with a specific, essential expertise and to decline could put the hospital or clinic at risk of incomplete coverage in the case of a smallpox outbreak. To decline vaccination could lead to rumors about the health status of decliners or their family members. Thus, a vaccinee who would otherwise decline to volunteer for vaccination might feel coerced into participation.

A second concern is more fundamental. It is standard practice to request consent to an intervention, such as vaccination, but highly unusual for an intervention, other than in clinical trials, to have known risks but unknown benefits. Yet, that is the nature of this program, within the broader context of national security. The committee suggests explicitly stating that the benefit of the vaccination program is to increase the nation's public health preparedness, but that the benefit of vaccination to any one individual might be very low (given the current threat assessment). Vaccinees must have a clear understanding of the real risks of the vaccine and of the consequences of developing smallpox, tempered by the best estimate of the risk of a smallpox release. The informed consent materials that are given to vaccinees must clearly lay out the risks and benefits to receiving the vaccine. Vaccinees should be quizzed verbally and in writing to assess their knowledge and understanding about the vaccine and should be asked in a structured and standard way about their decision to be vaccinated. Communication and materials designed to obtain and ensure informed consent should avoid "Yes/No" questions, offering ample opportunity for potential vaccinees to make a thoughtful, well-informed decision. Furthermore, the screening process should include questions about household contacts and other close personal and professional contacts, and vaccinees should be provided with educational material for their contacts. To be certain that the consent is truly voluntary, **the committee recommends that all consent documents include a statement that the risks of the smallpox vaccine, while very low, are predictably higher than the risks associated with most other vaccines, but that the benefit is at present unknown—possibly very low (absent exposure to smallpox) or very high (in the event of exposure).**

The committee further recommends that informed consent forms include explicit notification of the availability, or lack thereof, of compensation for adverse reactions. The prototype information sheets provided by CDC for the post-event vaccination program guidance clearly state that CDC will NOT cover the costs of treating adverse reactions, other than the cost of vaccinia immune globulin (VIG) or cidofovir (Vistide), and that other medical costs must be borne by insurance or the vaccinee. A similar bold statement should be included in information and consent materials for the pre-event program as well. Many potential vaccinees may falsely assume that the provisions of the Homeland Security Act of 2002 or the federal Vaccine Injury Compensation Program would provide compensation for medical expenses or income loss experienced as a result of receiving or being exposed to the smallpox vaccine. This information may be an important factor that will weigh on a potential vaccinee's decision about whether to receive the vaccine. Understanding that the issues surrounding compensation for adverse reactions to the vaccine will most likely not be resolved before vaccinations are scheduled to begin, health care workers need to know this information before making a decision about whether or not to be vaccinated. If there are any developments in the availability of adverse reaction compensation for recipients of the smallpox vaccine (or their contacts), then the informed consent materials should be updated to reflect this change.

Given the many contraindications to receiving the smallpox vaccine, it is important to ensure that potential vaccinees have read and have thoroughly understood all of the material in the informed consent form. The committee suggests that the first page of the informed consent form contain a line for the vaccinee's signature, to acknowledge that the vaccinee has read all the forms and has had all questions answered. Subsequent pages of the informed consent form should contain a space for the vaccinee's initials.

The committee also encourages CDC to pretest the informed consent materials in populations with different educational, socioeconomic, and cultural backgrounds before these materials are used for the first phase of the pre-event smallpox vaccination program, if this is possible given the time frame. If not, then material should be evaluated after phase I and modified before phase II.

Screening Potential Vaccinees

The committee would like to commend CDC on all the hard work and planning that have already gone into developing effective, efficient, and equitable screening methods and guidelines for pre-event clinic operations. Much has already been accomplished, and everyone involved recognizes that additional issues need to be considered before vaccination of response teams begins.

CDC has stated that they will err on the side of caution in determining who should be vaccinated. The committee agrees that this is the correct approach and encourages practicing continued and enhanced caution in screening vaccinees.

Consistency in Screening Materials

The committee understands that CDC had to develop all of the screening materials and guidance on a very accelerated basis and thus had limited time to compare all documents for overall consistency. Since screening will be the first aspect of the vaccination program that response team volunteers will encounter, any confusion over screening guidelines could have a detrimental effect on the overall communications effort of the pre-event smallpox vaccination program. Consistent screening guidance will be paramount to ensuring the American public's trust in the vaccination program. The committee believes that it is very important to take the necessary time to ensure consistent guidance on contraindications and screening advice before the first member of a public health or health care smallpox response team is vaccinated. The chapter on smallpox that will be added to CDC's Epidemiology and Prevention of Vaccine-Preventable Diseases (CDC, 2002b), as well as all screening materials and guidance, should be examined for consistency.

Comprehension of Screening Materials

How successfully this first phase of vaccination is conducted will depend in part on how well potential vaccinees comprehend the educational and screening materials that are provided to them. **Understanding that**

different populations may interpret the educational and screening materials somewhat differently, the committee recommends that CDC pretest the educational and screening materials in populations with different educational, socioeconomic, and cultural backgrounds before these materials are used for the first phase of the pre-event smallpox vaccination program, if this is possible given the time frame. If not, then material should be evaluated after phase I, and modified before phase II.

The committee encourages CDC to evaluate the educational and screening materials on an ongoing basis and evaluate them as formally as possible following implementation of the first phase of the program. CDC should determine whether the educational and screening materials used for the first phase of the program also would be appropriate for the second phase. If revisions are indicated, the committee encourages CDC also to pre-test these revised materials on different populations.

Educating Household Contacts

Because the smallpox vaccine provides an increased risk of adverse events to household members of vaccinees (Neff et al., 2002), every effort must be made to screen out potential vaccinees whose household members have contraindications to the vaccine. The potential for household members to not disclose certain contraindications (e.g., pregnancy, HIV status) must be acknowledged. Therefore, it can be assumed that some potential vaccinees will not know if there is a contraindication in their household. **The committee recommends that CDC develop specific educational materials for household contacts of potential vaccinees.**

Potential vaccinees should be given such educational materials at the first visit to the vaccination clinic and instructed to give them to all their household members. The educational materials should urge household members to disclose to the potential vaccinee any condition that could be considered a contraindication. It is important to develop such materials (like all the educational materials given to vaccinees) in languages other than English, to test them for comprehension and readability at different literacy levels, and to target them to specific user populations. When vaccinees return to the clinic to receive their vaccine, the informed consent materials should double-check whether the vaccinee discussed all of the contraindications with all members of his household and determine that no contraindication in a household member was identified. **The committee recommends that the materials also include instructions about how household members can avoid accidental infection with vaccinia, should the household member choose not to disclose the contraindication to the vaccinee.**

The committee heard preliminary data that a significant proportion of those with contraindications were intending to take the vaccine (Everett et al., 2002). In so far as it is possible, this should be avoided. The committee thus spent considerable effort considering alternative means of screening, which might be more effective than simple provision of information. Ideally, the vaccine would not be administered at the place of work, to avoid peer pressure, and peer knowledge, about the decision made by a potential vaccinee, though this may be unavoidable in phase I.

Commonly used blood donation forms provide multiple confidential opportunities for donors to opt-out of the blood donation process if they believe that their blood is not safe to be given to someone else. The committee believes this model could be considered for the pre-event smallpox vaccination program. Vaccinees should not feel any pressure to receive the vaccine, for fear that a medical condition that they do not want to disclose may be discovered by the vaccination clinic or potentially, by their employer. By offering multiple opportunities to optout of vaccination, CDC can help ensure that the program is carried out in the most ethical manner possible. **The committee recommends that CDC consider using the blood-donation opt-out and informed consent processes as models for the pre-event smallpox vaccination program.**

Reasons for Declining Vaccine

Potential vaccinees will have different reasons for declining the vaccine, ranging from personal contraindications, contraindications in household and other close contacts, fear about adverse reactions of the vaccine, or apprehension about the benefit of receiving the vaccine. **The committee recommends that CDC collect data on the reasons why potential vaccinees choose not to be vaccinated.**

One way of doing this would be to provide a form to all potential vaccinees at the first visit to the vaccination clinic asking permission to follow up with them at a later date for a survey. A survey that could contain data from both vaccinees who chose to be vaccinated and potential vaccinees who decided against vaccination would be extremely valuable. Such a survey would be able to have a representative cohort of potential vaccinees as its study population, assuming that the nonresponse rate is similar in both populations. Being able to survey potential vaccinees who decided against receiving the vaccine will provide a representative control group (if nonresponse rates are similar) for any study of phase I vaccinees.

Another method for gathering data would be to add a carbon copy to the form that potential vaccinees complete regarding reasons for not receiving the vaccine. This method for gathering data would not offer representative cohort information (because it would not include the people who decided between the first and second visit to the vaccination clinic not to receive the vaccine and never returned to the clinic for the second time), but it would at least provide detailed information on the reasons why some vaccinees decided against receiving the smallpox vaccine. Though not representative, these data could be used to inform revisions to educational materials for subsequent phases of the vaccination program. The carbon should only be included in the area of the page that collects data on the reasons for not receiving the vaccine and not in the area of the page that would include personally identifiable information. Potential vaccinees should be informed that completing the form is entirely voluntary, and should be told that this information will be used for contrast group purposes.

Should either of these methods be employed, the committee encourages CDC to pretest the survey and response materials in populations with different educational, socioeconomic, and cultural backgrounds.

Assessment of Safety Profile

CDC has obviously spent much time and effort in designing and planning for the comprehensive Smallpox Immunization Safety System (SISS). Ensuring that adverse reactions are identified, treated, quantified, and evaluated will be critical to the success of the pre-event smallpox vaccination program. The committee offers a few recommendations to help ensure that the SISS is as comprehensive, efficient, and effective as possible.

Early recognition, evaluation, and appropriate treatment of adverse reactions to the smallpox vaccine will be critical to limiting the adverse consequences of the smallpox vaccination program and to ensuring the public's continued acceptance of the program. Detecting adverse reactions and evaluating them early will be the first step in this process.

The committee has had limited time to explore the interaction between CDC and the Food and Drug Administration (FDA), but hopes to turn to this important matter subsequently. CDC has capably assembled the necessary expertise to design the SSIS and the other components of the vaccination program. However, the committee believes that it is necessary to have the FDA fully engaged (to the extent which it is not already), and as quickly as possible, in all aspects of the program, and the SISS in particular. FDA involvement is important for ensuring that the requirements for the Investigational New Drug (IND) protocols for use of VIG and cidofovir are met. FDA's involvement also is critical to ensuring that FDA's surveillance systems become fully integrated into the overall surveillance for smallpox vaccine adverse reactions. CDC has been working extensively with FDA in determining how Vaccine Adverse Event Reporting System (VAERS) reports related to the smallpox vaccine will be shared with CDC and their state and local partners. The committee urges continued and enhanced CDC collaboration with FDA.

Identifying Adverse Reactions

The committee encourages CDC to work with the personnel who are already in place to provide local vaccination care, since they can be an important component of the evaluation of adverse reactions. Since the personnel who will be changing bandages will see vaccinees on a daily or very frequent basis, they also should be trained to recognize serious adverse reactions and advised on how to report these reactions to the appropriate data system. CDC should provide specific definitions for each serious adverse reaction to facilitate accurate data collection. Having these health care personnel trained to evaluate serious adverse reactions also would permit evaluation of vaccinees' rates of common adverse reactions (e.g., fever, malaise, sore arm). To facilitate this process, CDC should distribute widely information distinguishing between common adverse reactions and serious adverse reactions (e.g., generalized vaccinia, progressive vaccinia, encephalitis) that require further clinical evaluation.

Using the Pre-Event Vaccination System (PVS) to Collect Data on Adverse Reactions

Considering the anticipated risks of the vaccination program and the currently unknown benefit, it is extremely important that all adverse reactions from the smallpox vaccine (both known and suspected) be identified in a timely manner. Relying on passive systems that are dependent on vaccinees and their clinicians to bring the adverse reaction to the attention of the smallpox vaccination program managers will not capture all serious adverse reactions. The current guidance from CDC states that all adverse events (i.e., known serious adverse reactions and serious adverse reactions that are suspected to be related to the vaccine) should be reported to VAERS (CDC, 2002d). Relying primarily on a passive surveillance system (i.e., VAERS) is useful for identifying adverse reactions but creates the possibility that many smallpox vaccine adverse reactions may not be reported. The committee believes it is important to confirm the response of every vaccinee to the vaccine (i.e., determining whether there is an adverse reaction and gathering data on common adverse reactions), rather than relying solely on VAERS and other passive surveillance systems, which will underestimate the incidence of adverse reactions.

When all Dryvax vaccine was still unlicensed, detailed adverse reactions reporting was part of the IND requirement and would have been captured in a standardized manner to support the IND (CDC, 2002c).

However, since licensed Dryvax vaccine is available for use in the pre-event vaccination program, it is expected that VAERS will now be used to capture adverse reactions data. The VAERS report will ask for the Patient Vaccination Number (PVN), a unique identifier assigned to each vaccinee, which will allow the VAERS report to be linked to the patient's record in the PVS. The PVS is a secure data exchange Internet-based system designed to collect information on those being vaccinated against smallpox. The PVS will only capture adverse reactions as descriptive text. Considering that the smallpox vaccine has not been routinely used in the last 30 years, and there is uncertainty as to whether the adverse reaction profile for today's population will be similar to what it was in the past, the committee believes that active surveillance must be employed.

The committee believes that active surveillance should be accomplished through the planned PVS. The states and CDC plan to use the information contained in the PVS to monitor vaccine coverage, vaccine immunogenicity, complications, and reports of adverse reactions. States can either use the Internet-based PVS or can choose to send the same data to CDC using a certified data exchange process. The PVS (and uploaded data from states that use the certified data exchange process) will contain demographic data on each vaccinee, the vaccine and diluent lot information of the reconstituted vaccine given to the recipient, the "take" reading, and limited information on adverse reactions. It would take but minor modification for PVS to be used to more fully record adverse reactions as well, so the presence or absence of adverse outcomes can be confirmed. **The committee strongly recommends that active surveillance for adverse reactions be employed, rather than relying exclusively on the passive surveillance systems that already exist (e.g., VAERS). The committee recommends that CDC use the Pre-Event Vaccination System (PVS) as the primary data collection system for adverse reactions.**

Enhanced in this way, PVS could provide accurate and rapidly ascertained quantification of known adverse reactions, in approximately 500,000 vaccinated individuals. It will be important for CDC to be the entity that compiles all surveillance data on adverse reactions that are possibly related to the smallpox vaccine. Furthermore, however the PVS is used in the end, it should be pretested to the extent possible before the first phase of vaccinations begin.

The PVS also may be useful in accomplishing other functions. Analysis of where the vaccine is distributed, how much is distributed, and how much vaccine is wasted will be intrinsic to making midcourse revisions to the implementation plan. The committee encourages CDC to use PVS for detailed monitoring of vaccine distribution, since this will be important for evaluating the overall implementation of the vaccination program. The committee suggests adding a field to PVS that would identify whether the vaccinee accidentally transmitted the vaccinia virus to a contact. The committee encourages full analysis of "take" rate data, especially considering that this may be the only measure of efficacy of the vaccine for the time being.

PVS data should be analyzed regularly during phase I, and the full set of PVS data should be evaluated at the end of the first phase and prior to the commencement of the second phase. This information will help the transition from phase I to subsequent phases of the vaccination campaign. The committee also encourages CDC to provide additional training on the PVS to state and local partners so that the quality of data contained in PVS can be maximized.

The committee also was asked to provide advice on whether the proposed telephone survey of 10,000-20,000 vaccinees is an appropriate mechanism to obtain data on common adverse reactions, vaccinee satisfaction with the vaccination program, and the effect of vaccination on time lost from work. The committee suggests that if CDC decides to modify the PVS to make it an active surveillance system and utilize it as the primary mode of gathering data on adverse reactions, the previously planned survey would become redundant. **The committee recommends a follow-up on a subset of individuals in PVS rather than a telephone survey of vaccine recipients. The follow-up survey could be used to gather information on long-term effects from the vaccine, as well as information on cases of accidental vaccinia infection in household members of vaccinees, rather than focusing on obtaining data on common adverse reactions.**

Evaluation of Risk Factors for Known Adverse Reactions

Data from the cohort of 500,000 vaccinated individuals who would be included in the PVS could be used to conduct a series of nested case-control studies, comparing those suffering from each serious adverse reaction to a random sample of unaffected patients who also had received the vaccine, in order to determine the risk factors associated with serious adverse reactions. This would be critically important information to have before embarking on phase II of the vaccination campaign, in order to be certain that those at risk of serious adverse reactions would not be given the vaccine. Thus, **the committee strongly recommends analysis of the phase I PVS data as a series of nested case-control studies, with results available before moving on to phase II of the vaccination program.**

Monitoring for Rare Adverse Reactions

Although the committee would like to see PVS used as the primary system for gathering data on adverse reactions, the committee recognizes that VAERS is an extremely useful tool, when used the way it was designed (i.e., for hypothesis generating for unusual and unexpected adverse reactions) rather than for quantification of expected adverse reactions. As such, VAERS should not be eliminated from the safety system. Rather, the committee suggests that VAERS be used as a backup system and a system for generating hypotheses.

To help identify the combination of VAERS, PVS, and other surveillance systems that offers the best opportunity for identifying all possible adverse reactions, the committee encourages CDC to continue consulting state epidemiologists, vaccine program managers familiar with tracking other vaccine-associated adverse reactions, and clinicians to address these issues.

Quickly identifying adverse reactions in vulnerable contact populations will be important for ensuring the safest vaccination program possible. The committee encourages CDC to explore the benefit and feasibility of using data from surveillance systems for vulnerable contact populations (e.g., Medicaid data, cancer registries) as an ancillary approach to monitoring adverse reactions.

The committee suggests that CDC consider using mortality surveillance to supplement the adverse reaction surveillance occurring through VAERS and PVS. To reach this end, the committee encourages CDC to reach out to and coordinate with medical examiners and coroners to educate them about the pre-event smallpox vaccination program and to provide guidelines that can be used for determining whether a death was the result of a serious adverse reaction from the smallpox vaccine or from a random unconnected cause. Mortality surveillance also might help identify an otherwise unrecognized actual smallpox case.

CDC mentioned plans to develop a pregnancy registry, to track the outcomes of any pregnancies in recent vaccinees. The committee agrees that the development of a pregnancy registry would be a prudent step and could add to the limited body of knowledge that currently exists on the risk of spontaneous abortions to recent smallpox vaccinees and the incidence of fetal vaccinia.

Gathering Data on Background Rates of Conditions That Could Be Confused with Adverse Reactions

The nature of any large population experience is that there will be substantial numbers of unusual adverse reactions that, in fact, do not relate to vaccine administration but simply represent background rates of disease. Thus, of the approximately 500,000 vaccine recipients in phase I, it is likely that there will be reports of acute diseases such as influenza or local outbreaks of viral gastroenteritis. Surveillance would be useful in identifying illnesses in vaccinees that may be misattributed as vaccine adverse reactions. It also is possible that unproven associations will be suggested as long-term adverse reactions of the smallpox vaccine, as has occurred with other vaccines. When it comes to the more difficult long-term problem of diseases such as multiple sclerosis and Guillain-Barré syndrome being potentially misattributed to the smallpox vaccine, there are currently no data systems to use for comparison. As with the swine influenza studies, observations of any long-term sequelae from individual observations of alert practitioners, or from VAERS, should be treated as signals and prompt more formal epidemiologic studies to refute or validate them. There also is the possibility, if and when the vaccination program is expanded in phase II, that cohort studies could be set up in the sites using the Vaccine Safety Datalink, a CDC system already in place to evaluate adverse results of childhood immunizations. The committee encourages CDC to utilize surveillance systems that already exist (e.g., health care utilization rates from the National Hospital Discharge Survey and the National Ambulatory Medical Care Survey) to determine baseline rates of disease and place the data that will be obtained from PVS and VAERS into perspective.

Establishment of a Data and Safety Monitoring Board (DSMB)

The committee also considered CDC's plans for monitoring the safety of the smallpox vaccine. The committee briefly heard about plans for the establishment of a smallpox vaccine data and safety monitoring board, jointly operated between CDC and the Department of Defense (DoD) (Winkenwerder and Grabenstein, 2002). Since military vaccinations commenced soon after the President's smallpox policy announcement on December 13, 2002, the military should already have some safety data available. Where possible, the committee encourages CDC to share with their state and local partners any data or lessons learned from the DoD smallpox vaccination experience thus far. The committee first describes what it perceives to be the special considerations for such a board involved in the pre-event smallpox vaccination program.

Such boards are most commonly referred to as data and safety monitoring boards (DSMBs) or data safety and quality monitoring boards (DSQMBs), although data monitoring committee also is a term of reference. DSMBs are defined in essence by their membership, their relationship to the clinical intervention being monitored, their rules of operation, and the scope of their responsibilities. There are, in fact, no hard and fast rules for these entities, but a standard of practice exists and is codified in particular by the rules used by the National Institutes of Health for their DSMBs. The common feature of all DSMBs is independence—real and perceived—sufficient to protect the privacy and safety of the participants.

Many fine details of DSMB organization and function relate to their most common and important use—oversight of double-blinded research-oriented clinical trials. The smallpox vaccination program is neither blinded, research-oriented, nor a trial. It is a public health program. Given the risk of the vaccine and the nation's lack of familiarity with the vaccine and its adverse reactions, the committee applauds CDC's plans nonetheless to establish a monitoring committee in the spirit of a DSMB. It also applauds the intent to have the board jointly oversee the data emerging from the military vaccination program and the civilian program. This sharing of information and pooling of scientific resources can only improve the success of the vaccination program and increase the chances of the safest smallpox vaccination program possible.

The committee has concerns about the organizational arrangements proposed for the DSMB and their influence on independence. Currently it appears that the DSMB will operate as a working group of the Advisory Committee on Immunization Practices (ACIP), a CDC advisory committee. This concern is in no way a reflection on either the competence or integrity of the ACIP members, its chair or executive secretary, the members of the military, or military advisory committees suggested for inclusion on the smallpox vaccine DSMB. Nevertheless, this close organizational tie to the government entities (DoD and CDC) responsible for the program violates one of the key attributes of all DSMBs—both real and perceived independence from the organizing group. A perception that the scientists overseeing the actual data on safety (who will have a responsibility for advising CDC whether the vaccinations are as safe as possible and for advising CDC whether to request the administration to halt an unsafe program) are not truly independent of those setting or overseeing policy could quickly imperil the smallpox vaccination program, not to mention the unintended consequences of eroding trust in all vaccination programs or all public health programs. The DSMB's purpose should be perceived first and foremost as protection of vaccinees. If there are plans that could ensure independent function, this should be communicated in detail to this committee immediately. **If CDC is unable to assure this independent functioning of the DSMB, the committee recommends that the proposed organizational arrangement be reconsidered.**

Given that there will likely be serious adverse reactions, including death, from the vaccine, the committee believes that public trust in the management of the program is essential. It is important to preserve another key attribute of a traditional DSMB—the ability of the board to review data and deliberate in private. This is important for ensuring that the DSMB works in the best interest of the vaccinee, protected from any possible undue influence of the sponsoring agency. However, there will be great interest on the part of program managers, vaccinees, and the public in the safety assessments made by the DSMB. CDC has a responsibility for regular communication to the public about the findings from the DSMB.

Treatment of Vaccine Complications

CDC asked the committee for advice on whether the proposed safety system provides timely access to VIG. The system that CDC is currently proposing instructs the treating physician to contact the designated state official; the state would inform CDC of a request for VIG and/or cidofovir (Vistide); the CDC clinical team would assess the request with the state and treating physician; CDC Drug Services and the National Pharmaceutical Stockpile would coordinate release of VIG and/or cidofovir; and the treating physician would be designated as a co-investigator on the IND protocol. The committee generally believes that the currently proposed system is adequate in this regard, although the potential variability of cases requires case-by-case consideration and treatment. The committee encourages CDC to assemble a group of national experts that could be consulted on serious vaccinia adverse reactions and could provide individualized treatment regimens where necessary. The committee would like to gain more information about the details of the VIG and cidofovir distribution plans, in particular, the criteria for distribution. CDC should carefully monitor the characteristics of the requests for VIG and cidofovir and use these data as a form of passive surveillance.

CDC Safety System Guidance to States

CDC asked the committee to provide advice on whether the proposed safety system will provide for the development of state capacity, such that states will be able to manage smallpox vaccine adverse events if smallpox vaccination becomes routine. The committee felt that they did not have enough detailed information about the state plans to adequately address this question.

Without more specific information on the state plans, it is unclear to the committee if the states are sufficiently prepared to manage adverse reactions in phase I or phase II. But based on the perspectives of state and local public health organizations (Hardy, 2002; NACCHO, 2002), **the committee recommends CDC evaluate each state's capacity for managing adverse reactions before indicating that a state is ready to begin vaccinations.**

Evaluation of states' experiences with management of adverse reactions during phase I should shed more light on their level of preparedness to implement phase II. Should routine vaccination of the general population commence, states' preparedness will have to be evaluated again.

Training and Education

CDC's five training focus areas in preparation for the first phase include smallpox vaccination clinics processing, adverse events training for designated physician experts, data management for safety/VAERS, laboratory diagnostics for rash illness and smallpox, and surveillance for rash illness (Quick et al., 2002). Based on its review of planning material, the committee noted a need to broaden the audiences for certain training, expand the range of material covered, and most important, extend the timeline of training itself. The committee's overriding concern is that the preparation and implementation of training (of vaccinators and health care providers) and education (of vaccinees and the general public) appear to require a more generous time frame than what is permitted by the late January planned start date (Young, 2003). The readiness of vaccination sites and staff should be among the primary criteria for initiating implementation. A hasty launch may mean insufficiently trained vaccinators and uninformed vaccinees, leading perhaps to an increased likelihood of poor outcomes.

Focus Areas of Training and Education

Recommendations made in the screening and safety discussion in preceding pages of the report are relevant to the first training area identified by CDC—smallpox vaccination clinics processing. It is hoped that training will include more than just county health officers and nurses or will strongly emphasize the training of trainers, potentially to include health educators and others. During phase I, vaccination clinic workers need the knowledge and resources to educate the entire range of vaccinees, from professional to nonprofessional hospital workers of various cultural, linguistic, and educational backgrounds, about adequate hand washing technique and proper site care. Local health department trainees (health officers and nurses) will probably benefit from CDC assistance in the form of structured and detailed training modules for local vaccination clinic staff, focused educational materials for vaccinees, educational materials for all local health care providers, and plans to reinforce the learning of vaccinators and vaccinees.

In the area of educational materials, additional work is needed to ensure such items are highly effective. For example, the committee believes that the draft Vaccine Information Statement on smallpox is not sufficient as a tool for vaccinee education, and additional training and informational material should be customized, well-designed, and when possible, pretested to ensure functional relevance (to a vaccinee's work duties), readability, and cultural competence. Training standards should include the development of training material appropriate for the functional status (e.g., emergency department nurse), literacy level, and culturally diverse needs of vaccinees. Also, both vaccination clinics and the workplaces of vaccinees might contribute to supporting vaccinee site care knowledge and practices by making plans to reinforce information, given that repeated exposure to educational messages may be more successful in ensuring protective behaviors, like hand washing and site care. Both health care workers who are vaccinees and the public health personnel vaccinating them may be engaged in training and retraining efforts.

The second training focus area refers to adverse reactions training for physician experts. Rapid and accurate identification of adverse reactions depends upon the ability of all clinicians—infectious disease specialists, primary care physicians, nurse practitioners, and others—to identify common and serious adverse reactions to the smallpox vaccine in their patients.

> **The committee recommends that CDC expand the scope of their training and education regarding the identification, treatment, and reporting of serious adverse reactions to all clinicians. Education and training also should provide clear guidance about how adverse reactions should be reported and what resources are available to aid in their management and treatment.**

Webcasts for clinicians are not enough; outreach must be conducted through multiple modes. The committee commends CDC on the development of the 16-page color brochure providing information on smallpox vaccination and common and serious adverse reactions to the vaccine, and encourages CDC to distribute this brochure as widely as possible. Furthermore, if guidance has not been developed already, the committee encourages CDC to develop guidance for vaccination clinics (some of which may not be located in hospitals) on how to respond to anaphylactic reactions immediately following vaccination.

The committee also was asked to provide advice on what smallpox vaccine safety information practicing physicians need and how this can be most efficiently transmitted. The committee would first like to encourage CDC to think more broadly about who needs this information, and any plan to accomplish this should include sufficient reiteration to answer the problems of busy clinicians being able to attend single sessions. Rather than just focusing on "practicing physicians," this information should be provided to all types of health care providers—physicians, physician assistants, nurse practitioners, nurses.

> **The committee recommends that the first communication clinicians should receive is basic information about the details of the pre-event smallpox vaccination program.**

Although CDC has recognized a need to reach out to clinicians throughout the country and develop specific training materials for them, the committee believes that CDC has possibly underestimated the importance of the primary care system in the implementation of the pre-event smallpox vaccination program. The committee has limited information of plans to provide training about the vaccine to all primary health care providers (e.g., physicians and nurse practitioners), in addition to specialists and others. Given that CDC is encouraging health care workers contemplating vaccination to discuss their questions and concerns with their own health care providers (Rotz, 2002), the committee notes the need to provide some basic training and education to all providers, not just to those selected to address serious adverse reactions. The committee encourages CDC to expand their consideration of how the primary care system may become involved in the vaccination program, and the variety of modes (in addition to website-based) that can be used to provide training to the primary care community.

Much confusion and misinformation exist in both the general public (Blendon et al., 2003) and the health care community (Everett et al., 2002) about multiple components of the smallpox vaccination program. The committee encourages CDC to provide more consistent and comprehensive information to as wide a distribution of clinicians as possible, enabling them, at a minimum, to:

- Counsel potential vaccinees when they are seeking information and assistance in deciding whether to be vaccinated;
- Effectively and sufficiently screen potential vaccinees (or their household contacts) who have contraindications to vaccination;
- Recognize adverse reactions, both common and serious;
- Report serious adverse reactions;
- Seek assistance with managing serious adverse reactions;
- Identify types of dressings to use on the vaccination site (and effectively educate their patients); and
- Care for the vaccination site, including proper hand washing technique (and effectively educate their patients).

Methods for training and communicating with providers may include, but not be limited to: communiques to all health care providers (e.g., state-based fax rapid delivery systems); take-home video and audio cassettes; website and telephone-based information as a backup to brochures and other written materials; and training trainers at the local level to conduct workshops on components of local implementation. Frequently asked questions (FAQs) or similar tools also may be useful for practicing clinicians, and such material may be disseminated electronically and in print.

Data management for safety, the third training focus area is discussed in an earlier section of this report. The fourth and fifth focus areas of the

CDC training plan refer to laboratory diagnostics for smallpox and rash illness and training for rash illness surveillance. The committee was unable to address these areas directly at this time, but believes that they are of great importance, and that the training principles outlined by CDC and the guidance provided in this report should be applied to these components of the training plan.

Additional Training Areas and Training-Related Planning Activities

The committee expressed concern that many aspects of smallpox vaccination planning seem to have occurred in isolation from broader public health activity, reinforcing the programmatic separation characteristic of much public health planning and funding (Boufford and Lee, 2001; IOM, 2002). Although this is an atypical program, similar preparedness and large-scale implementation would be expected to characterize local public health readiness to respond to other public health crises, such as other bioterror threats and emerging infectious diseases. Ideally, smallpox activities would be integrated into overall bioterrorism preparedness, and as much as possible, measures taken to strengthen surveillance, staff training, and communication would be more broadly conceived as dually applicable to smallpox and other public health efforts. A possible strategy to optimize resources and broaden the impact of smallpox vaccination preparations may be collaboration with Centers for Public Health Preparedness to enhance various dimensions of the smallpox program, an opportunity not explicitly considered by CDC planners at the time of the committee's first meeting (Strikas, 2002).

Over the next 2-6 months, in anticipation of phase II of training and education, CDC should provide additional guidance and models/templates for training and education materials to be used at the state and local levels and should develop a database of findings and evaluation materials. This may require activities such as conducting a survey or maintaining an evaluation site to assess the experience of vaccination clinics, hospitals, and health departments around the country. Furthermore, the committee hopes that CDC has been reviewing lessons learned from other mass events with public health implications (e.g., local governments' experience with mass campaigns, the expertise of organizations that routinely plan large events and the movement of large numbers of people).

The first phase of smallpox vaccination will provide unprecedented information about the training and education needs of vaccinators, public health and health care workers, prospective vaccinees and their close contacts. CDC may benefit from establishing mechanisms to collect such information throughout phase I that would be useful in the planning and implementation of expanded vaccination efforts.

Communication

Communication Planning

The committee agrees with the assumptions behind CDC's pre-event communication planning, and has noted that CDC has provided a substantial outline of the communication objectives to be met and activities to be conducted prior to beginning vaccination. However, the committee has noted the need for a more comprehensive, detailed, and strategic communications plan and, in the following pages, identifies some additional broad areas or issues that should be considered in communication planning, including:

- Timing;
- A single, expert voice to represent CDC in presenting science-based public health messages regarding smallpox;
- Audience specificity; and
- Clarity, appropriateness, and mode of delivery of messages (e.g., literacy level, pretesting, Internet).

First, communicating to the public about the vaccine, its benefits and risks should occur before vaccination of health care workers begins. Now is the time to shape messages and influence perceptions with honest answers and scientific evidence; once a serious adverse reaction occurs, attempts to control information or change public opinion will likely be too little, too late. The next steps in the development of a pre-event communication plan require greater clarity and more specific details about the methods and channels to be used and the outcomes expected.

Second, the committee believes it is important that the CDC communications effort strictly address the public health aspects of the smallpox vaccination policy and focus on providing public health and health care workers and the general public with the most complete and scientifically accurate information, while supporting informed decision-making regarding vaccination. Also, **the committee recommends that CDC's communication efforts about smallpox vaccination clearly separate public health issues from national security matters. The latter are best addressed by representatives of the administration more directly involved in such matters, and not by representatives of scientific agencies. Therefore, the responsibility of CDC is to deliver clear, consistent, and science-based public health communications.**

There is evidence from the risk-perception literature that the public expresses less fear when it receives its information from people it trusts (Gray and Ropeik, 2002), and trust is facilitated by honesty, transparency, and the transmission of consistently accurate, science-based information. **The committee recommends that CDC identify a single "voice" for the national vaccination program, a credible individual with a strong scientific background and an experienced communicator who can serve as the key CDC spokesperson. Additionally, the agency should develop several back-up sources for the media who can offer the same level of informed comment and thoughtful observation as the program's primary "voice."**

Such spokespersons should be trained in media techniques, as necessary, to respond to the wide variety of difficult questions that are going to arise during this challenging enterprise. Since the media also will refer to many well-informed critics of the vaccination effort, it is crucial that CDC's communications are based in strong science and communicated with authority. These are essential ingredients to foster public confidence in the program's direction and ultimate outcome. This cadre of health communicators must be able to speak authoritatively to both members of the general public and to health care providers who have anxieties and concerns that must be addressed. To safeguard the separation between political and public health communications, the key spokesperson should not be a politician. This spokesperson (and other key public health communicators) should address the public and be available for the media immediately and regularly after the occurrence of a serious adverse reaction or smallpox release crisis. Such a spokesperson may gain the public's confidence by constituting a credible and consistent source of information and reflecting the expert management of a public health crisis.

Third, if CDC has not done so already, its communication planning may be enhanced by developing specific objectives and strategies targeting each of the audiences that have been identified. As an example, the media, which itself informs the public and needs access to the best, science-based evidence, requires information and transparency that will enable their reporting on program status. Based on their enormous influence in shaping public opinion and disseminating information to the public, the committee believes that state and local efforts would be benefited by CDC-prepared communication objectives focused specifically on communicating with media professionals at the national, state, and local levels, with strategies intended to increase communication between the media and health officials at all levels. The nation's ability to prepare and respond to a smallpox attack or other potential bioterror threat depends heavily on the content and influence of media outputs before an outbreak occurs. A well-informed public also is essential to the success of the smallpox vaccination program, and to public health preparedness in general. Community leaders, community-based organizations, and local civic associations possess human and communications resources that can prove invaluable in assisting the CDC to develop, evaluate, and disseminate targeted public health information to the public.

The objectives outlined in CDC's Smallpox Response Plan and Guidelines (2002d: E-6) appear to combine the information needs of the general public, policy makers, and media, and the communication standards needed by health care workers. Some of the broad communication areas mentioned pertain to the knowledge and understanding of smallpox and immunizations concepts among health care workers and the public; ability of health care worker, public, media and policy maker audiences to respond appropriately to a smallpox case or outbreak; and protocols for surveillance and the communication of data needed after a smallpox case or outbreak. The first two areas are too broad, requiring much more detailed discussion of individual audiences and approaches, and the third is more accurately described as a matter of health informatics (e.g., surveillance, VAERS), discussed to some extent in this report.

A fourth area of great importance to communicating about smallpox has to do with message development and the delivery of information to the public. Methods for communicating to and with the public seem overly reliant on the Internet. Not all health care workers, and certainly not all members of the public, obtain their information online. Print materials should be made available through a variety of outlets, including professional associations, community organizations, and others. Information should be disseminated to the public broadly through a variety of methods, ranging from print materials tested for readability and cultural appropriateness, to public service announcements on television and radio. Given the public's limited and often incorrect knowledge about vaccines, communicating well and early about the smallpox vaccine is essential to support public confidence in the public health system. The public should be provided with pretested, targeted information about vaccines in general (how they are developed, how they work, their benefits and potential side effects), and about the smallpox vaccinia immunization in particular (i.e., the reality that the smallpox vaccine is different from other vaccines in its greater risk of adverse reactions and even death, though such risk is relatively low and may be minimized if appropriate screening, site care, and other precautions are taken). Primary care providers and nurses should be well-informed through communication activities since they are trusted sources of information for individuals and communities. Transparent, culturally competent, accessible, and understandable presentation of what is known and unknown is needed.

In general, CDC's communication plans reflect a greater focus on crisis management than on broader communication strategies. More emphasis should be placed on communications to help frame the public's initial awareness and knowledge and to build trust, which will be essential in dealing with a potential crisis. CDC has outlined four communication principles: (1) consistency and consensus; (2) acknowledgement of and tolerance for uncertainty; (3) communication research; and (4) importance of addressing diversity of communication needs. In addition to these principles, and as previously noted, the committee finds a need to differentiate between political and public health communications and to position CDC firmly in the realm of evidence-based public health communications. Finally, but perhaps most important, there is the principle of informed consent, mentioned above. All communication materials and strategies targeting potential vaccinees and the general public should emphasize the voluntary nature of the vaccination program.

The second through fourth communication principles are addressed to some extent throughout the report. In regard to the first communication principle of consensus and consistency, the committee was unclear about how communication between CDC communicators and their state and local health communicators will occur. What strategies will be employed to ensure standard language is used and that local, state, and national decisions and plans are well aligned?

The committee has concluded that CDC's communication strategy seems well developed in two broad areas: passive information (e.g., training materials, fact sheets) about the disease, the vaccine, and the vaccination campaign, available on the website; and crisis material, prepared to respond to a news event/vaccine crisis or smallpox release. Although the first phase of the vaccination program involves only health care workers, it is never too soon to begin educating the general public; therefore, **the committee recommends that more attention be given to developing a variety of materials and channels to inform and educate the public about the immunization program before vaccinations begin.**

Furthermore, communication planning and tools should differentiate between pre- and post-event information needs. Current training needs and news events are different from potential crisis response, and planning must take place to address each area individually.

A wide range of channels should be used to communicate to and with various audiences, from the media to the general public, from health care workers to policy makers. As the time to make the vaccine available to the general public nears, CDC may wish to consider a mass mailing to every U.S. household, in the style of former Surgeon General Koop's mailing on HIV/AIDS.

Some of the communications questions submitted by CDC to the committee were not answered, as they require empirical and formative communications research (e.g., message development, literacy-level testing). Other than recommending a candid, transparent communications approach that is sensitive to and appropriate for the range of literacy levels and cultural backgrounds among potential vaccinees and the general public, the committee hopes that CDC will seek other types of expert advice and resources.

The committee advises CDC to communicate frequently with the public focusing on consistency, transparency, and a balanced representation of what is known and not known. CDC should be very clear about its jurisdiction—questions about the likelihood of attack are national security issues that CDC is not able/qualified to answer. If asked about the risk of the smallpox vaccine, however, the agency should answer with the facts—that the risk of serious adverse reactions is relatively low, but still higher than any other vaccine in routine and mass use.

Guidance to States

With the exception of guidance on safety system issues, the committee is unable to comment on CDC's guidance to states due to lack of access to certain materials. The committee hopes to provide comments on other components of guidance to states in a future report, when it has received further information.

Overall Progress at Achieving the Goals of the Program

CDC's overall goal seems to be the successful implementation of an immunization program that is truly voluntary and as safe as possible but that establishes the response capacity necessary to protect the public's health in the event of a smallpox attack. Success would mean securing an adequate set of vaccinated teams of health care workers willing to participate in responding to such an attack. The committee is unable to assess CDC's progress at this time, but will do so as program implementation experience allows.

Areas of Potential Future Inquiry

There are a number of important matters the committee recognized but was unable to address in this report and some additional areas on which CDC may wish to request guidance as the implementation of the vaccination program begins and progresses. These matters and areas include, but are not limited to:

- Discussion of the optimal response to an immediate change in the determination of smallpox threat, with a focus on state and local preparedness;
- A review of local readiness for implementation and an assessment of opportunity costs and resource allocation issues;

- Assessment of the adequacy of the screening materials, based on experiences during the first phase;
- Assessment of the adequacy of the informed consent materials (particularly the information provided to vaccinees on the relation of risks to benefits and the range of possibilities for adverse reactions), based on experiences during the first phase;
- Assessment of secondary transmission to contacts, including an assessment of site care guidance and vaccinee's adherence to that guidance;
- Occupational safety issues, particularly related to bifurcated needles;
- A review of the organization and function of the DSMB; and
- Prioritization of recommendations, recognizing that multiple demands may be necessary and some of the committee's recommendations require resources.

CLOSING REMARKS

In closing, the committee wishes to thank you for the opportunity to be of assistance to the Centers for Disease Control and Prevention as it implements this important vaccination program. We look forward to finding out how the committee can help CDC address other program components as it works with state and local partners to move forward with implementation.

Brian L. Strom, *Committee Chair*
Kristine M. Gebbie, *Committee Vice Chair*
Robert B. Wallace, *Committee Vice Chair*
Committee on Smallpox Vaccination Program Implementation

REFERENCES

AHA (American Hospital Association). 2002. Statement to the IOM's Committtee on Smallpox Vaccination Program Implementation on December 19, 2002. Notes: Statement presented by Roslyne Schulman (Senior Associate Director for Policy Development, American Hospital Association).

Altman LK. 2002, December 10. Health Care Workers Union Wary of Smallpox Vaccinations. *New York Times*, A23.

Altman LK, O'Connor A. 2003, January 5. Health Officials Fear Local Impact of Smallpox Plan. *New York Times*, A1.

ANA (American Nurses Association). Statement to the IOM's Committee on Smallpox Vaccination Program Implementation on December 19, 2002. Notes: Statement presented by Cheryl Peterson (Senior Policy Analyst, American Nurses Association).

Associated Press. 2003, January 2. Texas Official Wants Delay in Smallpox Vaccinations. *Amarillo Globe-News*.

Blendon RJ, DesRoches CM, Benson JM, Herrmann MJ, Taylor-Clark K, Weldon KJ. 2003. The public and the smallpox threat. *New England Journal of Medicine* 348(5):1-7.

Boufford JI, Lee P. 2001. Health Policies for the 21st Century: Challenges and Recommendations for the U.S. Department of Health and Human Services. New York: Milbank Memorial Fund.

Burstein J. 2002. Statement of the American College of Emergency Physicians. Transcript from the IOM's Committee on Smallpox Vaccination Program Implementation Meeting One on December 19, 2002, Washington, DC: 267-271.

CDC (Centers for Disease Control and Prevention). 2002a. CDC Telebriefing Transcript: HHS Teleconference on Smallpox Policy. [Online] Available at htpp://www.cdc.gov/od/oc/media/transcripts/t021214.htm. Accessed January 10, 2003.

CDC. 2002b. Epidemiology and Prevention of Vaccine-Preventable Diseases, 7th Edition. [Online] Available at http://www.cdc.gov/nip/publications/pink/Full.htm. Accessed January 10, 2003.

CDC. 2002c. Pre-Event Vaccination System Webcast Questions and Answers. [Online} Available at http://www.bt.cdc.gov/agent/smallpox/vaccination/vaccination-program-qa-pvs.asp. Accessed January 8, 2003.

CDC. 2002d. Smallpox Response Plan and Guidelines (Version 3.0). [Online] Available at http://www.bt.cdc.gov/agent/smallpox/response-plan/. Accessed January 9, 2003.

CDC. 2002e. Summary of October 2002 ACIP Smallpox Vaccination Recommendations. [Online] Available at HtmlResAnchor http://www.bt.cdc.gov/agent/smallpox/vaccination/acip-recs-oct2002.asp. Accessed January 9, 2003.

Connolly C. 2002a, December 15. Bush Plan for Smallpox Vaccine Raises Medical, Fiscal Worries. *Washington Post,* A33.

Connolly C. 2002b, December 24. Smallpox Plan May Force Other Health Cuts. *Washington Post*, A01.

Everett W, Coffin S, Zaoutis T, Halpern S, Kim J, Strom B. 2002. Smallpox Willingness: A National Study of Emergency Department Personnel. Presented to the IOM's Committee on Smallpox Vaccination Program Implementation on December 19, 2002.

GAO (General Accounting Office). 1977. The Swine Flu Program: An Unprecedented Venture in Preventive Medicine. Washington, DC: GAO.

Gray GM, Ropeik DP. 2002. Dealing with the dangers of fear: the role of risk communication. *Health Affairs* 21(6):106-116.

Hardy G. 2002. Statement of the Association of State and Territorial Health Officials. Transcript from the IOM's Committee on Smallpox Vaccination Program Implementation Meeting One on December 19, 2002, Washington, DC: 284-291.

IOM (Institute of Medicine). 2002. The Future of the Public's Health in the 21st Century. Washington, DC: The National Academies Press.

Lane JM, Ruben FL, Neff JM, Millar JD. 1969. Complications of smallpox vaccination, 1968: national surveillance in the United States. *New England Journal of Medicine* 281(22):1201-1208.

Lane JM, Ruben FL, Neff JM, Millar JD. 1970. Complications of smallpox vaccination, 1968: results of ten statewide surveys. *Journal of Infectious Diseases* 122:303-309.

McDonough M. 2003. A Pox on It! Health Lawyers Worry About Smallpox Vaccine Liability. American Bar Association Journal eReport. [Online] Available at http://www.abanet.org/journal/ereport/j10pox.html. Accessed January 10, 2003.

McKenna MAJ. 2002, December 17. Atlanta Hospital Declines to Vaccinate Workers Against Smallpox. *Atlanta Journal-Constitution.*

Mitchell M. 2003, January 2. Cost of Smallpox Vaccinations Prompts Call for Delay in Texas. *Fort Worth Star Telegram*, Metro, 1.

NACCHO (National Association of County and City Health Officials). 2001. Local Public Health Agency Infrastructure: A Chartbook, 51.

NACCHO. 2002. Statement to the IOM's Committee on Smallpox Vaccination Program Implementation on December 19, 2002. Notes: Statement presented by Patrick M. Libbey (Executive Director, NACCHO).

Nakamura D, Weiss EM. 2002. Local Workers Weigh Benefits and Risks of Vaccination. *Washington Post*, A9.

Neff JM, Lane JM, Pert JH, Moore R, Millar JD, Henderson DH. 1967. Complications of smallpox vaccination: national survey in the United States, 1963. *New England Journal of Medicine* 276(3):125-132.

Neff JM, Lane JM, Fulginiti VA, Henderson DA. 2002. Contact vaccinia—transmission of vaccinia from smallpox vaccination. *Journal of the American Medical Association* 288(15):1901.

Neustadt RE, Fineberg HF. 1978. The Swine Flu Affair: Decision-Making on a Slippery Disease. U.S. Department of Health, Education, and Welfare.

Orenstein W. 2002. Transcript from the IOM's Committee on Smallpox Vaccination Program Implementation Meeting One on December 19, 2002, Washington, DC: 311-318.

Price JH. 2002, December 20. Health Workers Resist Smallpox Vaccinations. *The Washington Times*, A1.

Quick L, Nelson R, Strikas R. 2002. Training and Education Overview. Presented to the IOM's Committee on Smallpox Vaccination Program Implementation on December 19, 2002.

Richmond T. 2003. Money Needed for Vaccinations. *The Duluth Superior [Minnesota].*

Rotz L. 2002. Transcript from the IOM's Committee on Smallpox Vaccination Program Implementation Meeting One on December 19, 2002, Washington, DC: 112-147.

SEIU (Service Employees International Union). 2002. As Bush Plan for Mass Smallpox Vaccination Stirs Controversy . . . Nation's Largest Health Care Organization Says Hospital Workers, Patients Will Face Unnecessary Risk. [Online] Available at http://www.seiu.org/media/press_releases/press.cfm?ID=1096. Accessed January 8, 2003.

Strikas R. 2002. Transcript from the IOM's Committee on Smallpox Vaccination Program Implementation Meeting One on December 19, 2002, Washington, DC: 38-81, 172-173.

Vogel S. 2003. No Serious Problems in Military Inoculations. *Washington Post*, A7.

White House. 2002, December 13. President Delivers Remarks on Smallpox. [Online] Available at http://www.whitehouse.gov/news/releases/2002/12/20021213-7.html. Accessed January 8, 2003.

Winkenwerder W, Grabenstein J. 2002. DOD Smallpox Vaccination Program. Transcript from the IOM's Committee on Smallpox Vaccination Program Implementation Meeting One on December 19, 2002, Washington, DC: 235-267.

Young J. 2003. Public Health Departments Will Offer Vaccine Directly to Hospital Workers if Employers Decline. Washington Fax.

C

Review of the Centers for Disease Control and Prevention's Smallpox Vaccination Program Implementation, Letter Report #2

March 21, 2003
Dr. Julie Gerberding
Director
Centers for Disease Control and Prevention
1600 Clifton Road, NE
Atlanta, GA 30333

Dear Dr. Gerberding:

The Committee on Smallpox Vaccination Program Implementation is pleased to offer you our second letter report. We appreciate your timely response to our first report issued on January 17, 2003 (Gerberding, 2003). In particular we note that a number of recommendations have been implemented or their implementation is planned, including, but not limited to:

- creating and implementing active surveillance for adverse events;
- developing an information sheet for contacts of vaccinees;
- adding information about the status of compensation issues in the Vaccine Information Statement; and
- enhancing evaluation efforts.

We hope that our second report proves useful to you and your partners. We also realize that the Centers for Disease Control and Prevention's (CDC) planning and implementation activities have been advancing rapidly while the committee has been developing its report, and it is possible that at the time of the report's release, CDC will have already made changes congruent with some of our recommendations.

CURRENT PROGRAM CONTEXT

At the time the committee met on February 13, 2003, the vaccination program was 3 weeks old. Approximately 1,000 vaccinations had taken place in the civilian population, and the military program reported well over 100,000. Within 1 week, the number of civilian vaccinations had more than doubled. As of March 14, 2003, the total number of civilians vaccinated by the states was nearly 22,000 (CDC, 2003d). On March 6, 2003, the secretary of the Department of Health and Human Services (DHHS) announced a proposal for a compensation program for vaccinees who are injured as a result of receiving the smallpox vaccine. On the same day, states were instructed that they could expand voluntary vaccination to all health care workers and first responders (e.g., firefighters, law enforcement, and emergency workers) as a continuation of the first phase rather than as a distinct second phase of vaccinations (Connolly, 2003c). Also, vaccinations were to be offered to certain federal employees (e.g., Commissioned Corps of the Public Health Service, CDC staff). Despite the plan for expansion, many impediments to participation remain as they were in December 2002. Many health care workers and the officials of health agencies or organizations:

- do not consider themselves (or their institutions) at high risk of a smallpox attack;
- are confident that, in the event of an attack, vaccinations can take place quickly enough to protect them and the public;
- are troubled about the possibility, however small, of transmitting the virus to their patients, particularly those who are immunosuppressed;
- remain concerned about the lack of comprehensive, no-fault adverse event compensation (The committee is pleased that the administration has attempted to remove this barrier by proposing a smallpox vaccination compensation plan to Congress, in the hope that a resolution of this issue will lead to greater willingness to receive the vaccine. However, at the time of this writing, Congress had not yet made a decision regarding compensation.); and
- remain concerned about the implications of possible administrative leave or duty reassignment.

In this report, the committee addresses several important issues: the vaccination program's need for evaluation (including program safety) and clearly defined objectives; a needed emphasis on defining preparedness against smallpox attack; CDC's communications plans; CDC's training and education efforts; the systems for monitoring the safety of the vaccine; the need for a compensation program; and matters of resource allocation.

CDC completed an enormous amount of work between the committee's first and second meetings. The committee extends its congratulations and expresses its admiration to CDC and the thousands of state and local partners in health departments, hospitals, and elsewhere involved in this program. The vaccination program has thus far progressed cautiously and with great deliberation, with states, local jurisdictions, and hospitals taking locally appropriate steps (Henderson, 2003). It is fitting that the beginning, scale, and pace of each local program have been dictated by considerations of the safety of participants and their families and close contacts (who may be vulnerable to spread of vaccinia from an improperly cared for vaccination site) and by local decisions and analyses about what smallpox preparedness requires.

SUMMARY OF KEY MESSAGES

The committee urges CDC to:

1. Carry out all aspects of ongoing discussion, planning, and analysis of the smallpox vaccination program with the intent to advance the goal of smallpox preparedness.
2. Conduct comprehensive evaluation of the program and its outcomes in order to improve its implementation and to protect the vaccinees and the public.

OVERARCHING ISSUES: PREPAREDNESS AND EVALUATION

Plans for implementation of the vaccination program have evolved in a way that precludes the firm demarcation between what were initially intended as two distinct phases or stages of the program. The committee hopes that this turn of events will not impair efforts to ensure the safest vaccination program possible, but steps must be taken to (1) define and progress toward smallpox preparedness, and (2) evaluate the effectiveness of implementation and the safe use of the vaccine as extensively as the mandates and realities of the vaccination program will allow. Thus, evaluation at the national level might not take place before the program progresses (although some state and local jurisdictions may be able to pause for evaluation before expanding their program activities) but at least should occur simultaneously, to ensure that lessons are learned from phase I even in the face of a rapid expansion.

In its first report (IOM, 2003:5), the committee observed that generally, "public health interventions are undertaken with recognition of some benefit to some individuals, no effect on others, and the possibility of some risk to a small percentage of the population . . . , with expectation of overall benefit to the population receiving the intervention." The committee believes it is important to reiterate the risk-benefit context of the smallpox vaccination program.

"Based on the administration's statement[1] that the risk of a smallpox attack is indeterminate (not zero but currently assumed to be very low) (White House, 2002), the benefit of the vaccination program to the public also is not zero but is assumed to be very low. The benefit to any individual might indeed be zero if the individual never encounters the smallpox virus. However, in the event of exposure to smallpox virus, the benefit to individuals may be very high. Given this profile of high vaccination risk and likely very low to zero benefit, the administration's policy to offer vaccination to public health, medical, and emergency workers must be implemented in a most prudent and cautious manner."

Understanding this complex reality highlights the importance of both preparedness to ensure optimal benefit to the public (i.e., rapid vaccination in the event of smallpox attack) and evaluation to ensure the lowest risk from the vaccine (i.e., overall program safety, including safe use of the vaccine).

A Focus on Preparedness

The expressed intent of the expansion, as the committee understands it, is to make the vaccine available to greater numbers of relevant personnel. However, it is important to retain a focus on smallpox preparedness as the goal of the program. Increasing the number of vaccinated persons might contribute to meeting that goal, but it does not mean preparedness to respond to a smallpox attack has been achieved. Having more vaccinated individuals is only as effective as the plans for deploying these individuals in a potential smallpox bioterrorist event and the collaboration and communication among the various agencies responsible for aspects of smallpox preparedness. This means that a jurisdiction needs not only sufficient workers to vaccinate the public, diagnose and treat cases, and conduct other needed activities (e.g., identify and protect immediate contacts), but also well-

[1]The president's statement was made on December 13, 2002. Although there has been no public statement about an increase in the risk of smallpox attack specifically, at the time of this writing, the Homeland Security Department has elevated the national threat level to Level Orange, or high risk of attack, and the U.S. campaign in Iraq has begun (White House, 2003).

defined roles for all auxiliary agencies and workers, such as law enforcement, firefighters, and emergency personnel. Communities, in partnership with state and federal public health agencies, will need to define smallpox preparedness, assess how close they are to attaining it, and decide what additional actions are needed to ensure they are prepared.

At its February 2003 meeting, the committee heard from CDC and its partners that the success of program activities should not be judged solely by number of vaccinees reached, but by what has been a principal goal since the beginning—preparedness, in terms of safely building capacity to respond effectively to a potential smallpox bioterrorism event (Anderson, 2003; Henderson, 2003). It is important to note that the president's statement on December 13, 2002, gave no numerical goal, but later statements by the administration and DHHS offered between 400,000 and 500,000 vaccinees as a possible total (CDC, 2002). Although based on assumptions and very rough calculations,[2] these figures quickly became the symbolic target for phase I of the program, but as was noted in the February 6, 2003 CDC telebriefing, the program "goal is achievement of a preparedness capacity" (CDC, 2003a).

The committee strongly agrees with the emphasis on preparedness. Although original estimates were useful in planning and initiating the program, the practical experience acquired by states and localities in the first several weeks of the program suggests that other benchmarks are equally if not more important. CDC will now be able to consider both the realities of operationalizing the vaccination program and a more careful view of how many vaccinated individuals, and in what roles, it would take to achieve preparedness to respond to a smallpox attack.

Defining Preparedness

In general, state and local jurisdictions will be able to determine when they are prepared to respond to a case of smallpox in their region, but due to the movement of populations across state boundaries and to geographic,

---

[2]The June 2002 Advisory Committee on Immunization Practices (ACIP) recommendation was for the creation of at least one public health response team per state or territory and for health care teams in designated hospitals to serve as referral centers for initial smallpox cases. Rough estimates made at that time indicated that approximately 15,000 vaccinees would be required. That recommendation was revised in October 2003 due in part to concerns that no one hospital would volunteer for what could be viewed as the stigma of "the smallpox hospital" in that state. Thus, the recommendation was amended to offer all acute-care hospitals the opportunity to create smallpox health care teams. Rough estimates made at that time indicated that this approach would result in approximately 500,000 vaccinees (AMA-CSA, 2003). In practice, it appears that the reality of the program will result in a number of vaccinees somewhere between these two estimates.

program, and resource variations among states, there is an undeniable need for leadership and coordination at a national level. Also, agreement on local, state, and national definitions of smallpox preparedness would be helpful in evaluating the program's success. (An outbreak in one state has implications for that state's neighbors, and all states need the assurance that neighboring jurisdictions are sufficiently prepared and have the capacity to assist in an emergency if needed.) The Public Health Competencies for Bioterrorism and Emergency Preparedness and the state and local Emergency Preparedness and Response Inventories may be useful resources in developing smallpox-specific inventories and checklists of competencies to guide action and enable evaluation (Columbia University, 2002).

CDC and its state and local partners face the need to determine how to best and most rapidly integrate a new set of potential vaccinees into efforts toward smallpox preparedness. CDC's goals for the entire vaccination program (i.e., preparedness/capacity to respond, protection of those who will investigate and treat suspected cases, and gaining experience with vaccination, [Anderson, 2003]), suggest that states may determine that once each local jurisdiction: (1) has ready access to both a public health and a health care response team;[3] (2) is capable of investigating an outbreak and caring for cases;[4] and (3) is ready to rapidly and safely vaccinate anyone else necessary—from additional health care workers to the general public—it can conclude that it has completed precautionary smallpox vaccination of critical personnel, thus accomplishing one component of overall preparedness. Clearly, the contribution of additional vaccinees to this profile of preparedness can best be assessed by each jurisdiction in partnership with CDC.

As the committee noted in its first letter report (IOM, 2003), state and local officials working to approach smallpox preparedness goals would benefit from taking into account program sustainability, particularly in terms of staff turnover. At the state level, program management and leadership could be affected by turnover in state health commissioners, and at the local level, the ability of a jurisdiction to rapidly vaccinate great numbers of people could be affected by changes in the employment status of members of public health and health care response teams. The prospect of such changes requires planning, recruitment, training, and education for volunteers needed to replenish the smallpox response teams, and training and education of new state public health officials, to help ensure program continuity.

---

[3]Note: this does not require that each jurisdiction should contain a public health or health care smallpox response team.

[4]October 2003 ACIP recommendation states that a health care team should be sufficient to provide "continuity of care" for 2 days.

Thus, **the committee recommends that CDC work with states to decide what more is needed to achieve smallpox preparedness, if anything. Further, given the routine turnover in personnel, each state should evaluate what it needs to maintain this preparedness.**

Concerns About Program Expansion and Implications for Preparedness

The committee has a number of significant concerns triggered by the program's rapid expansion to make the vaccine available to all health care providers, emergency responders, and others (Connolly, 2003c). First, the program's swift expansion may inhibit CDC and state efforts to evaluate the program with a focus on strengthening the systems that promote the safest and most effective vaccination program possible. These systems include analyzing vaccine adverse event data, the effectiveness of training and education materials, the ability of screening and informed consent measures to protect vaccinees, and the effectiveness of clinical care setting–based processes (e.g., bandages and leave) in preventing spread. In other words, expanding the program before conducting a thorough evaluation may preclude the opportunity to learn from the first phase or stage of the program before proceeding.

The committee's second concern pertains to funding. As discussed later in the report, some public health agencies and hospitals participating in the program have described serious difficulties in making limited resources adequately address general public health prevention needs, overall bioterrorism preparedness, as well as the requirements of the smallpox program (Libbey, 2003; NACCHO, 2003). Expanding the vaccination program may negatively affect other aspects of smallpox preparedness, bioterrorism preparedness in general, and even the delivery of essential public health services. At the time this report is being written, it is not clear when or even if additional funding will be made available to state and local programs for the expansion of smallpox vaccination.

Third, the committee is concerned about the opening of the program to more potential vaccinees before guidance pertaining to this expansion is available and before many states and localities have had the opportunity to develop new objectives and more detailed plans about the integration of new types of workers into overall smallpox preparedness. Furthermore, many states and localities may not have had the chance to initiate or enhance linkages with the agencies (e.g., local police and fire departments, emergency management, etc.) that will be involved in the expansion. New populations of potential vaccinees imply at a minimum new training and education needs, novel types of occupational and contact issues, and additional communication to the general public.

The committee's concerns are further informed by the clear unease expressed at the committee's February 13, 2003, meeting by the liaison panel to the committee—a group of organizations invited to inform the committee of the real-world implications of the program—about the plan for one continually expanding vaccination effort. They asserted that this did not seem consistent with the way the program was described at its launch and expressed great concern that such an attempt to seamlessly blend the two phases would pre-empt and prevent attempts to evaluate the first phase before embarking on wider vaccination.

The committee will hold its third meeting on May 1, 2003. At this meeting, leaders of state, local, and hospital-based vaccination programs will discuss the lessons learned and best practices demonstrated in the first 3 months of the vaccination program and also will discuss how the communities are defining and measuring smallpox preparedness. The committee expects that sufficient experience will have been gained by that time to help create a significant contribution to the smallpox vaccination program evaluation for CDC and its partners.

A Need for Evaluation

As the administration and CDC likely anticipated, and the committee observed in its first report (IOM, 2003), the program has evolved. Although our understanding of existing threat assessments has not changed, the vaccination program has moved from the tabletop into the field, where things have progressed in ways determined by state and local circumstances and decisions. **The committee recommends that CDC conduct comprehensive evaluation of the program and its outcomes in order to improve its implementation and to protect the vaccinees and the public.** This would ideally occur before program expansion, but present circumstances may require creative ways to evaluate during expansion.

Ongoing evaluation at the national and state levels should include (1) learning about best practices and process issues in implementing the program (including an assessment of program costs), (2) a determination of smallpox preparedness, and (3) an assessment of the program's safety. Evaluating the ways the program has been conducted might include the logistical and administrative issues addressed by states and localities, from clinic management to communication methods and messages. Determining whether preparedness has been reached might include comparing outcomes to objectives identified in planning, such as number of response teams, and measures for wide-scale vaccination, such as the number and distribution of mass vaccination clinics, and security and transportation issues. Evaluating program safety might include, but not be limited to, careful data collection about adverse events following vaccination, accurate clinical descriptions that are integrated with laboratory data, taking advantage of the national experience to determine modern incidence rates for vaccine reactions, and identifying risk factors for these reactions. Since the Department of Defense (DoD) has vaccinated a much larger cohort than the civilian vaccination program to date, it is hoped that data on adverse events in DoD's vaccination program will be incorporated, to the extent possible, in the overall evaluation of vaccine safety.

As the committee has stated previously, evaluation is a matter of data analysis, not specifically of time, and would entail, among other issues, the necessary reasoned analysis of the strengths and weaknesses of the procedures used to ensure patient and contact safety in the first phase. Because vaccination programs in most jurisdictions by early March 2003 are unlikely to be of sufficient size for a full evaluation, an evaluation of national scope is needed to ensure that the analysis is powerful enough to provide meaningful information as the program progresses. Although present realities may make it impossible to conduct a national evaluation at a particular point in time, efforts must be made to analyze data on a national scale as soon as sufficient data are available. Based on the findings of such an evaluation, supplemented with state-level evaluations, states may deem that preparedness goals have been reached. If more vaccinees are needed, the evaluation will be important in guiding efforts to make the program better, faster, and safer.

Any effort to assess the level of smallpox preparedness must be linked with an analysis of the threat of a smallpox attack. Accurate communication (discussed in the next section) about the current threat assessment is critical, and the federal government has a responsibility to communicate any change in that threat assessment, whether an increase or decrease, to the American public. Ensuring both preparedness (capacity to extend the benefits of the vaccine to the public) and the lowest possible vaccine risk to the public's health is only possible if decisions and informed consent are based on the best available information about the level of threat.

PROGRAMMATIC ISSUES

Communication[5]

CDC is to be congratulated for greatly expanding its communication efforts in a short amount of time and demonstrating recognition of the importance of communications in the implementation of the smallpox vaccination program. Below, the committee will address broad issues related to

[5]Communication, training, and education have overlapping meanings. For the purpose of clarity and brevity, this report will generally use "communication" to describe activities that target the media and the general public, and "training and education" when the audiences are public health and health care response team members and other vaccinees with functional roles in smallpox preparedness.

CDC's communication planning, as it has been presented to the committee, and later will address specifics, including answers to questions asked by CDC about its communications.

Overarching Communication Issues

The communication effort could be strengthened if CDC defines the objectives for the program's expansion, and for smallpox preparedness in general, and then determines the communication strategies that will help meet these objectives. As in its first report (IOM, 2003), the committee urges CDC to focus on defining audiences, developing clear messages for each, determining best and multiple channels for communication, and explaining to each audience its present role. Media coverage of the program may leave members of the general public confused about the immediacy of the threat, the need to get vaccinated, and other issues. It is critical that CDC, as the nation's trusted public health authority, inform the public about what steps are being taken to protect them against smallpox and other bioterror threats. Ultimately, despite the novel challenges of our time and this particular program, CDC is still engaged in carrying out what has always been its defined and historic mission of safeguarding the public by promoting health and preventing disease.

In addition to the need to strengthen communication capacity, the committee believes that communication means much more than dissemination. It also involves listening to the public to assess their level of knowledge about smallpox (disease and vaccine), as well as their opinions and attitudes. Efforts to survey the public should be ongoing, to help refine communication materials and diversify channels for communication. The planning, implementation, and evaluation of strategic communication activities for the smallpox vaccination program could begin to form a foundation for broader communication about bioterrorism.

Communication Specifics

Communicating with the General Public

Print and broadcast media interest in the program has been a constant since the program began. However, it also has become apparent that smallpox vaccination is a subject of greater complexity than many health issues in the public dialogue, due to its emergence out of national security considerations, its relationship to other bioterrorism preparedness measures, and persisting concerns about liability and compensation. This complexity may make it more difficult to communicate clearly and accurately. The program's expansion to other categories of responders highlights the fact that communication will continue to be an area of critical importance, in relaying information about the evolving program to the public and gauging public understanding and opinion about the issues.

Media reports provide a wide range of on-the-ground perspectives and informal program implementation updates. Some media reports about the vaccination program have reflected the concerns of organizations, agencies, and individuals, others have conveyed reassurance about the public health system's readiness to respond to bioterror threats. Some adverse events following smallpox vaccination have been reported in the media before CDC has formally described these adverse events. There seems to be a range of perceptions, both reflected in and by the media, about the program and the vaccine. Some concerns about and attitudes toward the vaccination program may be in part related to the current lack of clarity about the program's objectives mentioned above. For example, because the parameters for the program are unclear (e.g., timelines, definitions, and evaluation of preparedness), it is possible to conceive of each hospital that declines to participate as a blow to preparedness, or of vaccinee numbers that are far from target as a detriment to the first line of response. Such conclusions may not be warranted but are somewhat understandable in the existing information environment. Therefore, **the committee recommends CDC revisit and communicate to the public the program's objectives in view of state-level realities, and provide a preliminary perspective on the national and state success in reaching those objectives. The CDC should continue to support, as well as build on the experience of state and local health departments who are developing their communication strategies about state and local program implementation.**

The committee is aware of CDC's forthcoming public service announcements and looks forward to additional communication activities targeting the general public. A great range of groups are important to consider as audiences and as partners in communication, including schools, religious congregations, local community organizations, and professional associations, among others. Local resources, such as community leaders and other trusted individuals could be mobilized in addition to national spokesperson(s) for the vaccine, and a wide range of communication channels employed to reach the broadest constituencies.

States have begun to develop and disseminate public communications (e.g., newspaper inserts) on the subject of bioterrorism, including information about smallpox disease, vaccine, and the vaccination program. Although national and state efforts to keep communities informed are needed, the committee expressed some concern that the messages given to the public may not be timely, may be too broad, and may provide a great deal of unfocused, undifferentiated information.

The committee recommends that CDC and its state and local partners develop communications strategies that:

- **Provide adequate quality and quantity of information.** Communication to the public should consist of well-developed, consistent messages that provide scientific and public health information specifically relevant to the current assessment of disease risk (Covello and Sandman, 2001). Although pages of small print and dozens of facts and details are useful in some cases and with some audiences, public communication would be most effective using clear, concise, and focused language, in an easy-to-read and culturally appropriate format, with instructions for accessing more detailed information (e.g., through a website, toll-free information hotline). Also, it may be helpful to generate core messages for nationwide use, to which information relevant to local circumstances may be added.
- **Are timely.** The timing of messages is important to promote a realistic understanding of current risk. For example, vaccinations are not recommended for the general public at this time, and communication efforts should carefully reflect this. However, other messages and information should be finalized and ready for release in the event circumstances require a change in communication content.
- **Reassure the public that efforts are in progress to protect them in the event of a smallpox attack.** People should be informed that the public health system is increasing its capability to protect them, with response teams ready to vaccinate, and identify and treat cases. However, such communication can occur only if program objectives are defined and supported by adequate resources and preparedness is demonstrated by subsequent evaluation efforts. Clearly, jurisdictions can only reassure the public about their readiness to respond to a smallpox attack if they indeed are ready; thus, communication is contingent on achieving an adequate degree of preparedness. Information should be made available about post-event readiness as part of the pre-event communication strategies.

As is the case with training and education efforts, discussed later in this report, messages about smallpox (disease, vaccine, and vaccination) call for careful planning, design, and pretesting to ensure comprehension, and require evaluation to determine whether anticipated knowledge and behavior changes have occurred. Several polls and surveys (Blendon et al., 2002; Nowack et al., 2002; NNii, 2003) have demonstrated that many people, including health professionals, have inaccurate or incomplete understanding about matters related to smallpox, and such misinformation can be easily spread, creating unnecessary anxiety. It also is possible that confusion over smallpox vaccination could have an adverse effect on public attitudes and behaviors regarding childhood immunization, unless communication is very carefully planned.

It is not easy to reconcile the program's present focus on public health and health care response teams with the need to communicate with and to the public. Although the public needs information and education on the subject of smallpox, this would ideally be accomplished without creating or confirming a sense of crisis and anxiety, hence the need for sufficient, but focused information. Current vaccination policy, based on a threat assessment that is believed to be low but not zero, and possible but not imminent, states that it is not necessary for the public to receive smallpox vaccine at this time. Therefore, the public should receive enough information that will reassure them that these actions are appropriate at this time.

Communicating with the Media

Furthermore, while media reports provide the valuable service of informing the public about the vaccination program's progress, they sometimes include inaccurate information (e.g., misrepresenting the severity of adverse reactions). For example, generalized vaccinia is a condition that may result from smallpox vaccination, and it consists of a generalized, benign rash. Although this is not considered a life-threatening adverse reaction to the vaccine, it might sound like one, and without adequate explanation in media reports, the public may perceive it as such. In order to facilitate accuracy in media reports, **the committee recommends CDC develop and offer journalists training materials and opportunities specifically designed for the media, explaining the program's clinical components, providing the best available scientific evidence, and dedicating staff experts to provide technical support to media representatives.**

CDC asked the committee to provide advice on the level of investment that should be committed to communication efforts. It is clear that communication is one of the core aspects of the program, not a marginal, disposable component, and the effectiveness of communication activities in the smallpox program will build a foundation for other bioterrorism activities. Ensuring the public has basic accurate knowledge about the disease and the vaccine and informing the public about the public health system's efforts to prepare itself to protect the public's health could strengthen the credibility of CDC as a trusted source of health information.

Communicating with Health Care Workers and Others

In addition to communicating with the media and the general public, it is important that CDC and its state and local public health partners maintain regular communication with health care entities, as well as law enforcement, fire, emergency response, and other relevant agencies. Local governments should ensure that public health, health care, and emergency responders are well-informed about post-event vaccination plans and, should the threat level of smallpox attack rise, about the processes by which the state would reconsider and communicate its decision about expanded precautionary vaccinations and widespread vaccination.

Training and Education

The committee applauds CDC's efforts to develop partnerships with professional organizations and clinician networks to provide a forum for education, training, and clinician communication with CDC. The committee noted the stratification of information for clinicians into "Just in case" and "Just in time"—demonstrating readiness both to provide essential information broadly to all clinicians and to release additional information for immediate clinician access in the event of a suspected case or outbreak. The committee also is pleased to see that CDC has enlarged the circle of clinicians to include others, such as nurses and physicians' assistants. However, the evidence base used to develop training and education for clinicians must go beyond how physicians learn to include nurses and physician's assistants. CDC's intention to utilize a broad array of methods is likely to be of assistance in educating and training.

Given the program's expansion, great care should be given to developing training and education materials to be delivered through a wide range of channels to the potential vaccinees, who may include other health care workers, as well as emergency, law enforcement, and fire personnel. This may require functional modules addressing the occupation issues of all possible areas of practice. Training and education efforts also should include continuing broad dissemination of information to and dialogue with all health care providers around the country, as well as evaluating the effectiveness of training and education. It is important to note that carrying out this component of the program might require resources.

Broad Issues Relevant to Training and Education

CDC has produced a vast array of training and education tools, and is disseminating them widely. The committee believes it would be of great value, however, to conduct outcome evaluation and not just process evaluation of these activities. Some excellent learning tools have been developed, but an assessment of the effectiveness of educational materials in increasing knowledge is needed. Such an assessment might evaluate the dissemination of materials (e.g., are they easily accessed) and their effectiveness in increasing target group knowledge (e.g., increasing familiarity with CDC smallpox site care in clinicians and vaccinees, clinician and vaccinee knowledge of expected reactions to vaccinia, health care provider familiarity with local smallpox response plans and their personal roles, and clinician awareness of clinical resources, such as the CDC Clinician Information Line).

Specific Issues in Training and Education

It is not apparent from the materials and information available to the committee whether educational products and training activities for other health care providers (e.g., respiratory therapists and radiology technicians) and other members (e.g., security and housekeeping staff) of hospital response teams are available at the time of the writing of this report. Furthermore, the committee's liaison panel expressed a need for educational materials that are relevant to professional practice and the circumstances of vaccination (for example, health care providers working with recently vaccinated patients, or emergency medical technicians and other first responders who may be exposed to newly vaccinated individuals). Each of these groups, as well as the functional groups within public health response teams, requires customized materials and information, and the committee encourages CDC to assess and respond to their needs for training and education utilizing a range of materials and channels of dissemination most appropriate for each group.

The committee was pleased to find out that CDC has been taking steps to increase the readability of materials developed to provide important information about smallpox vaccine and vaccination, and even to translate many into other languages (Nowak, 2003). **The committee recommends that all print materials addressed to a diverse audience (e.g., the public) should be easily read and understood by all members of that audience. Also, all communication materials in other languages should be culturally appropriate.**

Simple translation may not be enough in cases where illustrations, format, and other facts are not culturally appropriate for the target audience. States will likely request materials in languages that correspond to the profile of their potential vaccinees.

Although CDC has thoughtfully developed its process for informing and educating potential vaccinees and their contacts, more is needed to ensure an adequate level of comprehension is reached.

For this reason, **the committee recommends that educational and training materials be tested for ease of comprehension with samples representing a cross-section of the sex, race, ethnicity, and level of education.**

This should be done for all current materials and should routinely be done prior to wide dissemination of all newly developed material, though time constraints might make this more difficult. Special attention is needed to highlight uncertain compensation for adverse reactions, and simplifying legal explanations currently provided on the Informed Consent form.

The dissemination of training and education materials to physicians and other health care providers is a vitally important component of the vaccination program, and CDC should take steps to determine the most effective ways to reach clinicians. For example, mailed materials may not even get past the administrative office and may not be effective in changing clinician knowledge or behavior. Diverse and interactive means of reaching physicians and other clinicians may be needed (e.g., use opinion leaders, professional associations). Furthermore, tallying the number of materials (brochures, videos, CD-ROMs) sent out to physicians and others is not sufficient to evaluate the effect of education and communication efforts; this is only an evaluation of the process, but not of its outcomes. Developing ways to measure change in level of knowledge and translation of knowledge to action is necessary to demonstrate effectiveness and determine where further attention is needed.

The committee was asked to provide recommendations to guide CDC's tracking of state training activities and evaluating the effect of training initiatives. Given their geographic, cultural, and social diversity, states are likely to use a wide range of strategies to train vaccinators, inform clinicians, and educate vaccinees and their contacts. The ongoing weekly discussions between states and CDC can capture some of this information, but CDC also could develop a format states can use to summarize their training activities and encourage states to complete it on a regular basis online. That may facilitate the sharing of best practices and the evaluation of phase I discussed above. With some additional planning, the effect of training activities (related to their quality, quantity, dissemination) could be linked to better program outcomes, such as better screening for contraindications, enhanced vaccinee education and reinforcement of good site care and hygiene practices, and improved clinical diagnostic ability.

Data to Assess Vaccine and Program Safety

Pre-Event Vaccination System

The committee was pleased to hear that the Pre-Event Vaccination System (PVS) is being revised, and that the system will be fully operational relatively soon. Data gathered through PVS will be extremely useful for evaluating vaccine take rates, vaccine distribution, and vaccine immunogenicity. The ability to create clinic-specific, state-specific, and national reports from PVS data will enhance overall evaluation of the pre-event smallpox vaccination program.

Through the Smallpox Vaccine Adverse Events Monitoring and Response System (which includes the Hospital Smallpox Vaccination Monitoring System, the Smallpox Vaccine Adverse Event Active Surveillance

System [both described in detail below], the Vaccine Adverse Events Reporting System, inquiries received through CDC's Clinician Information Line, and requests for vaccinia immune globulin and cidofovir), data on adverse events will be linked to a vaccinee's record in PVS using the vaccinee's Patient Vaccination Number (PVN). A case investigation of the adverse event will involve a reevaluation of whether the vaccinee had any contraindications that were not disclosed initially or were not recognized at the time. Because contraindications will be part of the case investigation, and it is possible that revisions will be made to the list of contraindications as the vaccination program moves forward, it will be necessary to know which version of the Pre-Vaccination Information Packet the vaccinee received. **The committee recommends that a data field be added to PVS to indicate which version of the Pre-Vaccination Information Packet was provided to the vaccinee, in order to document what information was given to the vaccinee prior to consent.**

Survey to Assess Common Adverse Reactions

CDC has proposed conducting a telephone follow-up survey of 10,000 vaccinees in eight states to study the rate of common adverse reactions in vaccinees and the average amount of time lost from work due to reactions to the vaccine. CDC plans to use a stratified sampling scheme to ensure adequate representation of men and women and primary vaccinees and revaccinees. The planned survey should provide valuable information about the rate of common adverse reactions in vaccinees, and the committee is pleased that CDC has designed a method for gathering these data.

CDC proposes to use an internal comparison/"control" group to control for the rates of common health events that will be observed during the course of this study. Since, in the context of the smallpox vaccination program, the health status of unvaccinated persons may differ significantly from vaccinees (i.e., due to contraindications), CDC proposes to use a comparison group exposed to the vaccine as a "control" group. CDC assumes that common adverse reactions associated with the vaccine will resolve by day 30 post-vaccination. Working under this assumption, the "control" group will be drawn from vaccinees who agreed to participate in the survey but were not selected for the sample. These "controls" will be observed for 21 days (the same length of time that the "treatment" group will be observed) following day 30 post-vaccination. The "controls" will receive the same diary card (for recall purposes) that is used by the "treatment" group (updated to reflect the different observation period), and will be observed for the 21 day period when they are assumed to experience "normal" health events (i.e., not due to the vaccine, since health events due to the vaccine are assumed to resolve by day 30 post-vaccination).

The committee suggests that CDC consider using an unvaccinated control group as well, especially if there are insufficient vaccinees to provide both an exposed (i.e., exposed to the vaccine) group of 10,000 and a control group that can be studied prospectively from the time the survey is scheduled to begin (currently expected to be late March). The use of an unvaccinated control group may provide insights into the effect of vaccination on common potential problems such as rates of work loss, febrile and rash illnesses, and temporary decreases in physical and social function. The committee agrees that it may not be appropriate to draw the control group from the complete pool of potential vaccinees that could not be vaccinated due to contraindications, since their health status may significantly differ from the health status of those who were vaccinated. However, this control group could perhaps be drawn from those potential vaccinees that could not be vaccinated because of secondary contraindications (e.g., contraindications in their close personal contacts).

The committee notes that the data gathered through the Hospital Smallpox Vaccination Monitoring System (HSVMS, discussed in more detail below) may supplement the data obtained through the survey. The HSVMS collects data on workdays lost due to illness, workdays with restrictions on work duties (e.g., no patient contact), the presence and severity of symptoms reported by the vaccinee, the type of dressing covering the vaccination site, the condition of the dressing, physical findings at the vaccination site, and vaccine take. Depending upon how many monitoring sites (i.e., hospitals, health departments, clinics) decide to use HSVMS, HSVMS could be considered as a means for gathering real-time monitoring data on common adverse reactions and days lost from work for a large proportion of vaccinees.

Active Surveillance for Serious Adverse Events and Monitoring Common Adverse Events

The committee congratulates CDC on developing so quickly a comprehensive active surveillance system for serious adverse events associated with smallpox vaccination. In its first letter report, the committee recommended that active surveillance for adverse events be employed. CDC has designed the Smallpox Vaccine Adverse Event Active Surveillance System (hereafter called the "Active Surveillance System") to accomplish active surveillance for serious adverse events following smallpox vaccination among all vaccinees during phase I of the vaccination program. The Active Surveillance System (and other coordinated data systems) will build upon the data that were gathered in the Pre-Event Vaccination System (described in detail in the committee's first letter report). The coordinated use of the Active Surveillance System with the Vaccine Adverse Events Reporting System

(VAERS), the HSVMS, inquiries received through CDC's Clinician Information Line, and requests for vaccinia immune globulin (VIG) and cidofovir will allow CDC to systematically collect information on vaccinees' experiences following vaccination and will greatly increase the likelihood that all serious adverse events following smallpox vaccination will be detected.

Active Surveillance System

The Smallpox Vaccine Adverse Event Active Surveillance System is designed to collect data on all vaccinees at the "close-out" of the vaccination process (this is usually 21 to 28 days after vaccination, when the scab falls off). The Active Surveillance System is a web-based system that is accessible through CDC's Secure Data Network (SDN). State and local health departments, hospitals, and vaccination clinics can enter data into the Active Surveillance System as long as they have been given authorization to access the SDN. The Active Surveillance System will collect information on:

1. Whether contraindications to vaccination among the vaccinee, or contacts of the vaccinee, were identified since the time of vaccination;
2. Whether the vaccinee received medical care for an adverse event; and
3. Whether vaccinia transmission to contacts of the vaccinee occurred.

Information from the Active Surveillance System will be supplemented with information from PVS, VAERS, the Clinician Information Line, and requests for VIG and cidofovir to help give a complete picture of the details of each adverse event.

Both PVS and HSVMS (discussed in more detail below) will include a link to the Active Surveillance System. When the Active Surveillance System is accessed through these means, many of the fields in the Active Surveillance System will be pre-populated with data from PVS or HSVMS. By the pre-population of as many data fields as possible with data from PVS or HSVMS, the risk of data entry error will be reduced.

By its nature, the Active Surveillance System is designed to obtain a confirmed outcome on every vaccinee. To ensure that the Active Surveillance System is truly "active," CDC instructs vaccination monitors to make at least three attempts at contacting the vaccinee before the vaccinee is designated as "unable to contact vaccinee for follow-up." The percentage of vaccinees that will be lost to follow-up should be relatively low, considering that phase I vaccinees are affiliated with a particular smallpox response team and monitors are instructed to make at least three attempts to contact the vaccinee for follow-up. However, it will be important to specifically identify any vaccinees that are lost to follow-up due to death or hospitalization. CDC is planning to track how many vaccinees are lost to follow-up.

To monitor the effectiveness of contraindications screening, the Active Surveillance System will seek to determine if any contraindications were missed during the initial screening of vaccinees. If the Active Surveillance System identifies a vaccinee or a close personal contact of a vaccinee that has a contraindication to vaccination not identified during pre-vaccination screening, an epidemiologist at CDC will follow up with the local Adverse Events Coordinator to determine why the contraindication was not identified during the initial screening process.

For serious adverse events that are identified through the Active Surveillance System, CDC requests that a VAERS report be filed (if one was not filed already). The Active Surveillance System includes a field for indicating the VAERS report number.

The Active Surveillance System also specifically asks whether transmission of vaccinia virus to contacts of the vaccinee occurred. If vaccinia virus was transmitted to a contact of the vaccinee, CDC requests that a VAERS report be filed for each contact to whom transmission of vaccinia occurred. The Active Surveillance System includes a field for indicating the VAERS report number for each contact.

The committee notes that the Active Surveillance System is designed to obtain a confirmed outcome on every vaccinee in the short term. However, it should be recognized that long-term side effects from the vaccine are possible. The committee encourages CDC to begin thinking about ways to monitor for long-term side effects from smallpox vaccination.

Hospital Smallpox Vaccination Monitoring System (HSVMS)

Another system that CDC will use for gathering data on vaccinees' experiences following smallpox vaccination is the HSVMS. The HSVMS is a voluntary, web-based system designed to assist hospitals and other vaccination monitoring sites (e.g., vaccination clinics and health departments) in real-time monitoring and tracking of vaccinees following vaccination. The HSVMS will provide a link to the Active Surveillance System.

As was mentioned in a previous section, the HSVMS collects data on workdays lost due to illness, workdays with restrictions on work duties (e.g., no patient contact), the presence and severity of symptoms reported by the vaccinee, the type of dressing covering the vaccination site, the condition of the dressing, whether the health care worker is wearing long sleeves, physical findings at the vaccination site, medications that were prescribed, and vaccine take.

To use HSVMS, monitoring sites only need to have Internet access (with 4.0 or higher Internet Explorer or comparable Netscape) and obtain a digital certificate and password from CDC. HSVMS was ready for use beginning February 18, 2003.

Name and social security number will not be collected in HSVMS. This system will, however, collect the PVN (or state equivalent), gender, year of birth, occupation, and clinical specialty (for physicians). It also will include an optional category for race and ethnicity.

The HSVMS allows monitoring sites to create reports on all vaccinees seen at their site, vaccinees who are due for a take reading, vaccine symptoms seen at their site, physical findings for vaccinees, and the status of site care and dressings at their site, as well as summary reports by day and by each vaccinee seen at their site. Health departments can access HSVMS to view and obtain data from their specific state or jurisdiction. HSVMS data also can be exported into Excel or Access.

The committee supports CDC's plan to use these data to evaluate progress and outcomes of phase I of the pre-event smallpox vaccination program. The HSVMS data will be only one component of the overall evaluation plan, but these data will be essential to the analysis and evaluation of the ongoing vaccination program.

The Active Surveillance System, HSVMS, and VAERS will all provide valuable data on vaccinees' experiences following vaccination. Since these data systems are designed to work together, by offering one more place that serious adverse events can be identified, the likelihood of missing a serious adverse event following vaccination will be reduced even further. **The committee recommends that CDC consider adding a data field to HSVMS to indicate whether a serious adverse event occurred or whether a VAERS report was filed (understanding that more complete information about circumstances surrounding the adverse event will be entered into VAERS and the Active Surveillance System).**

Implications of Program Expansion for Collection of Data on Adverse Events

The relatively quick expansion of the vaccination program to include all health care workers, firefighters, law enforcement, and emergency workers creates a number of implications for the capacity to collect data on serious adverse events, common adverse events, and vaccinees' experiences following smallpox vaccination. Up until now, CDC has designed the data systems for the smallpox vaccination program primarily for the logistical circumstances of the first phase of the program. CDC will have to consider if and how the data systems will need to be adapted for the expansion of the program (formerly "phase II") and beyond.

Conducting active surveillance of vaccinees from the recently expanded vaccination program (vaccination offered to all health care workers, firefighters, law enforcement, and emergency workers) may be more difficult. Since vaccinees in this category may not be members of a particular smallpox response team, and there may not be enough vaccination site care monitors available to contact and follow up with each of these vaccinees (let alone conduct "take" readings and monitor their vaccination sites on a daily basis), the ability of the Active Surveillance System to determine a confirmed outcome on each of these vaccinees currently is uncertain.

Accordingly, it also will be more difficult to collect data on common adverse reactions and vaccinees' experiences following smallpox vaccination. Because of the much larger number of vaccinees that will be included in the recently expanded vaccination program, there may not be enough vaccination site care monitors available to monitor vaccinees on a daily basis. If monitors are not designated or available to follow all of these vaccinees, and consequently, no data are entered into HSVMS for these vaccinees, valuable data could be lost. This could hinder the ability to evaluate the vaccination program on a national scale, since this expansion of the program would provide the majority of the sample size needed for significant results in an evaluation.

Collection of data on serious adverse events, common adverse events, and vaccinees' experiences following smallpox vaccination is important not only for "phase I" but also for any expansion of the program. Only with larger sample sizes can significant results be obtained from the data. **In order to assure the continued integrity and safety of the expanded vaccination program, the committee recommends that CDC work to ensure that a qualified health professional monitors, conducts a "take" reading, and provides a regular vaccination site inspection for each vaccinee in the program and enters the relevant data into the appropriate smallpox vaccination program data system.**

ACIP Working Group on Smallpox Vaccine Safety

In its first letter report (IOM, 2003), the committee recommended that CDC ensure the independent functioning of the group charged with monitoring data and vaccine safety. (The smallpox vaccine data and safety monitoring board now is formally called the Advisory Committee on Immunization Practices [ACIP] Working Group on Smallpox Vaccine Safety, which will hereafter be referred to as the "ACIP working group.") The committee is pleased that CDC already has taken some steps to address its concerns.

Adverse events reported following smallpox vaccination may be causally associated with the vaccine, or they may be coincidental illnesses that would have occurred anyway. Adverse events also may be interpreted as more serious than they actually are (e.g., generalized vaccinia).

The ACIP working group was charged with (1) evaluating data on vaccine safety, and the vaccine safety monitoring and treatment system, of the civilian National Smallpox Vaccination Program and DoD's Smallpox Vaccination program, and (2) monitoring safety data for use of VIG and cidofovir (both of which are under an investigational new drug protocol).

There are two competing concerns that surround the disclosure of the data that are reviewed by the ACIP working group: (1) the need for confidentiality of vaccinees' medical data and for private deliberations of the working group to analyze those data, and (2) the need for public disclosure of the ACIP working group's findings based on analysis of these adverse event data. Both of these concerns are extremely important, and one must not be jeopardized for the sake of the other.

Private deliberations of the ACIP working group are necessary for ensuring that adverse events that are coincidental illnesses rather than reactions to vaccination do not alarm the public needlessly about the safety of the vaccine or the safe use of the vaccine. These private deliberations also are necessary for ensuring confidentiality of vaccinees' medical data. Even if vaccinees' personally identifiable information is not discussed during the working group meetings, a vaccinee's particular circumstances could lead to identification if disclosed to the public (e.g., living in a state that only vaccinated a small number of response team members, unique characteristics of the adverse event that would be evident to the vaccinee's personal or professional contacts, unique job description).

The committee notes that reports of adverse events often appear in the media very early and may be unverified. Conducting case investigations of adverse events and designating them as suspected or probable are vitally important activities for all reported adverse events, whether or not they appear in the media before being formally described by CDC. The ACIP working group plays a valuable role in this process by conducting the final assessment of the putative adverse events.

Although recognizing that protection of the confidentiality of vaccinees' medical data and private deliberations of the ACIP working group are paramount to ensuring free discussion of data surrounding each reported adverse event, the committee also strongly believes that the working group should be able to freely issue findings or recommendations once they have reached a conclusion. Should the American public come to believe that relevant vaccine and program safety data are not being completely disclosed, the committee fears that lack of public trust in the implementation of the pre-event smallpox vaccination program could become an impediment to continued successful operation of the program. **The committee recommends that whenever the ACIP working group issues findings/recommendations to the ACIP and through it to the director of CDC, it carefully consider concurrent release to the public, and do so if it would be in the interest of transparency and maintaining the public's trust in the program.**

Maintaining public trust in the smallpox vaccination program also entails assuring the public that the ACIP working group is functioning independently from its sponsoring agency. To more fully understand the operating procedures of the ACIP working group and the implications of these procedures on the working group's independence, the committee requests that more information be provided about the working group's specific operating procedures and the criteria that the working group will use to decide when to issue findings/recommendations. The committee has much confidence in the ability and integrity of the members of the ACIP working group. However, given that the ACIP working group is participating in a very high profile activity, the committee has concerns that the close organizational tie of the ACIP working group to the government entities responsible for the pre-event smallpox vaccination program (i.e., CDC and DoD) could affect the appearance of independence of the data monitoring group from the vaccination program managers. The issue is one of perceived independence, rather than actual independence. The committee is confident that the ACIP working group will deliberate and issue their findings/recommendations in a scientific and unbiased manner, but the committee encourages CDC to be forthcoming and proactive in sharing information about the working group's operating procedures and publicizing any findings/recommendations issued by the working group. Once the committee gains more information on the ACIP working group's operating procedures, it will consider suggesting other processes that would not impair the working group's work or confidentiality, while assuring the public that its processes are being conducted without interference.

Reporting Adverse Events

Adverse events following smallpox vaccination often have appeared in the media before being formally described by CDC (Melton, 2003; Richardson, 2003). Currently, formal descriptions of adverse events following smallpox vaccination in the civilian population are reported in the *Morbidity and Mortality Weekly Report* (MMWR) every Thursday. Because the *MMWR* is released on a weekly basis, there is sometimes a delay between the time that a supposed adverse event is reported in the media and the release of a formal description of the adverse event in the *MMWR*. This delay can pique the media's and the public's interest and lead to confusion about why CDC is not reporting the adverse event immediately. **Considering the confusion that can arise from the timing of reports on adverse events and the multiple sources of adverse event data that are available, the committee recommends that CDC be very clear about what types of adverse events will be reported to the public and when.**

The committee understands that the *MMWR* will be the definitive source for information about adverse events reported following smallpox vaccination. However, the information distributed on adverse events by CDC's Office of Communication (CDC, 2003d:8) is presented in a different format from the information presented in the *MMWR*. **The committee recommends that the vaccination report webpage use categories that correspond to the categories presented in the *MMWR* adverse event reports.**

The committee also is pleased to see that CDC and the DoD are planning to provide regular updates on adverse events reported following smallpox vaccination. (The reports can be found at http://www.cdc.gov/od/oc/media/smpxrprt.htm and http://www.smallpox.army.mil/ media/pages/SPSafetySum.asp, respectively.) The committee encourages CDC and DoD to commit to a regular schedule for reporting adverse events, and to adhere to that schedule. Regular disclosure of adverse events could assure the public that the vaccination program is worthy of their trust. (As of March 19, 2003, CDC has updated its adverse event report web page every Thursday; DoD has not updated its adverse event report web page since February 12, 2003.)

Along with preparedness, safety has always been a paramount goal of the pre-event smallpox vaccination program. Effective and comprehensive screening for contraindications to vaccination is the first way to ensure safety. Breakdowns in the contraindications screening process could be considered "adverse" and could point to places where improvements could be made in the implementation of the pre-event vaccination program. It is important for both program managers and the public to know where improvements could be made in the contraindications screening process. **The committee recommends that CDC report on a regular basis how effective screening practices have been at identifying contraindications (e.g., pregnancy, HIV status, eczema or atopic dermatitis) prior to vaccination.** This should be done in a method that accomplishes the dual goals of protecting patients' confidentiality while also being forthcoming with the public.

Recent press reports (Richardson, 2003) have highlighted an adverse event reporting issue that may need to be resolved. It was reported that a civilian in Los Angeles county acquired an eye infection through close contact with someone vaccinated in the military's smallpox vaccination program. If the case investigation determines that this is indeed transmission of vaccinia to a contact of a vaccinee, then this would be considered an adverse event.

Although both civilian and military vaccination data have been reviewed by the ACIP working group, CDC and DoD have publicly reported civilian and military adverse events separately. For such a situation where a military vaccinee inadvertently inoculates a civilian, or vice versa, it is not clear how this adverse event would be reported—whether by CDC or by DoD. **If protocols governing such a situation have not yet been developed or finalized, then the committee recommends that CDC work with DoD to**

decide how adverse events that involve both the civilian and military populations will be reported.

Compensation

In its first letter report (IOM, 2003), the committee noted its concern that the lack of compensation for adverse reactions "could seriously affect achievement of the stated goal of the program—to increase the nation's bioterrorism preparedness." Recently, there has been a steady increase in evidence that the lack of compensation for adverse reactions to the smallpox vaccine is impeding full implementation of the pre-event smallpox vaccination program as originally envisioned (Connolly, 2003a; Denogean, 2003; Geraghty, 2003; Meckler, 2003). On March 6, 2003, the secretary of the Department of Health and Human Services proposed a plan to create a smallpox vaccination compensation program to provide benefits to public health and hospital response team members who are injured as a result of receiving the smallpox vaccine (DHHS, 2003). The proposed compensation program, modeled on the Public Safety Officers Benefit Program, would include:

- a $262,100 permanent and total disability benefit for disability caused by administration of the smallpox vaccine;
- a $262,100 death benefit for deaths caused by administration of the smallpox vaccine;
- a temporary or partial disability benefit, providing two-thirds of lost wages after the fifth day from work, up to a maximum of $50,000; and
- a health care benefit for reasonable out-of-pocket medical expenses for other than minor injuries.

The proposed program also would provide compensation to third parties who contract vaccinia from public health and hospital response team workers who have been vaccinated. Rep. Henry Waxman (D-CA) has introduced a bill (H.R.865) that proposes an alternative compensation program. At the writing of this report, a smallpox vaccine compensation bill had not yet been passed by Congress (Pear, 2003).

Workers' Compensation

Some of potential vaccinees' concerns about compensation may be addressed by workers' compensation coverage. However, as noted in the committee's first letter report (IOM, 2003) and again in this report, since it appears that this issue has not yet been resolved in most states, workers' compensation coverage is heterogeneous across states and not all vaccinated workers in all states will be eligible for compensation through their state's workers' compensation program, should they experience an adverse reaction to the smallpox vaccine.

Workers' compensation coverage is an uncertain solution for a number of reasons. Workers' compensation often only provides coverage for a percentage of the worker's salary, rather than the full salary. Workers often have to use a certain number of days of sick leave before they can receive compensation for days lost from work due to reaction to the vaccine. For vaccinees who experience common adverse reactions, they may only feel sick enough to take sick leave for one or two days (Lane et al., 1969, 1970). Some states' workers' compensation programs may not provide coverage if they deem the vaccination to be a "voluntary" component of work duties. Workers' compensation programs may not provide coverage for contacts of vaccinees who acquire vaccinia through contact transmission.

In some states, a provisional decision about coverage for smallpox vaccine adverse reactions by a state workers' compensation board may not be tested until an initial case is decided by the courts (ASTHO/NACCHO, 2002; Juffras, 2003). A vaccinee involved in the first case in a state may have to undergo months, or even years, of administrative and/or judicial proceedings before a final decision is made. Without a national compensation program in place, the possibility of months or years of legal action to resolve a workers' compensation claim may be more of a risk than many potential vaccinees are willing to take.

Lack of Compensation Impeding Program Progress

State health departments, hospitals, and individual vaccinees have expressed concern over the past 2 months about the lack of a national compensation program to cover medical expenses for adverse reactions, time lost from work, and (in the worst possible outcomes) permanent disability or death (McNeil, 2003). The committee is concerned that lack of compensation will be a continuing barrier to full implementation of the pre-event smallpox vaccination program if a smallpox vaccination compensation program is not created. Consequently, the nation's preparedness to respond to a smallpox attack could be hindered.

The voluntary pre-event smallpox vaccination has started off more slowly than originally anticipated. This is not necessarily a problem, given that the most recent statement of the president on the risk of a smallpox attack stated, "[o]ur government has no information that a smallpox attack is imminent" (White House, 2002). **However, if CDC and the states determine that there are insufficient response teams to ensure preparedness to respond to a smallpox attack, then the committee recommends that CDC gather data on the reasons why potential vaccinees are declining vaccina-**

tion and document the extent to which lack of compensation is identified as a barrier, among other possible barriers (e.g., uncertainty surrounding risk of smallpox, fear of transmitting virus to contacts, extent to which local programs are encouraging vaccination).

Notification About Availability of Compensation or Lack of Compensation

CDC implemented the committee's recommendation from its first letter report (IOM, 2003:13) that "informed consent forms include explicit notification of the availability, or lack thereof, of compensation for adverse reactions." The January 16, 2003 version of CDC's revised Vaccine Information Statement (VIS) includes the statement, "Treatment of severe reactions can be very expensive. Workers' compensation or health insurance may not cover these expenses. There is no federal program to reimburse you for time lost from work, either because of illness due to vaccination or concern about spreading the virus to others. Your employer can tell you if they, or workers compensation, will cover these expenses" (CDC, 2003e).

The committee commends CDC for more clearly describing the compensation situation to potential vaccinees. However, the committee believes that the language used for this statement should be in bold type and should be simpler, so it can be more easily understood by a wider cross-section of potential vaccinees, especially considering the recent expansion of the program to a more diverse pool of vaccinees. The committee believes that it is very important that all vaccinees have a clear understanding of what types of coverage and protection they can or cannot expect from their employer, their state, and the federal government. More readable compensation language could take the form of:

- "Right now, if you get sick or have to take time off from work, you cannot expect compensation." or,
- "Right now, if you get sick or have to take time off from work, the availability of compensation is uncertain." or,
- "Although other federal and state compensation proposals are under discussion, they have not yet been approved and you should not assume that you will be compensated for any injuries or illnesses that result from vaccination."

No matter what specific language CDC decides to use, the committee recommends that the compensation language be easy to read and understandable to a wide range of audiences.

CDC has included the notification about the availability, or lack thereof, of compensation in the VIS. It is expected that potential vaccinees will have read the VIS before signing the informed consent form. The informed consent form asks vaccinees to confirm that they have, "[r]eceived, read and understand the Smallpox Pre-Vaccination Information Package, including 1) the Vaccine Information Statement (VIS), 2) the VIS Supplements (A-E) on reactions after smallpox vaccination, vaccination site appearance and care, skin conditions, weakened immune system, pregnancy and breastfeeding, and 3) the pre-event screening worksheet" (CDC, 2003c). The availability of compensation for adverse reactions due to the smallpox vaccination may be an important factor affecting a potential vaccinee's decision to be vaccinated. **The committee recommends that potential vaccinees be reminded of the current compensation situation before they formally give their consent to be vaccinated.** It is possible that Congress will pass a smallpox vaccination compensation package soon; until then, the committee suggests that CDC include an explicit, bold print statement about the compensation situation directly on the informed consent form.

It also will be important for vaccinees to know that compensation may not be available to any contacts to whom they may accidentally transmit the vaccinia virus. This knowledge will be another important component of informed consent. The committee encourages CDC to expand the notification about compensation to address this issue. Such an addition could take the form of: "Should you accidentally transmit the vaccinia virus to someone else, that person cannot expect compensation."

The committee believes that it also would be helpful to test vaccinees' comprehension of this statement, in addition to other statements contained in the Pre-Vaccination Information Packet. Such a test could involve testing for a vaccinee's comprehension of a short list of key facts (e.g., decision is voluntary, major contraindications, types of adverse events that are possible, current lack of compensation for adverse events, what to do if a suspected adverse event occurs).

Funding

As reflected in media reports about health departments and hospitals around the country, and as anecdotally or formally documented by some organizations themselves, the smallpox vaccination program has produced significant financial worries among states and local health departments, and also in hospitals whose participation in forming health care response teams has been solicited (Connolly, 2003b; personal communication, R. Schulman, AHA, February 27, 2003; NACCHO, 2003). At the health department level, such worries appear to have resulted in the shifting of substantial financial and human resources from essential public health services to smallpox related activities (Connolly, 2003b; NACCHO, 2003). Hospitals also could incur costs by having health care response teams immunized, and there is reason for concern that this may overburden hospitals that are under strain already, such as public hospitals (NAPH, 2002; Health Leaders, 2003). Community health centers and public health clinics also may incur cost burdens. Since local health departments report that cost issues constitute a difficulty in program implementation, expanding the program as much as 20-fold may be unfeasible, unless additional resources are provided to states, local health departments, and their hospital partners.

Moreover, the committee remains very concerned about opportunity costs created by the program (including staffing-related costs), as well as redirecting resources from other areas, such as other disease prevention activities, and even broader bioterrorism preparedness. The committee was pleased to find out that CDC intends to conduct an assessment of the smallpox vaccination program's costs. **However, the committee recommends that this inquiry be broad in scope and include not only cost to local and state health departments, but also the financial impact on the provision of other essential public health services, the costs incurred by participating hospitals, and cost estimates of expanding the vaccination program to additional health care and public health workers and emergency first responders.**

Additional Data That Should Be Gathered

The committee applauds CDC for preparing a plan for phase I evaluation and research (CDC, 2003b). Many of the data and information needs that the committee raised in its first letter report (IOM, 2003) are addressed in this plan.

The committee understands that CDC has plans for estimating and evaluating the actual costs of the smallpox vaccination program and reasons for regional cost variations, the cost of diverting public health staff, and the opportunity costs of the smallpox program to other public health programs (CDC, 2003b). The committee believes that these studies will be extremely important for determining how the smallpox vaccination program should proceed in the future. The committee is very interested in these studies, in particular, and offers its assistance in designing these studies in any way that CDC deems useful.

To help provide ongoing advice to CDC about implementation of the smallpox vaccination program, the committee requests to see further details of the plans and protocols for the evaluation and research that CDC is proposing, (e.g., the plan for the proposed case-control study nested within the cohort of vaccinees). The committee applauds CDC for developing the evaluation and research plan so quickly and looks forward to receiving further communication from CDC about these issues.

CONCLUDING REMARKS

In closing, the committee reiterates its key recommendations.

- Advancing the smallpox vaccination program should occur with a focus on defining and then achieving national and local preparedness against a possible smallpox attack.
- Every effort should be made to evaluate on a national scale the program's implementation and, most important, its safety.

The committee wishes to thank you for the continuing opportunity to be of assistance to the Centers for Disease Control and Prevention as it works to protect the nation's health.

Brian L. Strom, *Committee Chair*
Kristine M. Gebbie, *Committee Vice Chair*
Robert B. Wallace, *Committee Vice Chair*
Committee on Smallpox Vaccination Program Implementation

REFERENCES

American Medical Association (AMA) Council on Scientific Affairs (CSA). 2003. Report 2 of the Council on Scientific Affairs—Smallpox: A Scientific Update. [Online] Available at http://www.ama-assn.org/ama/pub/article/2036-7063.html. Accessed March 20, 2003.

Anderson LJ. Smallpox Preparedness. Presented to the American College of Preventive Medicine Meeting on February 19-23, 2003.

ASTHO/NACCHO Smallpox Liability and Compensation Working Group. 2002. Smallpox pre-event vaccination: liability and compensation concerns (unpublished).

Blendon RJ, DesRoches CM, Benson JM, Herrmann MJ, Taylor-Clark K, Weldon KJ. 2002. The public and the smallpox threat. *New England Journal of Medicine* 348(5):426-432.

CDC (Centers for Disease Control and Prevention). 2002. CDC Telebriefing Transcript: HHS Teleconference on Smallpox Policy. [Online] Available at http://www.cdc.gov/od/oc/media/transcripts/t021214.htm. Accessed January 10, 2003.

CDC. 2003a. CDC Telebriefing Transcript: Smallpox Vaccine Adverse Events Monitoring and Response System on February 6, 2003. [Online] Available at http://www.cdc.gov/od/oc/media/transcripts/t030206.htm. Accessed March 11, 2003.

CDC. 2003b. DRAFT: Smallpox Vaccination Program Plans for Phase 1 Evaluation and Research Update, pp. 1-7.

CDC. 2003c. Smallpox Pre-Vaccination Information Packet: Contents and Instructions. [Online] Available at http://www.bt.cdc.gov/agent/smallpox/vaccination/infopacket.asp. Accessed January 29, 2003.

CDC. 2003d. Smallpox Vaccination Report Status and Adverse Events. [Online] Available at http://www.cdc.gov/od/oc/media/smpxrpt.htm. Accessed March 7, 2003.

CDC. 2003e. Smallpox Vaccine Information Statement (VIS): What You Need to Know. [Online] Available at http://www.bt.cdc.gov/agent/smallpox/vaccination/pdf/smallpox-vis.pdf. Accessed March 7, 2003.

CDC. 2003f. Smallpox vaccination and adverse reactions. *Morbidity and Mortality Weekly Report* 52(RR04):1-28. [Online] Available at http://www.cdc.gov/mmwr/preview/mmwrhtml/rr5204a1.htm. Accessed March 19, 2003.

Columbia University School of Nursing's Center for Health Policy. 2002. Bioterrorism and Emergency Readiness: Competencies for All Public Health Workers. [Online] Available at http://cpmcnet.columbia.edu/dept/nursing/institute-centers/chphsr/btcomps.pdf. Accessed March 19, 2003.

Connolly C. 2003a, February 24. Bush Smallpox Inoculation Plan Near Standstill. *Washington Post*, A06.

Connolly C. 2003b, March 10. Smallpox Campaign Taxing Health Resources. *Washington Post*, A04.

Connolly C. 2003c, March 7. Smallpox Vaccination Campaign Bolstered. *Washington Post*, A31.

Covello V, Sandman P. 2001. Risk Communication: Evolution and Revolution. In: Wolbarst A, ed. *Solutions to an Environment in Peril.* Baltimore, MD: Johns Hopkins University Press, pp. 164-178.

Denogean AT. 2003, February 3. Health Officials Weigh Smallpox Vaccination Pros, Cons. *Tucson [Arizona] Citizen.* Local News.

DHHS (U.S. Department of Health and Human Services). 2003. HHS Proposes Smallpox Vaccination Compensation Plan. [Online] Available at http://www.hhs.gov/news/press/2003pres/20030305.html. Accessed March 7, 2003.

Geraghty J. 2003, January 30. Fears, Questions Over Employee Compensation Slowing Smallpox Vaccine Program. *States News Service.*

Gerberding J. Letter to Brian Strom Dated February 13, 2003. Available from the National Academies Public Access Records Office, pulicac@nas.edu.

Health Leaders. 2003. Smallpox Scare: Hospitals May Incur Costs, Downtime from Vaccinations. Green Sheet, February. [Online] Available at http://www.healthleaders.com/magazine/2003/feb/greensheet.php. Accessed March 11, 2003.

Henderson J. 2003. Transcript From the IOM's Committee on Smallpox Vaccination Program Implementation Meeting Two on February 13, 2003, in Washington, DC:4-62.

IOM (Institute of Medicine). 2003. Review of the Centers for Disease Control and Prevention's Smallpox Vaccination Program Implementation: Letter Report #1. Washington, DC: The National Academies Press.

Juffras DM. 2003. Does the North Carolina workers' compensation act cover injuries resulting from smallpox vaccination? *Public Personnel Law Bulletin* (28):1-7. Institute of Government, University of North Carolina at Chapel Hill.

Lane JM, Ruben FL, Neff JM, Millar JD. 1969. Complications of smallpox vaccination, 1968: national surveillance in the United States. *New England Journal of Medicine* 281(22):1201-1208.

Lane JM, Ruben FL, Neff JM, Millar JD. 1970. Complications of smallpox vaccination, 1968: results of ten statewide surveys. *Journal of Infectious Diseases* 122(4):303-309.

Libbey PM. 2003. Testimony on Behalf of NACCHO (National Association of County and City Health Officials) before the Subcommittee on Labor, Health, and Human Services, Education and Related Agencies, Committee on Appropriations, U.S. Senate on January 29, 2003.

McNeil Jr. DG. 2003, January 30. Health Care Leaders Voice Doubts on Smallpox Inoculations. *New York Times*, A13.

Meckler L. 2003, February 5. Concerns About Compensation for People Injured by the Smallpox Vaccine Are Hampering Inoculation Program. *Associated Press State and Local Wire*. State and Regional.

Melton RH. 2003, March 6. VA Woman Hospitalized After Receiving Smallpox Vaccine. *Washington Post*, A4.

NACCHO (National Association of County and City Health Officials). 2003. Impact of Smallpox Vaccination Program on Local Public Health Services. NACCHO Research Brief No. 9.

NAPH (National Association of Public Hospitals and Health Systems). 2002. Annual Survey Results Reveal Extraordinary Financial Strains on Nation's Public Hospitals and Health Systems. NAPH Issue Brief. July 2002.

NNii (National Network for Immunization Information). 2003. Nurses Perceptions and Intentions Regarding Smallpox Vaccine: A National Survey. [Online] Available at http://www.immunizationinfo.org/features/index.cfm?ID=51. Accessed February 3, 2003.

Nowak G. 2003. Transcript from the IOM's Committee on Smallpox Vaccination Program Implementation Meeting Two on February 13, 2003, Washington, DC:240-294.

Nowak G, Janssen A, Tardif R, Herring R. 2002. A Qualitative Assessment of Physician and Public Perceptions of Smallpox Disease, Vaccine, and Immunization Strategies. Presentation given on May 9, 2002. [Online] Available at http://dccwww.bumc.bu.edu/smallpox/images/Part%204/NOWAK.PPT. Accessed March 29, 2003.

Pear R. 2003, March 19. Anti-Germ Bill Advances, But a Related One Stalls. *Washington Post*.

Richardson L. 2003, March 1. Infection Tied to Smallpox Vaccine. *Los Angeles Times*, California Metro, 3.

White House. 2002. President Delivers Remarks on Smallpox. [Online] Available at http://www.whitehouse.gov/news/releases/2002/12/20021213-7.html. Accessed January 8, 2003.

White House. 2003. Homeland Security: National Threat Level Raised to Orange. [Online] Available at http://www.whitehouse.gov/homeland/. Accessed March 20, 2003.

D

Review of the Centers for Disease Control and Prevention's Smallpox Vaccination Program Implementation, Letter Report #3

May 23, 2003
Dr. Julie Gerberding
Director
Centers for Disease Control and Prevention
1600 Clifton Road, NE
Atlanta, GA 30333

Dear Dr. Gerberding:

The Committee on Smallpox Vaccination Program Implementation is pleased to offer you our third letter report in a series of brief reports providing advice to the Centers for Disease Control and Prevention (CDC) on the implementation of the pre-event smallpox vaccination program. In addition to some general comments about program activities, the committee would like to draw your attention to two main issues:

1. Considerations for next steps in the pre-event vaccination program, and
2. The smallpox components of the Continuation Guidance for the Cooperative Agreement on Public Health Preparedness and Response for Bioterrorism—Budget Year Four detailed in Program Announcement 99051 (DHHS, 2003a).[1]

[1]The guidance was issued on May 2, 2003, after the release of the committee's second report on March 27, 2003. State applications are due July 1, 2003.

In particular, the committee would like to reaffirm the need for a pause in the program, before the vaccine is offered more widely, and also make some specific suggestions about the recently issued guidance. In a forthcoming report, the committee intends to focus on issues surrounding definitions and measurements of smallpox preparedness and its integration into broader bioterrorism readiness. The committee also will discuss screening and follow-up issues relevant to the continuation of the vaccination program, and answer specific questions asked by CDC and its partners at the May 1, 2003, committee meeting.

GENERAL COMMENTS

The committee reiterates its high regard for CDC and its partners and the remarkable amount of work completed in the national smallpox vaccination program, especially in the context of additional strain on all resources caused by the emergence and spread of Severe Acute Respiratory Syndrome (SARS). In fact, the committee heard from program administrators that the effective response to SARS both at the national and local level was at least in part facilitated by smallpox preparedness efforts, in particular the improved communication and collaboration among parties.

The committee has noted that the safety system implemented by CDC worked as intended, bringing the cardiac adverse events to the immediate attention of the Advisory Committee on Immunization Practices (ACIP) Smallpox Vaccine Safety Working Group and program administrators at CDC who responded promptly by modifying screening procedures and informed consent materials. The program has progressed with deliberation and caution. Thus far, the screening of potential vaccinees may have played a role in preventing several of the historically expected moderate-to-severe adverse events (e.g., eczema vaccinatum, progressive vaccinia) to the vaccine in 36,217 people vaccinated in the civilian program as of May 9, 2003 (CDC, 2003c). Also, it appears that vaccinee education on the risk of vaccinia transmission to contacts and measures taken to prevent it with appropriate bandaging and site care have worked well and may in part account for the absence of reported cases of vaccinia transmission from civilian vaccinees to either health care or personal contacts.

Although safety data to date have not revealed many of the moderate-to-severe adverse events or transmission that historically have been associated with smallpox vaccination, this does not necessarily mean that more robust trends will not be discovered later in the process, as vaccination numbers increase and more occupationally diverse volunteers consider vaccination.

The enactment of the smallpox vaccination compensation legislation (Smallpox Emergency Personnel Protection Act of 2003; P.L. 108-20) is likely to remove one of the barriers to vaccination identified by the committee and others (APHA, ASTHO, and NACCHO, 2003).[2] As this is a complex matter, the committee notes the need for additional clarification by CDC to the states on the provisions of the law and for fact sheets or other explanatory materials for potential vaccinees. These fact sheets should clearly explain the provisions of the legislation and protections enacted and refer potential vaccinees to additional information sources, such as their own state health department.

CONSIDERATIONS FOR NEXT STEPS IN THE VACCINATION PROGRAM

It is imperative that before continuing to expose individuals to a vaccine that is effective, but not without some risks, the national and state programs determine what level of pre-event vaccination is needed for preparedness. In its first report (IOM, 2003a), the committee recommended that "sufficient time should be allowed between the two phases to ensure adequate assessment and plan revision by CDC and its partners" and in its second report (IOM, 2003b), it recommended that the evaluation of "the effectiveness of implementation and the safe use of the vaccine" be carried out as extensively as allowed by "the mandates and realities of the vaccination program." At the program's beginning, it appeared that a wide variety of data about the process and the outcomes of the first phase of vaccination would be available and that comprehensive evaluation could be conducted between phases. Although the initially expected civilian numbers have not been reached, pausing to evaluate remains an important component of the overall program of safely building smallpox preparedness. Also, by combining the safety data from both civilian and military vaccinations (totaling over 460,000 vaccinees) a great deal can be learned, shared, and disseminated (CDC, 2003a; DoD, 2003). CDC acknowledges that there is "a natural pause that occurs between stage one and stage two" (Henderson, 2003).

The committee recognizes that pausing also involves potential risks. A pause implies slower vaccination of the number of responders a jurisdiction may require for preparedness, a loss of momentum, and perhaps vulnerability in the event of a potential smallpox event. However, given that the smallpox threat level, as it is publicly described, has not changed, the committee continues to believe that the benefits of the pause likely out-

[2]At the time of the writing of this report, the compensation language in CDC's Vaccine Information Statement had not yet been updated to reflect the newly enacted legislation.

weigh the risks. The committee is aware that some jurisdictions have already begun offering the vaccine to a wider population of potential vaccinees, but it reaffirms the need for a pause.

The committee recognizes that it is important for states to finish the vaccination of volunteers to complete health care and public health response teams according to state plans. However, in reiteration of its previous recommendations, **the committee recommends CDC facilitate the efforts of states that wish to pause to evaluate the process and outcomes of their vaccination efforts to date and plan for next steps before deciding whether and when to begin vaccination of new personnel. CDC should provide states with a target date for when CDC expects to have completed its revision of materials, data systems (adding new occupational categories, etc.), and guidelines. States that have identified a need for more vaccinated volunteers to carry out specific smallpox response functions will then be able to set their own timeline for vaccinating these new groups.**

The pause is important for three programmatic reasons.

1. **Safety.** First, a pause is needed to evaluate the vaccination program's processes and outcomes to date and thus ensure that expanded vaccination continues to be as safe as possible for both vaccinees and their contacts. The fact that by April 29, 2003, only 34 percent of vaccinees[3] were included in the Smallpox Vaccine Adverse Event Active Surveillance System (Mootrey, 2003) is an example of the additional work needed to help provide more data for a national view of the program. Some adverse events might not arouse concern on a state level, but aggregated nationally, new patterns could emerge. The cardiac complications were unexpected adverse events, and there may be others. That is why it is important to ascertain whether or not the vaccine played a role in the cardiac events and rule out any other reasons for concern before vaccination is expanded to other populations.

2. **Changing circumstances.** Second, a pause would allow time for CDC and the states to modify vaccination plans, data systems, and materials in response to changing circumstances (i.e., a new population of potential vaccinees). At the committee's second and third meetings, states commented on the need to revise educational materials before expanding vaccination to new types of volunteers (Bresnitz, 2003; Pezzino, 2003; Toomey, 2003). Furthermore, the Pre-Vaccination Information Packet has not been updated since March 31, 2003 (CDC, 2003b). It would be helpful for many states if these changes and revisions were made before they pro-

[3]Of vaccinees at 28 or more days post-vaccination.

ceeded with vaccination, in part to avoid the difficulty of implementing changes midcourse (ASTHO, 2003; Pezzino, 2003).

3. **Overall smallpox preparedness.** Third, vaccination is not a goal in itself, but a component of overall smallpox preparedness. Therefore, a pause is needed to re-evaluate the vaccination program's implications for and integration into overall smallpox preparedness nationally and locally (i.e., to determine what level of pre-event vaccination is needed and what personnel should be vaccinated to play specified roles in smallpox response).

Some issues to be addressed before deciding whether and how to proceed with vaccination include tasks to be accomplished in the short term, before moving on to new types of vaccinees:

- The completion of an in-depth analysis and investigation of all known serious adverse events to date and possible risk factors;
- The determination of what numbers and types of vaccinated personnel are needed to achieve preparedness;
- The update of educational and training materials by CDC;
- The revision of program data systems to include new types of vaccinees and to account for differences in data entry anticipated in expanding to a wider range of occupational contexts and personnel; and
- The development of guidelines regarding vaccine "take" readings, vaccination site checks and site care, and other issues related to vaccination follow-up of new types of vaccinees.

There also are tasks to be addressed on an ongoing basis and that also are significant to smallpox preparedness in general:

- The establishment of communication and collaboration with other partners (e.g., first responders, security personnel, health care and hospital systems, community-based health care providers);
- The revision by state and local programs of response plans that lay out clear roles and activities for teams responding to a potential event; and
- The need for strategic planning and reconciliation of the smallpox vaccination program with other bioterrorism programs and other public health priorities.

A break in the course of the vaccination program may help prevent vaccinating potentially large numbers of additional volunteers (e.g., health care workers, traditional first responders, and others) less safely than in the first phase of vaccinations, without adequate time to implement or update safeguards (e.g., screening, training and education) that would be appropriate to new types of vaccinees and their contacts.

COMMENTS ABOUT THE GUIDANCE

The continuation guidance issued May 2, 2003, outlines three elements of smallpox preparedness (DHHS, 2003b).[4] In its review, the committee has focused largely on the first element, "preparing key responders before an event occurs," and noted that jurisdictions may define both "preparing" and "key responders" differently (DHHS, 2003b).

Part of the "preparation of key responders" (DHHS, 2003b) occurred when health care and public health response teams were trained and vaccinated as part of what has previously been called "phase I" of the pre-event vaccination plan. As the committee has learned (ASTHO, 2003; Judson, 2003; Madlock, 2003; Selecky, 2003), state and local jurisdictions differ in their definitions of key responders, and the decisions about what preparation means. As noted, we will address this in a forthcoming report. The committee believes it is important that in addition to facilitating expanded vaccination if states conclude it is needed for preparedness, CDC also should facilitate the other smallpox preparedness activities (e.g., training, planning) of states that decide they have enough personnel vaccinated at this time.

The guidance contains several areas that may require clarification either because they provide insufficient direction for state programs, or may not be consistent with the overall tenor of the guidance documents. Several such items are found in Annex A of the guidance (DHHS, 2003b).

- First, page 2 states that since smallpox could appear in any hospital, "considerations must be made to ensure each facility has an acceptable number of teams vaccinated." Although many hospitals have formed and vaccinated response teams, this statement seems to imply that all hospitals need vaccinated response teams in order to be prepared, but this differs from the decisions and plans made by some jurisdictions and their partners. This guideline needs clarification or restating to call for planning to ensure each facility has the ability to train, and where applicable, train and vaccinate, identified individuals and teams pre-event, and that all facilities have access to vaccine and plans for vaccination of their employees post-event or if the threat level rises.

- Second, on page 5 the development of a comprehensive smallpox response plan is described as including post-event plans from "participating hospitals." It is unclear how "participating" is being defined. If it refers to hospitals that have vaccinated personnel, it also should be described how

[4]The three elements of preparedness are: "(1) preparing key responders before an event occurs; (2) rapid detection, identification, investigation and response to suspect or confirmed cases of smallpox; and (3) protection of the public including provision of mass vaccination clinics" (DHHS, 2003b).

hospitals that choose not to participate in pre-event vaccination will be included in the planning process.

• Third, page 3 provides a list of the types of personnel to be trained and vaccinated "in the following order." If these categories are indeed to be prioritized in this way, it is unclear why vaccinating security staff pre-event is more important than vaccinating health care providers. Furthermore, it is not clear in this section what type of staff should be trained as vaccinators.

• Fourth, on page 4, the guidance states that the public should be assured that public health has the capacity to "fully vaccinate the entire population within a short period of time once smallpox has been identified" and on page 6 of 7, that large-scale vaccination is to be "rapidly" executed. State programs might benefit from more specific guidance about the time frame for which they should aim.

The committee also noticed that the final enhanced capacity described in Focus Area B corresponds to one of the ingredients of smallpox preparedness identified in our phone discussions with local and state programs ("working links between health department staff and key individuals and organizations engaged in health care, public health, and law enforcement") (personal communications to staff, April 21-29, 2003). It is not clear why this important issue has not been identified as a critical capacity; preparedness appears to require working relationships with hospital administrators, fire, emergency and law enforcement officials, and many others.

In closing, the committee expresses its thanks for the opportunity to be of assistance to CDC and its partners. It would like to reiterate its call for a pause to facilitate evaluation and planning before moving on to more widespread voluntary vaccination of other types of personnel. Furthermore, the committee hopes its comments on the recently released guidance are helpful as states prepare their responses and as CDC evaluates those responses.

Brian L. Strom, *Committee Chair*
Kristine M. Gebbie, *Committee Vice Chair*
Robert B. Wallace, *Committee Vice Chair*
Committee on Smallpox Vaccination Program Implementation

REFERENCES

APHA (American Public Health Association), ASTHO (Association of State and Territorial Health Officials) and NACCHO (National Association of County and City Health Officials). 2003. National Public Health Associations Urge Legislative Action to Protect Smallpox Vaccine Volunteers. APHA/ASTHO/NACCHO Joint Press Release, March 7, 2003. [Online] Available at http://www.astho.org/templates/ display_pub.php?pub_id =618&admin=1. Accessed May 21, 2003.

ASTHO (Association of State and Territorial Health Officials). 2003. ASTHO Smallpox Preparedness Survey Results. [Online] Available at http://www.astho.org/pubs/spxsummaryb2.pdf. Accessed May 20, 2003.

Bresnitz E. 2003. Transcript from the IOM's Committee on Smallpox Vaccination Program Implementation Meeting Two on February 13, 2003, Washington, DC:73-130.

CDC (Centers for Disease Control and Prevention). 2003a. Update: adverse events following civilian smallpox vaccination—United States, 2003. *Morbidity and Mortality Weekly Report* 52(19):444-446.

CDC. 2003b. Pre-Vaccination Information Packet. [Online] Available at http://www.bt.cdc.gov/agent/smallpox/vaccination/infopacket.asp. Accessed May 21, 2003.

CDC. 2003c. Smallpox Vaccination Program Status by State. [Online] Available at http://www.cdc.gov/od/oc/media/spvaccin.htm. Accessed on May 21, 2003.

DHHS (Department of Health and Human Services). 2003a. Continuation Guidance for the Cooperative Agreement on Public Health Preparedness and Response for Bioterrorism—Budget Year 4. [Online] Available at http://www.bt.cdc.gov/planning/continuationguidance/index.asp. Accessed May 20, 2003.

DHHS. 2003b. Annex A: Summary of Smallpox Preparedness Activities. In Continuation Guidance for the Cooperative Agreement on Public Health Preparedness and Response for Bioterrorism—Budget Year 4. [Online] Available at http://www.bt.cdc.gov/planning/continuationguidance/index.asp. Accessed May 20, 2003.

DoD (Department of Defense). 2003. Smallpox Vaccination Program Summary, Department of Defense Smallpox Vaccination Program as of May 16, 2003. [Online] Available at http://www.smallpox.army.mil/event/SPSafetySum.asp. Accessed May 20, 2003.

Henderson J. 2003. Presentation to the Institute of Medicine Committee on Smallpox Vaccination Program Implementation Meeting Three on May 1, 2003, Washington, DC:13.

IOM (Institute of Medicine). 2003a. Review of the Centers for Disease Control and Prevention's Smallpox Vaccination Program Implementation: Letter Report #1. Washington, DC: The National Academies Press.

IOM. 2003b. Review of the Centers for Disease Control and Prevention's Smallpox Vaccination Program Implementation: Letter Report #2. Washington, DC: The National Academies Press.

Judson F. 2003. Transcript from the IOM's Committee on Smallpox Vaccination Program Implementation Meeting Three on May 1, 2003, Washington, DC:132-144.

Madlock Y. 2003. Transcript from the IOM's Committee on Smallpox Vaccination Program Implementation Meeting Three on May 1, 2003, Washington, DC:152-168.

Mootrey G. 2003. Presentation to the Institute of Medicine Committee on Smallpox Vaccination Program Implementation Meeting Three on May 1, 2003, Washington, DC.

Pezzino G. 2003. Transcript from the IOM's Committee on Smallpox Vaccination Program Implementation Meeting Three on May 1, 2003, Washington, DC:106-122.

Selecky M. 2003. Transcript from the IOM's Committee on Smallpox Vaccination Program Implementation Meeting Three on May 1, 2003, Washington, DC:82-96.

Toomey K. Transcript from the IOM's Committee on Smallpox Vaccination Program Implementation Meeting Two on February 13, 2003, Washington, DC:98-114.

E

Review of the Centers for Disease Control and Prevention's Smallpox Vaccination Program Implementation, Letter Report #4

August 12, 2003
Dr. Julie Gerberding
Director
Centers for Disease Control and Prevention
1600 Clifton Road, NE
Atlanta, GA 30333

Dear Dr. Gerberding:

The Committee on Smallpox Vaccination Program Implementation is pleased to offer you the fourth in a series of brief reports providing timely advice to assist Centers for Disease Control and Prevention (CDC) and its partners in their implementation of the vaccination program.[1] This report responds to issues raised by CDC at the committee's May 1, 2003, meeting. In particular, the report includes: (1) a discussion of smallpox preparedness and its integration into overall public health preparedness; (2) the committee's advice regarding offering vaccination to members of the general public who insist on receiving it; and (3) an examination of selected aspects of smallpox vaccination program implementation.

In a previous report (IOM, 2003c), the committee remarked on the

[1]As of July 25, 2003, 38,004 civilian volunteers have been vaccinated against smallpox (CDC, 2003l), and as of June 13, 2003, 2,125 hospitals have participated in the smallpox vaccination program (Strikas, 2003).

importance of working to attain a level of smallpox preparedness and not simply focusing on numbers of vaccinated individuals. Since then, CDC officials have remarked that the smallpox program is "not about a number, it is not about should we have 40,000 people or 400,000 or 4 million people. . . . It's about how do we get prepared" (CDC, 2003i). Furthermore, CDC plans to conduct an assessment of its smallpox preparedness efforts and recommend program adjustments to emphasize education and training and ways to facilitate reporting and test readiness (Connolly, 2003b).

The report is organized into three main sections: (1) Integrating Smallpox Preparedness into Overall Public Health Preparedness; (2) Vaccination of Members of the General Public Who Insist on Receiving Smallpox Vaccine; and (3) Selected Aspects of Smallpox Vaccination Program Implementation.

INTEGRATING SMALLPOX PREPAREDNESS INTO OVERALL PUBLIC HEALTH PREPAREDNESS

> State health departments have been actively involved in planning and preparing for the possibility of a bioterrorist event. We are now seeing that this level of preparation can also assist in unexpected natural outbreaks.
>
> Tommy Thompson, Secretary of the Department of Health and Human Services, in reference to the monkeypox outbreak (CDC, 2003a)

The discussion of integration of smallpox preparedness into overall public health preparedness is organized around four main topics: (1) Challenges in Defining and Assessing Public Health Preparedness; (2) Elements of Preparedness; (3) Testing Preparedness; and (4) Sustaining Smallpox and Overall Public Health Preparedness.

Challenges in Defining and Assessing Public Health Preparedness

There is significant agreement about the difficulties and flaws that characterize the public health infrastructure, and in the last 2 years there has been considerable discussion about the need for public health preparedness. Public health system leaders know the system is not sufficiently prepared based on the way it has responded to a number of threats and crises in recent years. However, the public health system is still in the early stages of developing consensus on defining preparedness and identifying evidence-based standards for planning for and evaluating preparedness. At a minimum, public health preparedness requires adequate and sustained funding based on priorities supported by evidence and a strong public health infrastructure, including surveillance, workforce, and communication (IOM, 2002).

Assessments of the public health infrastructure's capacity to respond to bioterrorism conducted after the events of September and October 2001 found a severe lack of financial resources and a great deal of fragmentation within the public health system, from surveillance systems (which were multiple, overlapping and duplicative, and incompatible in various ways) to communication (which was limited, reliant on obsolete, inefficient channels, etc.) both internal and with other sectors (IOM and NRC, 1999; Heinrich, 2001; Peters et al., 2001; IOM, 2002; Salinsky, 2002). It is unclear at this time whether the recent influx of funding aimed at strengthening the public health infrastructure is being used to reinforce public health capacity in an integrated way, responsive to local needs and epidemiologic evidence, or to simply create new funding and program categories, adding to existing fragmentation. The IOM Committee on Emerging Microbial Threats to Health in the 21st Century has described recent funding increases as opportunities for the nation to prepare to "protect against acts of bioterrorism and improve the U.S. public health response to all microbial threats" but expressed alarm that "some of these funds have been diverted from multipurpose infrastructure building to single-agent preparedness" (IOM, 2003a). In fact, smallpox may have "received the lion's share of attention and ... drawn attention away from the wide range of other agents that could be used" in a bioterror attack (Powers and Ban, 2002).

Vaccination: Only One Component of Smallpox Preparedness

In the early months of the smallpox preparedness program, preparations to respond to a potential smallpox attack have consisted largely of vaccination-related activities. These have been resource-intensive, giving rise to concerns about the opportunity costs (i.e., to essential public health services) of the smallpox vaccination program and about the optimal balance of investment of public health funds (e.g., are smallpox-related activities funded at the expense of a more wide-ranging kind of preparedness?) (APHA, 2002; Libbey, 2003; Madlock, 2003; NACCHO, 2003b; Nikolai, 2003). Surely, being prepared for a potential attack requires much more than just vaccination. It includes planning for a range of possible scenarios, including contingencies for crowd control, quarantine, and isolation; training, retraining, and management of response teams; education and training of health care providers, emergency responders, and many others to facilitate rapid surveillance, reporting, and notification; planning and coordination with many partners, including some at the state and federal level; and testing and continuous improvement of plans.

The smallpox vaccination program and associated activities implemented by CDC and its state and local partners have provided information and training about smallpox disease and vaccine to public health and health care workers, have probably improved clinician knowledge and rash illness diagnostic skills, and have led to vastly improved communication and collaboration among public health agencies, between the public health and clinician communities, and among public health, law enforcement, and emergency response agencies (Committee on Smallpox Vaccination Program Implementation Study Staff, 2003; Elliott, 2003; NACCHO, 2003b). However, much more is necessary to strengthen and test smallpox preparedness and to ensure that smallpox-related efforts are part of overall public health preparedness activities. The committee hopes that this report will provide some useful direction toward that end.

Smallpox Preparedness: Only One Component of Overall Public Health Preparedness

The national smallpox vaccination program may well be the first disease-specific test of implementing public health preparedness in a systematic and comprehensive manner and with some public visibility. The smallpox vaccination program has taken the notion of preparedness beyond the realm of public health professionals and academics and has brought it to the attention of a broader audience of health care workers, emergency responders, and even the general public.

Implementing the smallpox vaccination program, however, has also highlighted the need to integrate smallpox preparedness into readiness to respond to a vast range of public health challenges, including bioterror agents and other weapons of mass destruction, emerging or reemerging infectious diseases, natural disasters, and the insidious and growing threat of chronic diseases and their predisposing conditions (e.g., obesity). Smallpox is just one of a multitude of actual and potential threats to the public's health.

The Continuation Guidance for Cooperative Agreement on Public Health Preparedness and Response for Bioterrorism (CDC, 2003b), describes the capacities needed for smallpox response in the context of all other bioterrorism threats, even calling for coordination with the National Public Health Performance Standards, which guide public health activities in general. In practice, such integration has been lacking and has been difficult to accomplish, in part due to the intense emphasis on smallpox vaccination, which has been advanced perhaps at the expense of other aspects of smallpox preparedness, as well as overall public health preparedness to respond to any threat.

A Standard for Smallpox Preparedness

> The federal government should consider playing a more concerted role in providing resources and instituting unified standards for the common defense against the microbial threat, while giving state and local authorities the flexibility to implement programs in a manner that will best meet local needs.
>
> (Brower and Chalk, 2003)

The question of what exactly is involved in preparedness to respond to a smallpox attack has been a recurrent theme at committee meetings and in presentations to the committee. Many of the requirements for smallpox preparedness apply to preparedness in general; there are necessary components of the public health infrastructure including workforce, surveillance and laboratory capacity, information technology, legal authority, and communication networks. What remains to be clarified at the state level, with the guidance of CDC, are the specifics (e.g., vaccination sites; numbers of responders, vaccinated or not; strategies for training, communicating with, and mobilizing responders, etc.) needed to act effectively in each state and jurisdiction.

Before the occurrence of a public health emergency, such as a smallpox release, planning, coordination, and communication among local, state, and federal public health agencies must take place in order to establish leadership and responsibility (ASTHO, 2002; Salinsky, 2002). In the event of a bioterror attack, final authority in the matter must reside somewhere.

Similarly, leadership is required to establish a minimum standard against which preparedness may be tested. Having 50 or more different standards for preparedness seems inconsistent with a coordinated, effective response; for example, one state might prepare enough to mass vaccinate all residents in 10 days, while a neighboring state could be prepared to accomplish this in 2 days. Such variation may cause confusion and weaken confidence in the public health system's handling of a crisis. In the pre-event setting, CDC has been flexible in its guidelines to states and has advised states to define preparedness needs locally, in recognition of the fact that bioterrorism occurs at the local level. However, due to the infectiousness of certain agents, such as smallpox, the local quickly becomes national, and jurisdictional boundaries become less relevant. The regional planning required to prepare for a response to major fires is analogous to the preparedness planning required across jurisdictional boundaries for a response to a smallpox attack. Such circumstances would require stronger national (i.e., CDC) leadership to set some standards for preparedness while collaborating with state public health agencies in acknowledgement of the great variety in circumstances and resources across states and localities (ASTHO,

2002; Brower and Chalk, 2003; IOM, 2003c). **The committee recommends that CDC provide guidance to assist state public health agencies (and their partners,[2] as appropriate) in establishing a baseline level or a minimum standard of preparedness for a smallpox attack, after which, each state could individually assess its priorities and further expand its preparedness against smallpox and other threats to the public's health as needed.** The committee has been informed that CDC is developing metrics/indicators of preparedness to guide all state partners in implementing their cooperative agreements with CDC. The smallpox preparedness metrics/indicators will be the subject of the committee's meeting on September 4, 2003, and the committee hopes this effort will help to establish a minimum standard of smallpox preparedness.

Smallpox preparedness activities conducted in the first months of 2003 have enhanced the readiness of state and local public health agencies to respond to a potential smallpox attack (Committee on Smallpox Vaccination Program Implementation Study Staff, 2003; NACCHO, 2003a), but as noted above, vaccination alone—the focus of most of these activities—is not sufficient for preparedness. In fact, many states are pausing in their smallpox vaccination activities before proceeding to a broader group of potential vaccinees to evaluate their progress and ensure safety, to address changing circumstances by updating forms, materials, and processes, and finally, to consider what level of vaccination is needed for preparedness (ASTHO, 2003; IOM, 2003c). The deliberate and cautious implementation of the vaccination program to date testifies to the influence of lessons learned from the Swine Flu vaccination program of 1976 (Hardy, 2002; Strikas, 2002).

Attaining a high level of preparedness may well be possible without vaccinating any personnel pre-event. For example, Virginia Commonwealth University Health System, which presented its hospital preparedness plans to the committee at the May 1, 2003, meeting, has chosen not to have health care workers vaccinated pre-event (Edmond, 2003).[3] The health system's decision was based on considerations of hospital patient safety. Although no vaccinated teams of responders were formed, a policy on smallpox vaccination was developed, with plans to revisit the policy as needed. Furthermore, a working group on smallpox preparedness was established, facilities were modified in accordance with requirements for treat-

---

[2]State partners may include, but not be limited to, emergency management agencies, law enforcement, fire and emergency medical services, hospital and other health care associations.

[3]The ACIP estimated approximately 5,100 acute care hospitals would be eligible to participate in the smallpox vaccination program (ACIP, 2002). As of June 13, 2003, 2,125 hospitals have participated, with whole or partial teams of vaccinated response personnel (Strikas, 2003).

ing smallpox victims, training on smallpox diagnosis, treatment, and infection control measures was conducted, and plans were put in place to rapidly vaccinate hospital staff in a post-event scenario. The committee believes that Virginia Commonwealth University Health System's smallpox preparedness activities provide a good example of how an organization or jurisdiction can be well prepared to respond to a smallpox attack without necessarily having workers vaccinated pre-event.

CDC's initial attention to the numerical targets so well publicized in the media may have contributed to confusion and concern about goals and outcomes among the public health and health care communities, as well as in the general public (ASTHO, 2003; Connolly, 2003a; ENA, 2003; GAO, 2003; Russell, 2003; Solet, 2003). It has not been made completely clear to most audiences how national estimates of numbers of vaccinees were derived and how they relate to the publicly available threat assessment and to smallpox preparedness. Although the committee recognizes that the CDC has publicly acknowledged that preparedness is not about numbers (see page 1), it is clear that there is lingering confusion about the vaccination program's aims. This confusion is reflected in recent media reports that characterize the program as having fallen short of its goals (Connolly, 2003a; Snowbeck, 2003)—when comparing the fewer than 40,000 vaccinees in early July 2003 (CDC, 2003l) to the initially publicized target of vaccinating approximately 500,000 and 10 million individuals, in the first and in the second rounds of vaccination, respectively. There also is lingering confusion about how the 500,000 estimate described by CDC related to the 15,000 estimate cited by the ACIP in June 2002 (AAFP, 2002; CIDRAP News, 2002; Manning, 2002). Public confidence and clarity about preparedness efforts would likely be enhanced if the CDC explained how and why it came to view its earlier benchmarks as less than helpful (e.g., were early estimates of vaccinee numbers the upper bounds of what was needed for an effective response to a smallpox attack?). Given that CDC supports ongoing smallpox immunization (CDC, 2003m), there should be clarification about the goals and objectives being pursued (IOM, 2003c) to help reconcile the apparent incongruity between the claim that preparedness is "not about a number" and the stated intent to move forward with vaccination to ensure there are "enough people ... immunized" (CDC, 2003i). What number of vaccinees is needed for preparedness? Vaccinating many more than the number needed may waste precious resources that could be utilized to prepare against other threats to the public's health. Vaccinating fewer than what is needed to respond effectively and rapidly may leave the public vulnerable and unprotected.

The recent severe acute respiratory syndrome (SARS) and monkeypox episodes have provided CDC the opportunity to once again demonstrate its authoritative voice and competence as the nation's public health leader.

However, these serious infectious disease threats posed relatively straightforward public health challenges, without the national security issues that complicate the smallpox vaccination program. To maintain its credibility, CDC should demonstrate a sustained commitment to clarity and openness about its smallpox preparedness goals by working toward a concrete description of what preparedness entails (despite the complexities and unknowns involved), communicating regularly with the public, and discussing any specific numbers of vaccinees only within this broader context.

Elements of Smallpox Preparedness

At the committee's May 2003 meeting, one presenter described the essentials for improving smallpox preparedness as planning, training to the plan, exercising to the plan, and revising the plan (Selecky, 2003). In presentations and conversations with several state and local health departments, the committee heard similar comments about what program administrators believe are the "ingredients" of smallpox preparedness (Committee on Smallpox Vaccination Program Implementation Study Staff, 2003). Most programs remarked on the importance of:

- developing relationships with all relevant partners (might help enhance surveillance and reporting, as well as planning and implementation of smallpox response);
- engaging in regular communication with other local and state public health agencies;
- communicating openly, regularly, and consistently with the media and the public to create a foundation of optimal communication before a potential smallpox event;
- having a core of set of workers to provide initial response and vaccinate others;
- having concrete plans, including job descriptions and locations; and
- educating and training all participants before an event.

These themes are consistent with the three elements of smallpox preparedness identified in Annex A of the DHHS/CDC Continuation Guidance for Cooperative Agreement on Public Health Preparedness and Response for Bioterrorism (CDC, 2003b) and discussed in greater detail below:

1. **Preparing key responders**—with a section devoted to health care responders and preparedness in the health care sector (includes the relationship-building, training, and planning described above);
2. **Rapid public health response**—rapid detection, identification, in-

vestigation, and response to suspected or confirmed cases of smallpox (also includes the training, communication and relationships noted above, in addition to infrastructure capacity for surveillance, prompt reporting by providers, etc.); and

3. **Protecting the public (e.g., through mass vaccination)**—all ingredients described above contribute to the ability of jurisdictions to operate orderly, efficient mass vaccination clinics.

Two additional elements are discussed briefly below to address areas not directly covered by the three elements of preparedness listed above. These include the important role of the health care community in overall public health preparedness and the role of public and media communication.

Preparing Key Responders

The first element of smallpox preparedness described in the CDC/Department of Health and Human Services (DHHS) guidance involves preparing key responders. As the committee noted before, this does not necessarily involve vaccinating workers, but it would ideally include training and education of key responders, and even prescreening for vaccination in the event of a smallpox attack. It is unclear what level of pre-event smallpox vaccination is needed and how numbers of vaccinated personnel relate to the ability to respond effectively to a smallpox attack. This is a decision that must be made in the face of great uncertainty by each jurisdiction before deciding whether to vaccinate additional volunteers and, if so, the number and type of personnel to vaccinate. CDC and its partners have worked to strike a balance between vaccine risk and the benefit of having vaccinated health care and public health personnel pre-event, but it is difficult to determine when the line has been crossed between having insufficient people vaccinated to mount an effective and rapid response and exposing more people than absolutely necessary to a vaccine that is not free of risk, in the absence of imminent threat of disease.

It appears that most jurisdictions have chosen to address this dilemma by cautiously vaccinating at least a small number of volunteers, having apparently concluded that smallpox preparedness is served by having a cadre of vaccinated individuals, typically organized into health care and public health response teams (based either institutionally or regionally), in accordance with Advisory Committee on Immunization Practices (ACIP) recommendations regarding the organization of smallpox response efforts (CDC, 2002d). However, having a number of personnel immune to smallpox and ready to vaccinate, conduct public health investigations, and treat victims is not the sum of preparedness, especially if responders are scattered across the jurisdiction in multiple facilities. Whether vaccinated before an event or not, effective mobilization of key responders requires prior preparation to ensure, at a minimum:

- adequate size and composition of health care and public health response teams;
- regularly tested and updated plans known to all participants and relevant agencies;
- initial and periodic training, including training about response plan(s) (as well as training of vaccinators, case investigators, etc.);
- job assignments and descriptions for all responders (e.g., vaccinators, public health investigators, crowd control, and security), and consideration of relevant licensure or practice privileges should teams need to cross jurisdictional, state, or even national borders; and
- reliable and efficient channels of communication among all relevant parties, including methods for contacting team members (e.g., pagers), and for the movement of information between health care organizations and public health agencies and between the health sector and traditional first responder agencies such as law enforcement and emergency management (English et al., 1999).

Furthermore, having adequate workforce to respond to a smallpox (or other) event requires managing staff turnover (workers who leave or retire), and the ability to mobilize as many vaccinated personnel as possible. One recipient activity described in Annex A of the DHHS/CDC guidance is the development and maintenance by states and territories of a registry of all public health, health care, security, and other personnel who may be occupationally at risk and should receive vaccination immediately in the event of a smallpox release.

In addition to having identified such priority occupational groups to be vaccinated post-event, programs should take necessary steps to maximize the use of any available vaccinated personnel. For example, the Department of Defense (DoD) has vaccinated over 400,000 military personnel, some of whom are reservists, and others who will complete military service. The committee hopes that CDC and DoD could collaborate to maintain contact with vaccinees, particularly those who enter civilian life, and to link them to any mechanism developed to include as many as possible in planning for preparedness. Contact also should be maintained with health care or public health workers who received a smallpox vaccine because of exposure to a case of monkeypox, so they could be utilized for response to a smallpox event. **The committee recommends that CDC support the establishment of state and/or local and, if appropriate, national**

voluntary registries of individuals who have undergone vaccination to be mobilized, trained, and assigned as needed in the event of a smallpox attack. Such registries would include all willing vaccinated personnel not associated with a response team ranging from retired or relocated health care or public health workers to military reservists and former military personnel. Such registries might help supplement and enhance the personnel available to respond to public health crises (e.g., participating in the mass distribution of vaccines or other pharmaceuticals, caring for casualties, providing security, managing crowds). Establishing such registries will require consideration of issues related to confidentiality and privacy, among others. Ongoing efforts to organize volunteer personnel to help in emergencies (e.g., the USA Freedom Corps and the Public Health Service reserve corps) may serve as resources (Thompson, 2003).

Decisions also should be made about the vaccination activities needed to maintain a cadre of key responders immune to smallpox virus in the long term, but the evidence on the level of long-term immunity proffered by smallpox vaccination is mixed. Older data suggested that smallpox immunity lasts 3 to 5 years after vaccination (CDC, 2002a), while more recent research suggests possibly longer duration of immunity (Frelinger and Garba, 2002; Slifka, 2003). More conclusive research would undoubtedly assist in future policy decision-making regarding smallpox preparedness. Given the 454,856 personnel vaccinated through the DoD smallpox vaccination program (Grabenstein, 2003), many of whom have had and will have a series of serum specimens included in the Department of Defense Serum Repository, CDC should work with DoD to explore how the DoD Serum Repository can support research on smallpox antibody levels at different periods of time post-vaccination.

Whether a jurisdiction vaccinates traditional emergency responders, from law enforcement to firefighters, these parties should be considered partners in overall public health preparedness. Previously, emergency management officials, police, and fire departments had not considered public health agencies to be emergency responders, and health departments typically have not counted emergency and fire personnel among the ranks of public health responders. The committee has heard at every meeting about the importance of building relationships with a wide range of partners in the community; a common outcome of the smallpox vaccination program has been the forging of linkages between the public health and health care communities, and between public health and traditional emergency response agencies. Communication between all relevant partners is essential, including mechanisms for notification and information sharing.

Rapid Public Health Response (Rapid Identification and Investigation of Suspected and Confirmed Cases of Smallpox)

The second element of smallpox preparedness, rapid public health response, is defined in Annex A of the Guidance (CDC, 2003b) as "disease surveillance for rash illnesses and laboratory analysis to rapidly detect a single case of smallpox and any subsequent cases." Building capacity for rapid response requires strengthening communication and information networks, training and education of public health, health care and other relevant personnel, and the review of legal authority and public health law.

Communication and information networks needed for rapid public health response require many components, including connectivity among levels of the public health infrastructure (agencies and laboratories), a system for rapid reporting by practicing clinicians, a means for rapid notification of all relevant parties in the event a case of smallpox is confirmed, and a way to notify and mobilize all response team members. An additional aspect of communication that should not be overlooked is the provision of timely, clear, and accurate information to the media and public.

Because clinicians might well be the first to identify a potential smallpox case, training and education are needed to enable health care providers in all settings to assess and report rash illnesses. All clinicians, including primary care providers, infectious disease practitioners, emergency physicians, and those in other health care settings need to be familiar with the precautions to be taken and parties to be notified and consulted (local and state public health agency, CDC). At the public health agency level, public health response team members require regularly updated training and education about their agency's plans, about their roles, and about the knowledge and skills needed to rapidly identify and respond to suspected or confirmed smallpox cases.

Many aspects of public health surveillance and information systems and channels that operate both within and among states rely on public health law, which defines types of authority during public health emergencies (quarantine, evacuation, etc.) (Fraser and Fisher, 2001). Although the variation in public health statutes across states is understandable and to some extent inevitable, the Turning Point Public Health Statute Modernization Collaborative has been working to achieve a level of consistency and uniformity through a draft Model State Public Health Act (IOM, 2002; Turning Point Public Health Statute Modernizing Collaborative, 2003). Following this and other resources, states could review the requirements of legal authority that will be needed to meet all contingencies in the event of smallpox attack or other public health threats and facilitate any changes needed to ensure effective response.

Protection of the Public (Through Mass Vaccination, etc.)

The third element of preparedness described in the CDC/DHHS guidance is the protection of the public, through means such as mass vaccination. To ensure the public is protected, the location of vaccine stocks and logistic plans must support the most efficient distribution of vaccine to all local jurisdictions involved in smallpox vaccination. The location and operation of vaccination clinics also must be established before a potential event. To apply this element of smallpox preparedness to comprehensive public health preparedness for all threats, the same sites could be used to distribute other vaccines or countermeasures and provide other services in response to an outbreak or other threat. Furthermore, the circumstances of an attack and available resources may not allow the immediate vaccination of the entire population, so plans for prioritizing categories of vaccinees should be worked out pre-event, perhaps taking as guidelines the definition of essential personnel, the needs of medically at-risk groups, and those of groups at high risk of exposure (Fock et al., 2002). Furthermore, contraindications and screening criteria for smallpox vaccination in a post-event situation may be different, and these potential changes should be explored as soon as possible. Prospective vaccinees in a mass vaccination situation also might have different needs and rights for information and education, and they will require some degree of follow-up (e.g., vaccine take checks). Planning should include these and other considerations.

To facilitate rapid public health response and conduct efficient mass vaccinations, there are special subsets of the population that will require added consideration in the areas of planning, communication, and training of key responders. These include populations that have historically been negatively affected by government policies or programs, populations with special needs, and other hard-to-reach populations, including, but not limited to, immigrants, particularly those with limited English proficiency. To help ensure that these populations are included in preparedness planning and programs, pre-event communication and plans for post-event communication (including vaccination clinic site informational and screening materials and procedures) should emphasize social, cultural, and linguistic competence and, wherever possible, should include the participation of opinion leaders and community leaders, including those representing special populations, in planning, implementation, and testing of response plans.

The Role of the Health Care Community in Public Health Preparedness

Good communication and information systems (within and among public health agencies, and at the interface with the health care sector) form the core of smallpox and overall public health preparedness (IOM, 2002;

Fraser and Fisher, 2001). These include surveillance and reporting by health care providers (e.g., physicians, nurse practitioners, physicians' assistants) who identify unusual symptoms or patterns. On the one hand, the West Nile virus experience underscored the value of alert and knowledgeable health care providers who can respond rapidly to suspicious symptoms and of established and tested reporting mechanisms (GAO, 2000). On the other hand, analysis of the early response to the West Nile outbreaks showed that lines of communication between health care providers and public health agencies were unclear, and there was confusion about "what to report, when, and to whom" (GAO, 2000). In a more recent example provided by the monkeypox outbreak, local health authorities and CDC were apparently only notified about the initial rash 13 days later (Mitchell, 2003). The "disconnect" between the health care and public health communities is a detriment to readiness to protect the population's health against threats. The health care sector, including private health care practices, hospitals, health care systems, health care organizations, and insurers, constitutes a major stakeholder in bioterrorism preparedness because it often serves as the first line of defense in a disease outbreak and it employs a substantial proportion of potential responders to a public health threat (including the majority of personnel vaccinated against smallpox) (GAO, 2000; Covert, 2001; Fraser and Fisher, 2001; IOM, 2002). This explains why communication and collaboration between the health care and public health communities are essential to bioterrorism preparedness. The Health Resources and Services Administration (HRSA) National Bioterrorism Hospital Preparedness Program Cooperative Agreement Guidance for FY 2003 describes areas where collaboration is needed between public health agencies and hospitals, as well as other health care partners. The crosscutting guidance provided in this document also is included in the CDC Guidance (CDC, 2003b).

It was not entirely clear from the HRSA and CDC crosscutting guidance whether all hospitals and health care providers in a jurisdiction are expected to participate in planning for preparedness and in implementing and testing plans. Nevertheless, the preparedness efforts of state and local public health agencies should engage all hospitals and health care systems, not just those participating in the vaccination program (IOM, 2003d). Hospitals and health care systems that declined to participate in the vaccination program have cited valid reasons, such as concerns about liability and potential risk to patients. However, it is important that these organizations ensure that their emergency preparedness plans incorporate contingencies for responding to bioterrorism. It is necessary that the health care community (and any relevant partners), at a minimum, conduct or oversee the following activities:

- develop, implement, and exercise bioterrorism response plans as part of or in addition to their existing emergency preparedness plans;
- have clear protocols for interfacing with public health authorities (both routinely, such as common infectious disease reporting, and in emergencies, such as the first cases of a suspected outbreak) and for collaborating with other hospitals and health care systems;
- review and modify institutional policy as needed and call for changes in state licensure and accreditation protocols (Blank et al., 2003);
- provide ongoing staff training on bioterror agents, including smallpox;
- develop guidelines for identifying and managing suspicious cases (including suspected smallpox) in their outpatient clinics, emergency departments, laboratories, and other facilities;
- link with the local or state jurisdiction's public health preparedness efforts (including the acquisition and distribution of Strategic National Stockpile drugs, vaccines, and supplies, including smallpox vaccine, regionally); and
- exercise, test, and revise plan(s) as needed.

Although it is essential that public health agencies reach out and collaborate with professional organizations and the hospital industry, such efforts might overlook the increasing number of health care providers in private practices or ambulatory care settings who are not affiliated with professional organizations, but with entities such as the American Medical Group Association or the Medical Group Management Association. The public health community is responsible for finding ways to communicate with and integrate the widest possible range of health care providers in the planning, training for, and testing of smallpox and overall public health preparedness.

Public health agencies also are responsible for strengthening and updating information systems to facilitate disease surveillance and reporting by health care providers, for making efforts to familiarize the health care community with surveillance and reporting procedures, and for providing timely feedback to such reporting and enhancing all communication channels with the health care community, with particular attention to infectious disease experts and primary care providers (Teutsch and Churchill, 1994; Thacker and Stroup, 1994; Baxter et al., 2000; Elliott, 2002). These activities should be coordinated with CDC's existing internet-based resources.

At the federal level, CDC has conducted many activities to inform and educate providers about smallpox and smallpox vaccination, and these efforts must be sustained over time and must be enhanced to include the knowledge and skills required for a broader kind of preparedness. A range of training and education resources for clinicians are also available from the

American Medical Association (AP, 2003b), the Agency for Healthcare Research and Quality, the Association of Professionals in Infection Control, and from a number of university-based centers that study bioterrorism and disaster preparedness (e.g., the Centers for Public Health Preparedness).

In addition to the efforts of public health agencies, accreditation systems could be used to further the engagement of hospitals and health care organizations in bioterrorism and overall public health preparedness. In the area of accreditation, the Joint Commission on Accreditation of Healthcare Organizations (JCAHO) has been integrating bioterrorism and smallpox components into the requirements for emergency preparedness. The committee urges CDC to work with all health care accrediting bodies (JCAHO, National Commission for Quality Assurance, and American Accreditation HealthCare Commission [URAC]) to encourage the incorporation of emergency preparedness standards (i.e., for developing, implementing, and exercising plans for responding to a potential bioterrorist attack including, but not limited to, smallpox) into requirements for the accreditation of hospitals and health care organizations.

The Role of Public and Media Communication in Smallpox Preparedness

Public communication is an essential component of public health and smallpox preparedness. As detailed in the CDC guidance issued May 2, 2003, health departments should have communication plans in place and channels of communication tested to prepare for the possibility of an attack (CDC, 2003b). However, as with other aspects of preparedness, risk communication should be focused on all possible threats, including, but not limited to, smallpox. Public health officials and spokespersons should be familiar with all potential bioterror agents and also should have a clear understanding of other major threats to the public health.

Practicing good communication would suggest that before a potential event and the intense sense of crisis it would create, public health authorities communicate to the public about what preparations are being made (e.g., rapidly accessible vaccine and other pharmaceutical stocks, mass vaccination or point of distribution sites), and about the availability of prepared key responders in their jurisdiction. Having information about what is in place and what will be done before a crisis occurs will help to ease the public's fears and concerns. This includes communicating about the smallpox vaccine, its risks and benefits, its availability, and plans for its rapid distribution when needed, as noted above.

The media would play a vital role in a potential bioterrorist event; journalists and other media specialists should be included in scenarios and exercises (DiGiovanni et al., 2003). This will help educate the media about the nature of infectious agents, the capacity of the public health and health care systems to respond, and plans to protect the public's health. Also, community leaders and opinion leaders have been shown to have an important role in communicating with the public in a crisis (DiGiovanni et al., 2003). Such individuals should be included in communication plans and their roles well-described before a potential emergency.

Testing Smallpox and Public Health Preparedness

Evaluating the readiness of public health and health care systems to mount an effective response is challenging and requires a clear standard and indicators of preparedness to test against (as noted above) and tools with which to test preparedness. Helpful ways to examine and test preparedness systematically might include: (1) building hypothetical scenarios; and (2) analyzing the public health response to real-life situations such as recent outbreaks, as analogous, though perhaps on a different scale, to future potential threats.

Using Scenarios to Test Preparedness

Many types of smallpox attack scenarios could be developed to aid in exercising and testing preparedness. There are multiple variables to be considered, from ways in which the disease may be introduced, number of initial contacts, pattern of spread and number of geographical areas hit—just a few examples of the vast range of unknowns. What is the duty of the public health system in the face of such great unknowns, and what tools are available to help develop the capacity to respond to all or many possible scenarios?

Although no centralized collection or database of smallpox (or other public health threats) scenarios exists at this time, there are a number of related resources, including the Columbia University collaboration with the National Association of County and City Health Officials (NACCHO) in the Public Health Ready project (developing standards for planning and evaluating public health emergency scenarios), the NACCHO CD-ROM for scenario building, and expertise available from DoD (Columbia University School of Nursing, 2003; NACCHO, 2003a). **The committee recommends that CDC facilitate the development of a range of scenarios for potential smallpox attack(s), including one or more multi-threat scenarios, and urge states to use these to expand and continuously improve their plans to respond to a wide range of possibilities.** The committee offers its assistance in conceptualizing these scenarios, should such advice be needed.

For each scenario that is developed, state and local jurisdictions could assess their personnel and training needs, their infrastructure requirements (including legal authority), their communication plans and messages, the partners to be involved, etc. For example, local public health agencies could conduct their exercises in conjunction with local hospitals required to conduct exercises for JCAHO accreditation (Fraser and Fisher, 2001). Existing tools, such as the state and local assessment instruments developed by the National Public Health Performance Standards Program (CDC, 2003c) and the local and state Public Health Preparedness and Response Capacity Inventories (CDC, 2002b, 2002c), could be used as resources to develop a detailed and quantitative minimum standard (as recommended above) for assessing preparedness to respond to various scenarios. Resources also are available for specific components of preparedness capacity, such as a recently developed model for efficient mass smallpox vaccination campaigns (Hupert et al., 2003).

Using Lessons Learned to Test Preparedness

Another option for testing response capacity and processes and for identifying gaps in preparedness might be to conduct state and/or local systematic reviews of public health and health system performance in response to recent outbreaks, natural disasters, and other public health crises. It is likely that many or most jurisdictions have had experience with at least one potential or actual public health crisis in recent years.

Many jurisdictions who responded to West Nile virus or to the anthrax attacks described themselves as nearly overwhelmed; responding to a major public health threat left a slim margin of resources available for other essential public health services (GAO, 2000; NACCHO, 2001). More than one infectious agent may surface at the same time (e.g., the emergence of both SARS and monkeypox within weeks of each other), either through deliberate introduction or natural occurrence, and the public health system needs to be prepared to mobilize quickly and prioritize all its resources and respond as well as possible to more than one threat. A smallpox attack may occur in concert with other events, such as meningitis in a college population, a spike in West Nile infections, or a major food-borne disease outbreak. Health departments struggling with implementing smallpox preparedness report difficulties in conducting routine immunization activities, operating family planning clinics, or conducting other disease investigation (AP, 2003a; Cook, 2003). The added strain of SARS in some of these jurisdictions nearly overwhelmed their response capacity (Neergaard, 2003).

To test performance and identify lessons learned, a jurisdiction could examine, among other aspects of preparedness:

- the relationships and channels of communication between the public health and health care communities during the crisis, and in general;

- the speed and ease of health care provider referral, reporting, and request for technical assistance;
- the involvement of other parties when relevant (fire fighters, law enforcement);
- the training and education needs revealed by the incident, both in public health and health care communities;
- the public communication needs revealed by the incident;
- the gaps in the public health infrastructure uncovered by the incident, including in information systems, legal authority, surveillance, workforce deployment, and communication; and
- the implications of these findings for the jurisdiction's overall preparedness and, in particular, its ability to respond effectively to a smallpox attack.

Sustaining Smallpox and Overall Public Health Preparedness

The resurgence of tuberculosis (TB) as a public health threat in the last two decades strikingly illustrates the importance of sustaining public health capacity. In the early 1970s, funding for tuberculosis decreased dramatically, and tuberculosis control programs at the state and local levels were dismantled (IOM, 2000). As the disease was considered a waning threat, capacity to deal with TB was allowed to diminish, and as a result, the reemergence of TB exposed a public health system unprepared to respond effectively. Protecting the health of the public requires sustained readiness, and wherever possible, multipurpose readiness. Although threats to the public's health evolve, the structures, skills, and resources needed to address them are often the same, or overlap significantly.

Sustaining general public health preparedness requires an array of capabilities and resources, and strategic planning at all levels is needed for long-term smallpox preparedness, if this is determined to be a necessity. Maintaining specific elements of smallpox preparedness includes, but is not limited to, the following activities:

For key responders:

- Vaccinating and revaccinating select key responders as appropriate to address turnover and decreasing immunity; and
- Providing training and education on an ongoing basis to all key responders on the subject of smallpox response plans and on their functional assignments or roles, on smallpox disease and vaccine, etc.

For public health response:

- Sustaining the public health infrastructure to facilitate effective rash surveillance, syndromic surveillance, reporting, laboratory capabilities, and communication; and
- Re-training and communicating with health care workers and providers on identifying and diagnosing suspicious symptoms, reporting requirements and contact information regularly.

For mass vaccination:

- Testing the readiness of key responders responsible for mass vaccination (vaccinators, security, etc.) regularly;
- Maintaining adequate vaccine stocks; and
- Testing capacity to set up clinic operations and rapidly process large numbers of people regularly.

The first two key messages of the report are:

> Smallpox is not the only threat to the public's health, and vaccination is not the only tool for smallpox preparedness.
>
> To improve smallpox preparedness, it is essential to "plan, train to the plan, exercise to the plan, and revise the plan" (Selecky, 2003).

VACCINATION OF MEMBERS OF THE GENERAL PUBLIC WHO INSIST ON RECEIVING SMALLPOX VACCINE

On December 13, 2002, President Bush announced his policy on pre-event vaccination against smallpox. In those remarks, the president stated, "Our government has no information that a smallpox attack is imminent. . . . Given the current level of threat and the inherent health risks of the vaccine, we have decided not to initiate a broader vaccination program for all Americans at this time" (White House, 2002). Because of the possible threat, he said that "the military and other personnel who serve America in high-risk parts of the world" would be vaccinated and that "medical professionals and emergency personnel and response teams that would be the first on the scene in a smallpox emergency" could volunteer to receive the vaccine (White House, 2002).

During those remarks, the president also stated, "There may be some citizens, however, who insist on being vaccinated now. The public health agencies will work to accommodate them. But that is not our recommendation at this time" (White House, 2002). CDC has been charged with implementing this component of the president's policy, in addition to facilitating the vaccination of public health and health care response teams and vaccination of a broader group of health care, police, fire, and emergency response personnel. The committee appreciates the president's motivation to be responsive to the general public, particularly to those who are concerned for their personal and family's safety and who believe that a smallpox vaccination is the only way to ensure safety against the threat of smallpox introduction.

The committee notes, however, that public health programs do not proceed simply on the basis of an individual's request for medication, a vaccine, or any other intervention. The same is true of immunizations or prescription medications given by health care providers. Immunizations are not given unless the risk to the patient and population is believed to be outweighed by the benefit to be gained. In this case, smallpox vaccination not otherwise indicated by participation in smallpox preparedness efforts, exposure to monkeypox, or risk of disease from other orthopox viruses in the course of laboratory work and in the absence of identified risk for that individual of acquiring smallpox would be an extremely unusual circumstance outside of a clinical trial, as is discussed below.

CDC has asked the committee's advice on how to carry out this program (Henderson, 2003). The committee has several concerns about a vaccination program aimed at the general public at this time that need to be considered before determining how to launch such a program:

LOGISTICS: It is not clear how many members of the general public are seeking vaccination. As of early May, CDC's "hotlines have never been completely inundated by people from the public calling and wanting to know where to get the vaccine," but CDC also acknowledges that "there have been calls [about this issue] to some state and local health officials over time" (Henderson, 2003). CDC also has stated that "there's been relatively little clamoring" for the vaccine by members of the general public (McNeil, 2003). If few are seeking vaccination, the burden on public health agencies might be slight, but this might be counteracted by a possibly broad geographic distribution of those seeking vaccine. In addition, sporadic requests for vaccination from members of the general public, for whom different informational materials and medical oversight might be required, do not necessarily improve smallpox preparedness and could well be even more disruptive to public health agencies than a large-scale but concentrated set of requests. Other issues related to public or private insurance coverage for employment loss and medical care for adverse events or ensuing disability for members of the general public will have to be addressed.

RESOURCES: The committee has noted several times in previous reports that many public health agencies are stressed to their limits in trying to implement the smallpox vaccination program for the target professional populations, executing the other elements of preparedness, dealing with adverse events following vaccination, improving communication, enhancing the various vaccine surveillance programs, and addressing competing public health mandates, such as SARS. It is possible that the development and execution of a robust public vaccination program at this time would severely deplete human and fiscal resources from other high priority public health activities and even detract from the next expansion of the planned vaccination program or from a mass vaccination program in the event of an introduction of smallpox.

COMMUNICATION: Communicating about the public health system's readiness and ability to protect the public could greatly influence how many people feel it is necessary to receive the smallpox vaccine prior to any exposure or identified case. If the public is well-informed about the plans that CDC, states and localities have in place to respond to a smallpox attack (e.g., an adequate vaccine supply, plans for mass vaccination clinics, and development of a newer smallpox vaccine), there may be less demand. The committee encourages CDC and their state and local partners to describe to the public how the public health system is enhancing preparedness to protect them from the consequences of a smallpox attack and about the state of preparations. By learning about the range of preparations that are being made and the existence and distribution of prepared key responders in each jurisdiction, members of the general public will be better able to judge whether they want to pursue receiving the smallpox vaccine in a pre-event setting.

SAFETY: As with all smallpox vaccinees, vaccinated members of the general public would pose a risk to their families and other close contacts, due to the long period following vaccination when contact with the vaccination site can cause injury to third parties. Although the basic issues of potential spread to families and contacts are the same as among health care and public health workers, the level of vaccinee knowledge about adverse events and agency monitoring are likely to be substantially less when members of the general public are vaccinated. Thus, each new vaccinee poses additional risk to the general population without, in the absence of an actual outbreak of smallpox, any added benefit for the vaccinee or the general population. It also will be important to determine how much follow up for short- and long-term clinical outcomes would be appropriate, and who would be responsible for submitting follow-up reports needed for surveillance, since no institutional aegis would be present.

RISK-BENEFIT: In the absence of any current benefit to individual vaccinees and the remote prospect of benefit in the future (as such benefit would be realized only in the event of a smallpox outbreak, and the outbreak occurred in the vaccinee's region), the balance of benefit to the individual and risk to others (through contact with the vaccinee or through disruption of other public health initiatives) becomes unfavorable. This poor risk-benefit balance is particularly problematic here, where third parties have not consented to the risk of contact with a vaccinee. In the absence of other forms of benefit, therefore, offering vaccination to members of the general public is contrary to the basic precepts of public health ethics, which focus on a fair and reasonable balance of risks and benefits among individuals and for the population as a whole.

Two potential areas of benefit might alter this equation, however, in some circumstances. One is when, as with first responders, there is a possibility of greater personal need for the vaccination. In the general population, this may occur when individuals have been exposed to monkeypox or when they work with the smallpox virus (and other closely related viruses). For these individuals, their personal protection needs can appropriately be seen to outweigh the risk their vaccination would impose upon themselves and others.

A second circumstance would be one where vaccination of individuals offers a benefit to the general population, such as in a clinical trial, where participation facilitates scientific research that might lead to safer or more effective ways to guard against the disease. Clinical trials also offer a series of apparently effective techniques for minimizing risks to participants and third parties through careful attention to participant screening, education, and monitoring. Thus, here too, the combined benefits to the individual and society may outweigh the risks of proceeding with vaccination.

Given all of these concerns, **the committee recommends that CDC proceed with a deliberate and stepwise approach toward meeting the President's policy of offering vaccine to members of the general public who insist on receiving it by:**

1. Conducting brief quantitative surveys to determine public interest and desire for smallpox vaccine. These surveys should include public and private health agencies as well as the general public, in order to understand the potential scope of public interest.

2. Determining the budgetary and other requirements that would meet the demand noted.

3. Identifying, monitoring, and referring people to existing or planned smallpox vaccine clinical research trials or other well-structured clinical arrangements that meet the basic requirements of medical and public health ethics, including assurances for safety of vaccinees and their contacts, acceptable balance between risk and benefit, and acceptable distribution of scarce public health resources to meet all preparedness as well as other public health goals. The committee encourages CDC to consider utilizing a pilot program or some other means of evaluating the initial experiences with this effort.

The third key message of the report is:

> Vaccinating members of the general public beyond the key personnel states deem necessary for preparedness should proceed only under the aegis of smallpox vaccine clinical research trials or other well-structured clinical arrangements that meet the basic requirements of medical and public health ethics.

SELECTED ASPECTS OF SMALLPOX VACCINATION PROGRAM IMPLEMENTATION

In the following section of the report, the committee discusses several important components of the national smallpox vaccination program: (1) Communicating About and Coordinating the Response to Adverse Events; (2) Data Systems Used in Smallpox Vaccination Program; (3) Pregnancy Screening; (4) Advisory Committee on Immunization Practices Smallpox Vaccine Safety Working Group (ACIP SVS WG); (5) Evaluation and Safety Studies; and (6) Compensation Available for Smallpox Vaccine Injuries.

Communicating About and Coordinating the Response to Adverse Events

Communication among CDC, states, and local jurisdictions is extremely important for identifying every serious adverse event, conducting follow-up of the vaccinee who experiences the adverse event, and providing feedback to states and particularly local jurisdictions about how their reporting efforts help to ensure the overall safety of the national smallpox vaccination program. The committee heard that some local jurisdictions feel overburdened by the adverse event management and reporting requirements created by both the state and CDC (Committee on Smallpox Vaccination Program Implementation Study Staff, 2003; Nikolai, 2003). In many jurisdictions, there also seems to be confusion among local health departments, hospitals and health care systems, and treating physicians about who is supposed to report which type of adverse event to which system (Committee on Smallpox Vaccination Program Implementation Study Staff, 2003). The use of multiple data systems for the smallpox vaccination program has contributed to some of this confusion.

These observations highlight the need for greater communication and coordination among CDC, states, local health departments, hospitals, and health care providers with respect to adverse event reporting. Because state and local partners cite the need for improved coordination and reduction of the time burden for reporting and managing adverse events, the committee is concerned that partners in the smallpox vaccination program could be reluctant to report all adverse events or ill-informed about how to report them. **To help ensure that the adverse event reporting and follow-up procedures work as seamlessly as possible, the committee recommends that CDC coordinate better with their state partners and provide feedback to local partners who reported the adverse event.**

Data Systems Used in Smallpox Vaccination Program

With the rapid development of the national smallpox vaccination program, CDC has had to develop data systems for use during the program in a very short time frame. CDC should be congratulated for developing the Pre-Event Vaccination System (PVS), the Smallpox Vaccine Adverse Event Active Surveillance System (subsequently referred to as the "Active Surveillance System"), and the Hospital Smallpox Vaccination Monitoring System (HSVMS) so quickly. In conjunction with the Vaccine Adverse Event Reporting System (VAERS), these data systems have allowed adverse events following smallpox vaccination to be reported quickly and helped identify new patterns of adverse events (e.g., myo/pericarditis, myocardial infarction), which ultimately may or may not be shown to be causally associated with the smallpox vaccine.

Streamlining Data Collection

Of the multiple data systems being used concurrently during the pre-event smallpox vaccination program, PVS, the Active Surveillance System, and HSVMS were all created uniquely for the pre-event smallpox vaccination program; VAERS is a data system that was previously established to collect reports of adverse events following any vaccination. For the purposes of the smallpox vaccination program, these data systems have been designed to work together. PVS and HSVMS provide a link to the Active Surveillance System, and VAERS supplements the data gathered through the Active Surveillance System. (More detailed descriptions of these data systems are available in the committee's second report [IOM, 2003c].)

In an ideal world, one data system would have been created specifically for the smallpox vaccination program that could have worked in conjunction with VAERS. However, the timing of the vaccination program and the different types of users that need to access each system necessitated that these data systems be created in the manner that they were. Even so, the committee believes that there may be ways to integrate these systems better, so the data-reporting burden on all vaccination partners is reduced. The data-reporting burden also includes the weekly data reports that states are required to send to CDC, which are sometimes redundant with the data that states have already entered into PVS. **The committee recommends that CDC pursue ways to streamline the data systems that are used in the smallpox vaccination program, improving user-friendliness and integrating the multiple systems to avoid duplicate data entry, especially considering that any future expansion of the vaccination program would require a larger number and greater diversity of data system users, some of whom may be using these systems for the first time.**

When the vaccination program expands to include new types of vaccinees (many of whom do not work in a health department or hospital setting), there potentially will be many new users of PVS, HSVMS, the Active Surveillance System, and VAERS. To ensure continued collection of data on all vaccinees, new users of these data systems will have to be educated about existing data systems, their purpose, and how they are linked together. The committee encourages CDC to provide greater outreach and communication about the data systems used in the smallpox vaccination program to all the potential users of these systems in the expanded program, as well as a redoubling of outreach and communication efforts to partners involved in the first phase of the program who have not completely utilized these data systems. The committee also encourages CDC to plan for streamlining or limiting the data collected from vaccinees, should an outbreak occur, in order to keep things moving more efficiently.

Ease of Use and Value Gained from PVS

As effective as these data systems have been at helping to identify serious adverse events following smallpox vaccination, state and local vaccination programs appear to be experiencing continuing difficulty in using these systems. For example, the committee has heard during presentations at committee meetings and in discussions with state and local health departments that PVS is not user-friendly (Committee on Smallpox Vaccination Program Implementation Study Staff, 2003; Madlock, 2003; Nikolai, 2003). State and local health departments have reported that it takes inordinate amounts of time to enter data into PVS and that the CDC servers that host this system sometimes do not function properly. CDC has acknowledged these problems with PVS and has stated that it is working to resolve them. The committee encourages CDC to resolve these problems as quickly as possible, since the cumbersomeness of PVS threatens broad use of this system by state and local vaccination programs, potentially leading to a loss of useful information.

The data entered into PVS provide great value to overall evaluation of the vaccination program's progress. It is this value that counterbalances the burden placed on state and local vaccination programs to enter data into

PVS. However, the committee has heard that some state and local vaccination programs view the difficulty in entering data into PVS as outweighing the perceived benefits they receive from their participation (Committee on Smallpox Vaccination Program Implementation Study Staff, 2003). The committee encourages CDC to facilitate and support regular, timely data reports from PVS and other sources to its state and local partners so they can gain value from their participation in the range of data systems used for the pre-event smallpox vaccination program.

Utility of the Active Surveillance System

As described above, the data systems that CDC has utilized during the pre-event smallpox vaccination program seem to have been effective at identifying serious adverse events following smallpox vaccination. However, the committee cannot be completely certain of how effective the Active Surveillance System has been at identifying these serious adverse events until all vaccinees are entered into the system. An "active" surveillance system is effective when there is a confirmed outcome on virtually every vaccinee. As of June 11, 2003, only 10,835 (44 percent) of 24,781 PVS records of vaccinees that had at least 28 days elapse since the time of vaccination were included in the Active Surveillance System (Mootrey, 2003b). The recent reports of two cases of cardiomyopathy identified three months after smallpox vaccination (CDC, 2003n) also point to the need to continue active surveillance of all vaccinees, including follow-up of those vaccinees who report only mild symptoms in the weeks after vaccination. CDC conducted a survey of their grantees to gain a better understanding of their participation (or lack thereof) in the Active Surveillance System. The 48 grantees that responded to the survey identified four main reasons for data entry delay in the Active Surveillance System: (1) follow-up time is longer than anticipated; (2) data entry is slow because of general lack of personnel or infrastructure resources; (3) technical difficulties related to digital certificates; and (4) problems with PVS (Mootrey, 2003a).

The committee understands that CDC has diligently encouraged every state and local vaccination program to create an Active Surveillance System entry for every vaccinee. **Because the civilian smallpox vaccination program is a true partnership among CDC, states, and local jurisdictions, the committee recommends that CDC continue and expand their communication with states and local jurisdictions about the imperativeness of their participation in the Active Surveillance System, stressing that the safety of the vaccination program cannot be guaranteed without their full participation and cooperation.** In these communications, CDC should stress that the number of people vaccinated in the expanded vaccination program could be many times larger than the number of response team members vaccinated so far. Therefore, the consistent use of the Active Surveillance System would provide a rich source of data for detecting trends in reported adverse events.

In its first letter report (IOM, 2003b), the committee identified its reasons for recommending the creation and use of an active surveillance system:

> Considering the anticipated risks of the vaccination program and the currently unknown benefit, it is extremely important that all adverse reactions from the smallpox vaccine (both known and suspected) be identified in a timely manner. Relying on passive systems that are dependent on vaccinees and their clinicians to bring the adverse reaction to the attention of the smallpox vaccination program managers will not capture all serious adverse reactions.

The committee still believes in the value of the Active Surveillance System but recognizes the importance of doing an evaluation of the efficacy of the system so its role in the ongoing program can be assessed. Such an evaluation should involve getting data on every person vaccinated in the first phase of the program entered into the Active Surveillance System, and then evaluating the completeness, validity, and added value of the data gathered through the Active Surveillance System compared to other means (e.g., VAERS, the Clinician Information Line). Once such an evaluation is conducted (with as complete ascertainment as possible of data on all vaccinees, so reliable statistical analyses can be generated), the committee and CDC can have a better understanding of the relative value of the Active Surveillance System in the ongoing operation of the pre-event smallpox vaccination program. Regardless, such an evaluation would provide reassurance of the completeness of safety data, and correspondingly, the overall safety of the vaccination program.

It is important to recognize, however, that an evaluation of the Active Surveillance System during the first phase of the program may not necessarily be generalizable to the expanded program. In the expanded vaccination program, there may be a larger number of people vaccinated than in the first phase of the program. Because of this potentially larger number of vaccinees, there may also be a larger number of adverse events reported. The standardized data collection format used in the Active Surveillance System may make investigations easier for this potentially greater volume of reported adverse events and may allow determinations of probable causality to be made more quickly, potentially lessening the sense of alarm that would arise from the sheer volume of adverse events that could be reported. In addition, whereas the first phase of the program focused on public health and health care workers who already may have had knowledge of adverse event reporting mechanisms, workers vaccinated in the expanded vaccination program (and their fellow workers who may be entering data on this new pool of vaccinees) may not have the same knowledge about adverse event reporting mechanisms. Thus, the Active Surveillance System may have more value during the expansion of the vaccination program, especially if proactive communication about the specific data systems being used during the smallpox vaccination program, the purpose of each one, and how they are linked together is provided to those who will be responsible for data entry and management.

Pregnancy Screening

On May 2, 2003, CDC described women who had been exposed to smallpox vaccine during pregnancy and their enrollment in the National Smallpox Vaccine in Pregnancy Registry in an article appearing in the Morbidity and Mortality Weekly Report (CDC, 2003k). The registry includes women found to be pregnant when vaccinated, those who became pregnant within 28 days of vaccination, and those who, while pregnant, were in close contact with a person vaccinated within the previous 28 days. The registry will be used to monitor outcomes of pregnancy in these women. Women vaccinated through the military smallpox vaccination program, the civilian smallpox vaccination program, and recent clinical research studies are included in the registry.

In pregnant women, the smallpox vaccine can cause fetal vaccinia, a rare but serious condition that can lead to premature delivery, skin rash with scarring, stillbirth, or death of an infant after delivery (CDC, 2003o). Some infants who experience fetal vaccinia are born with skin scars but are otherwise healthy (CDC, 2003o). Fewer than 50 cases of fetal vaccinia have ever been reported in the world, and only three of these cases occurred in the United States (CDC, 2003o). From 1967 to 1971, when smallpox vaccine was routinely given in the United States, only one case of fetal vaccinia was reported among an estimated 90,000 to 280,000 pregnant women who received the vaccine (CDC, 2003o). Smallpox vaccine has not been shown to cause an increased risk of birth defects (CDC, 2003o).

In the military program, from December 13, 2002, to April 22, 2003, a total of 62,222 women of reproductive age were screened for smallpox vaccination, and 52,185 were vaccinated; 85 were inadvertently exposed to smallpox vaccine during pregnancy. (As of June 11, 2003, 125 women from the military program were enrolled in the registry [Grabenstein, 2003].) The median age was 22 years. On the basis of the estimated date of conception, 62 women conceived before vaccination and 23 conceived during the four weeks after vaccination. In the civilian program, from January 24, 2003, to April 24, 2003, a total of 6,174 women of reproductive age were vaccinated; 6 were inadvertently exposed to smallpox vaccine during pregnancy. (As of June 18, 2003, eight women from the civilian program were included in the registry [Mulinare et al., 2003].) The median age was 31 years. On the basis of estimated date of conception, two women conceived within 1 week before vaccination and four conceived during the 4 weeks after vaccination. Two of the civilian women had miscarriages during early pregnancy. In clinical studies of the smallpox vaccine, from November 2001 to April 24, 2003, a total of 12 women were inadvertently exposed to smallpox vaccine during pregnancy. The denominator for women of reproductive age for this population is not available. The median age was 28 years. Each of the women had a negative pregnancy test on the day of vaccination (CDC, 2003k). In all of these populations, the actual number of pregnancies exposed to smallpox vaccine could be expected to be underreported, since not all women will report their pregnancies to the registry and some pregnancies may end before a woman recognizes that she is pregnant.

Because exposure to smallpox vaccine during pregnancy can cause fetal vaccinia, a rare but serious condition, CDC and the Department of Defense (DoD) have provided education about the risk of smallpox vaccine exposure during pregnancy and advised women not to receive the smallpox vaccine if they are pregnant, to take a pregnancy test if they think they might be pregnant, and avoid pregnancy for four weeks after vaccination, and advised close contacts of pregnant women not to receive the smallpox vaccine (CDC, 2003h; DoD, 2003).

CDC has estimated that the expected rate of unknown pregnancy (i.e., pregnancies of <4 weeks' gestation or <6 weeks based on obstetrical dating) and the expected rate of conception during a 4-week period would be 12 per 1,000 women in the general population and 8 per 1,000 women in a population comparable to the older health care workers vaccinated in the civilian program, in the absence of screening and counseling (CDC, 2003k). The reported rate of pregnancies exposed to smallpox vaccine during the first phase of the civilian and DoD programs is approximately one per 1,000, which is substantially lower than the expected rates of unknown pregnancy and conception during a 4-week period (in the absence of screening and education) of 8 per 1,000 women in the population comparable to the civilian health care workers and 12 per 1,000 women in the general population (CDC, 2003k).

Even though some women have been inadvertently exposed to smallpox vaccine during the civilian vaccination program, the lower than expected rate of unknown pregnancies and conception in the 4 weeks after vaccination in women vaccinated in the civilian program reassures the committee that the pregnancy screening practices have been relatively effective thus far. Stronger advice about contraception during the 4 weeks after vaccination or greater emphasis on the need to conduct a pregnancy test on the morning of vaccination could help to reduce the rate of women inadvertently exposed to smallpox vaccine during pregnancy. It is impossible, however, to detect every pregnancy since pregnancy tests might miss very early pregnancies. Understanding this and recognizing that each woman has the right to decide for herself whether a pregnancy test is appropriate, the committee agrees with the October 2002 recommendation of the ACIP that "Routine pregnancy testing of women of child-bearing age is not recommended" (CDC, 2002d).

CDC has stated that they are considering expanding the questions and advice about pregnancy and intention to become pregnant (included in the Vaccine Information Statement Supplement E) (Mulinare et al., 2003). The committee believes that additional public health interventions to screen for pregnancy and provide advice on avoiding pregnancy could probably be beneficial, if they do not detract from other important screening and programmatic activities. **Considering that the rate of inadvertent exposure to smallpox vaccine during pregnancy is lower than expected and it is impossible to detect all pregnancies at the time of vaccination, the committee does not recommend extra pregnancy screening efforts at this time.** Data on the rate of pregnancies exposed to smallpox vaccine should be evaluated regularly, with the decision on whether to intensify pregnancy screening efforts also being reevaluated regularly.

On June 11, 2003, CDC recommended smallpox vaccination for persons investigating monkeypox outbreaks, involved in caring for infected individuals or animals, or who have had close or intimate contact with individuals or animals confirmed to have monkeypox (CDC, 2003a). Smallpox vaccination is recommended for persons who have contraindications to vaccination (e.g., pregnancy, eczema) if they have had close or intimate contact with a person with a rash illness, but CDC cautions that it is important to confirm suspected cases of monkeypox before recommending smallpox vaccination for a person with contraindications. Considering that there may be some pregnant women who will be advised to receive a smallpox vaccination because of their close personal contact with a confirmed case of monkeypox, the committee recognizes that it will be important for CDC to describe how such women will be incorporated into the National Smallpox Vaccine in Pregnancy Registry. These women will not have experienced an "inadvertent" smallpox vaccine exposure, because smallpox vaccination will have been recommended due to their contact with a monkeypox case. As these issues begin to be worked out, the committee encourages CDC to describe how data on them will be combined with or separated from the pregnancies exposed to smallpox vaccine stemming from the pre-event smallpox vaccination program, and how follow-up data on the pregnancies exposed to smallpox vaccine because of contact with monkeypox will contribute to evaluation of the other pregnancies included in the registry.

Advisory Committee on Immunization Practices Smallpox Vaccine Safety Working Group (ACIP SVS WG)

CDC and the Advisory Committee on Immunization Practices Smallpox Vaccine Safety Working Group (ACIP SVS WG; subsequently referred to in the text as "working group") have placed a high priority on safety in the national smallpox vaccination program. When safety concerns have arisen, CDC and the working group have responded promptly, as evidenced by the emergency meeting of the full Advisory Committee on Immunization Practices and the working group on March 28, 2003. The committee was reassured that CDC and the working group reported in a timely fashion and conducted further evaluation of the cardiac adverse events that came to light in March. The committee also commends CDC and the working group for modifying screening and education materials when it was recognized that there could possibly be an association between smallpox vaccination and the development of cardiac adverse events, and for communicating these changes to state and local partners in a rapid fashion. The committee notes that the working group has described CDC as being professional, timely with data, and responsive in their interactions with the working group (Neff, 2003).

As has been stated before, the charge of the working group is to (1) evaluate data on vaccine safety and the system for monitoring, treatment, and response and (2) monitor safety data for vaccinia immune globulin (VIG) and cidofovir made available under oversight of the U.S. Food and Drug Administration (FDA) through investigational new drug (IND) protocols (ACIP SVS WG, 2003a).

The committee appreciated receiving information on the operating procedures of the working group (ACIP SVS WG, 2003b). This helped reduce some of the confusion about how the working group was organized and structured. The Summary of the March 20-21, 2003 meeting of the working group by the working group chairpersons (ACIP SVS WG, 2003a) helped address many of the committee's questions and concerns expressed in previous reports (IOM, 2003b, 2003c). The committee was heartened to see clear descriptions of the case definitions for specific adverse events, trigger points for action on specific events, and actions that should be taken in response to specific triggers.

In assessing trigger points, the working group is (1) identifying appropriate data sets for use in estimating expected incidence, (2) developing statistical reference rates, and (3) determining what action should occur in response to triggers (ACIP SVS WG, 2003a). The working group has developed case definitions, trigger events, trigger points, and responding actions for neurologic, dermatologic, and cardiac adverse events; they also have developed case definitions, trigger points, and responding actions for different types of inadvertent inoculation (e.g., resulting from pregnancy, immune suppression, contact transmission). The committee endorses the general approach that the working group is taking for all of these actions. The working group has developed detailed plans for assessing different disease endpoints. However, understanding that the committee has not been privy to all of the working group's discussions, the committee would like to obtain more information about the working group's deliberations about death as an endpoint (as compared to the disease endpoints that are being considered).

The working group noted in the summary of the March 20-21, 2003, meeting that they still needed to define a trigger point for further action with regard to inadvertent vaccination of HIV infected persons. The committee looks forward to seeing the working group's definition of this trigger point when it is finalized.

The committee also endorses the working group's proposal for animal studies that investigate the basic pathophysiology of cardiac disease in relation to smallpox vaccination and the proposal to systematically observe and record how vaccine sites are managed and what outcomes result (ACIP SVS WG, 2003a).

As the working group has followed the safety data from the civilian and military smallpox vaccination programs, they have paid increased attention to the myo/pericarditis cases reported in both programs. In evaluating both the inflammatory (i.e., myo/pericarditis) and ischemic (e.g., myocardial infarction, angina) cardiac events, the working group was asked to evaluate a number of questions related to these events. Specific to the myo/pericarditis cases, the working group was asked, "Does a causal relationship exist between vaccination and inflammatory heart disease?" (Neff, 2003). The working group concluded, "DoD data support a risk for myocarditis after smallpox vaccination that is significantly higher than background rate, and suggest that a causal association is highly likely" (Neff, 2003).

This conclusion was one of the primary reasons that the majority (10 of 12) of the working group recommended that CDC "[c]ontinue with the current pre-event volunteer program, to vaccinate and maintain vaccination status of selected public health and first response health care workers with careful screening for known risk factors with a goal of meeting and maintaining state and local health department readiness needs," in addition to the entire working group recommending, "No member favors beginning phase 2 of the vaccination program" (Neff, 2003). After being presented with these recommendations of the working group, the full ACIP unanimously approved a draft resolution and later released a final statement recommending to CDC that it would be "unwise to expand beyond its current, pre-event smallpox vaccination recommendations because of the new and unanticipated safety concerns, i.e., myo/pericarditis, whose extent and severity, particularly of long term sequelae, are not yet known. Any smallpox vaccination that occurs should be carried out only within the context of the currently recommended response teams and state and local response plans and should be administered according to currently recommended vaccination procedures and protocols" (ACIP, 2003).[4] In their statement, the ACIP also reiterated "that it is critical for smallpox preparedness planning, within the context of broader terrorism and emergency response planning, to continue at the federal, state and local levels" (ACIP, 2003).

Evaluation and Safety Studies

The committee appreciated receiving the updated "Smallpox Vaccination Program Plans for Phase 1 Evaluation and Research" (CDC, 2003g) and found it very helpful to see all of the ongoing and planned evaluation and research activities in one document.

As CDC has acknowledged, evaluation of the cardiac adverse events reported following smallpox vaccination is very important to safely continue the smallpox vaccination program. CDC has been consulting with multiple experts in the field of cardiology and chronic disease epidemiology to investigate both the ischemic adverse events and the myo/pericarditis cases. To evaluate the cardiac adverse events, CDC's investigations have included: CDC-assisted epidemiologic field investigations ("epi-aids") in the states where deaths have occurred to obtain more comprehensive information on the cases; evaluation of case series data; collection of data on expected rates of cardiac events in comparable unvaccinated populations; and potential prospective studies that could provide information on biologic plausibility and rates of these events (CDC, 2003g).

Both CDC and the working group described considering the utility of animal studies that would investigate the basic pathophysiology of cardiac disease in relation to smallpox vaccination. CDC has stated that "studies to evaluate possible biologic mechanisms for cardiac adverse events following

[4]Less than a week after the ACIP released its statement on the national smallpox vaccination program, the National Vaccine Advisory Committee (NVAC) issued a letter to the acting assistant secretary for health and director of the National Vaccine Program containing a resolution that was unanimously passed by the NVAC: "The National Vaccine Advisory Committee reaffirms the necessity for the nation's health system to be prepared for biological threats, man-made or natural, and encourages continued efforts in this regard. With respect to the smallpox vaccination, the Committee recommends that the Assistant Secretary for Health in consultation with the Department's Office of Public Health Emergency Preparedness consider the recommendations of ASTHO regarding the routine smallpox vaccination program and that further smallpox vaccinations, beyond those of public health response and vaccination teams, should be delayed until a national consensus is developed on appropriate next steps" (NVAC, 2003).

smallpox vaccination are being considered" (CDC, 2003j). As stated earlier, the committee endorses carrying out such studies, and any other studies that could help elucidate possible biological mechanisms for the cardiac adverse events seen following smallpox vaccination. The committee also endorses the working group's proposal that a prospective protocol-driven case-control study be conducted to assess the association between cardiac adverse events and smallpox vaccination (ACIP SVS WG, 2003a).

To supplement the studies being planned by CDC, the committee suggests that CDC consider collecting data on which states are using screening criteria for cardiac events that are more stringent than those recommended by ACIP on April 4, 2003 (CDC, 2003d). Subsequently, CDC may want to consider using these data to determine if states that are using more stringent cardiac screening criteria are experiencing lower rates of cardiac adverse events in people vaccinated after April 4, 2003, than states adhering to ACIP's recommendations.

The committee has heard that some states are screening for positive HIV status more stringently than what was deemed necessary by ACIP and CDC. For example, Rhode Island is requiring proof of a recent (in past 45 days) negative HIV test before someone can be vaccinated (personal communication, A. Artenstein, June 13, 2003). As the committee noted in its first report, "Hospitals and health departments will implement the first phase of the pre-event vaccination program in slightly different ways, depending upon the circumstances and needs of their communities. Much could be learned from this differential administration of the program" (IOM, 2003b: 7). Knowing now that at least one state is using different screening criteria from what was recommended by CDC, the committee suggests that CDC collect data on the screening practices of other states and use these data to supplement the overall evaluation of the implementation of the civilian smallpox vaccination program.

DoD has stated that they will conduct follow-up of the myo/pericarditis cases seen among people vaccinated through the DoD program at six weeks, six months, and 12 months. After review of the 12-month data, DoD will determine whether additional follow-up is warranted (personal communication, J. Grabenstein, Department of Defense, June 16, 2003). At the May 1, 2003 committee meeting, CDC said that they intend to have continuing follow-up of the myo/pericarditis cases (including a standardized protocol and guidelines for how to conduct follow-up of those cases that have been identified), but the specifics have yet to be finalized (Mootrey, 2003c). Recently, CDC also has stated that "guidelines for evaluation and follow-up of patients with myo/pericarditis have been drafted" (CDC, 2003j). When the follow-up procedures and guidelines have been finalized, the committee looks forward to receiving this information.

The committee has some additional general comments on CDC's approaches and planned efforts for evaluation and safety studies related to smallpox vaccination. These issues may need to be addressed in order to have reliable findings from all the evaluation and research efforts. By listing these guiding principles, the committee is not saying that CDC is not already implementing such measures, but rather, that these principles should be considered for every evaluation or safety study undertaken by CDC to assess the smallpox vaccination program:

- Small, unrepresentative samples should be kept to a minimum. Small samples sizes could detract from the generalizability of the study.
- Sample sizes for many studies may be limiting for subgroup analyses. The majority of vaccinees in the first phase of the civilian program have been re-vaccinees. Considering the differential adverse reaction profile for primary vaccinees versus re-vaccinees, care should be taken to ensure that there are enough data on primary vaccinees.
- Since the vaccination program is moving to a more heterogeneous pool of vaccinees, evaluation efforts should focus on gathering data from people with less health knowledge than those vaccinated in the first phase.
- As with all studies, efforts should be taken to maximize participation rates in each study. Maximizing participation rates is not only important for generalizability, but also for the ability to validly compare rates (e.g., adverse event rates for the newer attenuated vaccines versus the old vaccines).
- CDC has made a specific effort to gather information from hospitals on their participation in the first phase of the smallpox vaccination program. However, the issues that are relevant to hospitals often also are relevant to health care systems. A concomitant effort should be made to gather information from health care systems.
- As has been noted in previous reports, the committee has stressed the importance of concurrent control groups for many of the studies. Control groups and cases should be studied using the same methods. The committee again encourages CDC to develop concurrent control groups for as many of their studies as possible, given the current realities of the pace of the smallpox vaccination program. The use of such control groups would greatly aid the investigations of the recently reported cases of cardiomyopathy (CDC, 2003n) and myo/pericarditis.
- There is a general need for longer follow-up in some of the vaccinee studies. Particularly, there is a need to follow those who experienced serious adverse events in order to learn about long-term outcomes, especially for those who experienced cardiac adverse events. Right now, this involves a relatively small number of people, but the information gained from long-term follow-up will be extremely important. There also may be value in long-term follow-up of a sample of vaccinees who experienced no adverse

events, as well as a sample of those vaccinees that experienced mild, less severe adverse events. This is particularly relevant now that two cases of dilated cardiomyopathy have been identified three months after vaccination (CDC, 2003n). (The DoD is planning on using the Millennium Cohort Study and the Defense Medical Surveillance System to compare and contrast people who have received the smallpox vaccine to people who have not received the vaccine [personal communication, J. Grabenstein, June 15, 2003].) Plans also should be made to assemble enough information so that follow-up can be done easily in the future.

- Follow-up also would be valuable for the pregnancies inadvertently and intentionally (i.e., in response to contact with a case of monkeypox) exposed to smallpox vaccination. The committee notes that DoD has an ongoing birth defects registry (covering all dependants of military personnel) that could contribute information on any concerns that might arise.

The committee also suggests that CDC and the ACIP consider holding periodic invitational workshops on the science of smallpox vaccine safety and efficacy to update and disseminate new findings in these areas. The results of these workshops could be actively disseminated to CDC's state and local partners in the smallpox vaccination program to update them on the latest research.

The committee encourages CDC to think long-term about the research agenda for the smallpox vaccination program. CDC has stated that the pre-event smallpox vaccination program will be an ongoing program (CDC, 2003i; CDC, 2003m), specifically in terms of vaccinating new people for maintenance of response teams, and broadly in terms of planning for a smallpox response. There will be many policy and implementation questions that will have to be answered along the way. **The committee recommends that CDC begin developing a structured, prioritized research agenda that can aid decision-making as the smallpox preparedness program moves forward.** The committee offers its assistance in refining this research agenda as the program evolves. Considering the extent of evaluation and research efforts that CDC could propose for the smallpox vaccination program as it moves forward, and the limited resources available to support all needed evaluation efforts, the committee encourages CDC to consider requesting the use of Public Health Service 1 Percent Evaluation funds for this purpose (if this approach has not been pursued already).[5]

[5]The Department of Health and Human Services is authorized under the Public Health Service Act to set aside up to one percent of appropriations for Public Health Service (PHS) programs for evaluation (directly, or by grants of contracts) of the implementation and effectiveness of PHS programs (42 USC 238(j)).

CDC has asked for the committee's assistance in prioritizing research and evaluation efforts specific to the smallpox vaccination program, given the limited resources available for these activities (personal communication, B. Gellin, CDC, March 26, 2003). **The committee recommends that in the short term, studies of the serious adverse events should receive the highest priority. For safety-related questions, in the longer term, studies examining long-term outcomes for those who experienced both serious and mild adverse events and studies of how mild adverse events contributed to lost work or social function should be a high priority. For system-related questions, in the longer term, studies of cost and opportunity costs should be a high priority.** The committee believes that, although still important, studies on the reasons why people declined vaccination, tracking rarer adverse events, improving adverse event classification, and tracking persons with missing data should be considered next-tier priorities.

Compensation Available for Smallpox Vaccine Injuries

As stated in the committee's third letter report, "the committee notes the need for additional clarification by CDC to the states on the provisions of the [Smallpox Emergency Personnel Protection Act of 2003 (P.L. 108-20)], and for fact sheets or other explanatory materials for potential vaccinees" (IOM, 2003d). CDC has since developed a summary of the Smallpox Emergency Personnel Protection Act of 2003 (SEPPA) benefits and compensation for smallpox vaccine injuries that is posted to its website (CDC, 2003e). However, at the time of the writing of this report, the compensation language in the Smallpox Vaccine Information Statement (VIS) (CDC, 2003f) had not yet been updated to reflect the newly enacted legislation. To ensure that potential vaccinees are aware of the compensation available to them for any adverse events that are determined to be connected to the smallpox vaccine, the committee encourages CDC to update the VIS as soon as possible and publicize the existence of the fact sheet. When the interim final rule implementing SEPPA is published, this fact sheet should be expanded with further information on what types of compensation are available, how to apply for compensation, the statute of limitations and statute of repose, and any other relevant information. The issue of compensation for live born children who were exposed to the vaccine in utero should be clarified as well.

To help publicize the existence of these materials, the committee suggests that CDC notify states when these updated materials are available. The committee also encourages CDC to send a postvaccination fact sheet or letter explaining the compensation available under SEPPA to every person who has been identified as experiencing an adverse event. CDC could also consider whether such information also should be sent to everyone who has already been vaccinated.

As of June 20, 2003, 17 suspected cases of myo/pericarditis and 4 probable cases of myo/pericarditis following smallpox vaccination were reported in the civilian population (CDC, 2003n). Because of the probable association of smallpox vaccination with increased incidence of myo/pericarditis, CDC is now including myo/pericarditis in the tables of "selected adverse events associated with smallpox vaccination among civilians" appearing weekly in the Morbidity and Mortality Weekly Report. The ACIP Smallpox Vaccine Safety Working Group has concluded that "Smallpox vaccination increases risk of myo-pericarditis" (Neff, 2003). The DoD has stated, "the observed rate of myopericarditis among primary vaccinees is 3.6-fold higher than the expected rate among personnel on active duty who were not vaccinated" (Halsell et al., 2003).

Research in non–smallpox vaccine settings suggests that some people who experience myocarditis may develop long-term sequelae such as left ventricular dysfunction (Hiroe et al, 1985) and cardiomyopathy (Hayakawa et al., 1984; Das et al., 1985; Drucker and Newburger, 1997). As of June 20, 2003, two cases of dilated cardiomyopathy were diagnosed in civilian smallpox vaccinees 3 months after vaccination (CDC, 2003n). CDC is now advising, "Because smallpox vaccination appears to be associated causally with myocarditis, which can cause [dilated cardiomyopathy], further evaluation is warranted" (CDC, 2003n). In one study, one-fourth of patients reporting to a major medical center with symptomatic dilated cardiomyopathy died within a year, and half died within 5 years (Dec and Fuster, 1994).

The possibility of long-term sequelae from the smallpox vaccine must be acknowledged. Whereas the acute smallpox vaccine injuries are relatively well understood, less is known about smallpox vaccine injuries that occur on a longer-term basis. SEPPA specifies that an individual who was administered the vaccine who is requesting a benefit under the law must file an initial request for benefits or compensation "not later than one year after the date of administration of the vaccine" (U.S. Congress, 2003). (Individuals who experienced accidental vaccinia inoculation, however, have up to "two years after the date of the first symptom or manifestation of onset of the adverse effect" [U.S. Congress, 2003] to file an initial request.) For individuals who received the smallpox vaccine, it currently is unclear to the committee how, if at all, any injuries that manifest themselves more than 1 year after vaccination will be addressed. It also is unclear how longer-term sequelae that result from an acute smallpox vaccine injury (e.g., cardiomyopathy that results from a "silent" case of myocarditis, with no initial request for benefits filed in the year after vaccination) will be handled. Also, in SEPPA, a "covered injury" is covered if it is "determined . . . to have been sustained by an individual the direct result of administration to the individual of a covered countermeasure during the effective period of the Declaration" (U.S. Congress, 2003). (The term 'Declaration' refers to the Declaration Regarding Administration of Smallpox Countermeasures issued by the Secretary on January 24, 2003, and published in the Federal Register on January 28, 2003.) The committee believes that it will be important to clarify and explain in the interim final rule the interpretation of "a direct result of . . . a covered countermeasure" (i.e., smallpox vaccine), since this will affect the level of evidence required for an injury to be covered. The committee encourages CDC to work with those who are developing the interim final rule for the smallpox vaccine injury table to clarify the conditions under which longer-term sequelae from the smallpox vaccine will be considered to be a direct result of smallpox vaccination.

The last two key messages of the report are:

> The safety system appears to be working well to date, but CDC and its partners should remain vigilant to ensure the continuing safe implementation of the program.
>
> The development of a research agenda for the smallpox vaccination program is important to ensuring the long-term success of smallpox preparedness efforts, as well as providing useful information for overall public health preparedness.

CONCLUDING REMARKS

The committee offers its assistance in the future in any areas that would prove useful to CDC. Two possible areas include developing a research agenda to support and evaluate the implementation of the smallpox preparedness program and exploring how to better integrate smallpox preparedness into overall public health preparedness.

In closing, the committee summarizes several of the key messages set forth in this report:

- First, smallpox is not the only threat to the public's health, and vaccination is not the only tool for smallpox preparedness.
- Second, to improve smallpox preparedness, it is essential to "plan, train to the plan, exercise to the plan, and revise the plan" (Selecky, 2003).
- Third, vaccinating members of the general public beyond the key personnel states deem necessary for preparedness should proceed only un-

der the aegis of smallpox vaccine clinical research trials or other well-structured clinical arrangements that meet the basic requirements of medical and public health ethics.

- Fourth, the safety system appears to be working well to date, but CDC and its partners should remain vigilant to ensure the continuing safe implementation of the program.
- Fifth, the development of a research agenda for the smallpox vaccination program is important to ensuring the long-term success of smallpox preparedness efforts, as well as providing useful information for overall public health preparedness.

The committee wishes to thank you for the continuing opportunity to be of assistance to the Centers for Disease Control and Prevention and its partners as they work to protect the nation's health.

Brian L. Strom, *Committee Chair*
Kristine M. Gebbie, *Committee Vice Chair*
Robert B. Wallace, *Committee Vice Chair*
Committee on Smallpox Vaccination Program Implementation

REFERENCES

AAFP (American Academy of Family Physicians). 2002. Panel calls for limited smallpox vaccination. *FP Report* 8(8).

ACIP (Advisory Committee to Immunization Practices). 2002. Record of the Meeting of the Advisory Committee on Immunization Practices—June 19-20, 2002. [Online] Available at http://www.cdc.gov/nip/acip/minutes/acip-min-jun02.rtf. Accessed July 30, 2003.

ACIP. 2003. Advisory Committee on Immunization Practices (ACIP) Statement on Smallpox Preparedness and Vaccination. [Online] Available at http://www.bt.cdc.gov/agent/smallpox/vaccination/pdf/acipjun2003.pdf. Accessed July 17, 2003.

ACIP SVS WG (Advisory Committee on Immunization Practices Smallpox Vaccine Safety Working Group). 2003a. March 20-21, 2003, Meeting of the Advisory Committee on Immunization Practices (ACIP) Smallpox Vaccine Safety Working Group, Chicago, IL: Summary of the Chairs.

ACIP SVS WG. 2003b. Operating Procedures of the ACIP Smallpox Vaccine Safety Working Group (ACIP SVS WG).

APHA (American Public Health Association). 2002. APHA Policy Statement on Smallpox Vaccination. [Online] Available at http://www.apha.org/legislative/policy/smallpox.pdf. Accessed June 17, 2003.

AP (Associated Press). 2003a, May 13. SARS Battle Strains U.S. Health System. *FOX News Channel*.

AP. 2003b, June 16. AMA Seeks to Standardize Training for Bioterrorism. *The Wall Street Journal*.

ASTHO (Association of State and Territorial Health Officials). 2002. Nature's Terrorist Attack: Pandemic Influenza. [Online] Available at http://www.astho.org/pubs/Pandemic%20Influenza.pdf. Accessed July 15, 2003.

ASTHO. 2003. ASTHO Smallpox Preparedness Survey Results (April 25, 2003). [Online] Available at http://www.astho.org/pubs/spxsummaryb2.pdf. Accessed July 7, 2003.

Baxter R, Rubin R, Steinberg C, Carroll C, Shapiro J, Yang A. 2000. Assessing Core Capacity for Infectious Diseases Surveillance. Final Report Prepared for the Office of the Assistant Secretary for Planning and Evaluation. Falls Church, VA: The Lewin Group, Inc.

Blank S, Moskin LC, Zucker JR. 2003. An ounce of prevention is a ton of work: mass antibiotic prophylaxis for anthrax, New York City, 2001. *Emerging Infectious Diseases* 9(6):615-622.

Brower J, Chalk P. 2003. The Global Threat of New and Reemerging Infectious Diseases: Reconciling U.S. National Security and Public Health Policy. Arlington, VA: RAND.

CDC (Centers for Disease Control and Prevention). 2002a. About the Vaccine: Immunity Against Smallpox. [Online] Available at http://www.bt.cdc.gov/training/smallpoxvaccine/reactionss/about_vac_Immunity.html. Accessed July 1, 2003.

CDC. 2002b. Local Public Health Preparedness and Response Capacity Inventory. [Online] Available at http://www.phppo.cdc.gov/od/inventory/docs/ Local%20Inventory%20version%201_1_FINAL.pdf. Accessed May 30, 2003.

CDC. 2002c. State Public Health Preparedness and Response Capacity Inventory. [Online] Available at http://www.phppo.cdc.gov/od/inventory/docs/State%20Inventory%20version%201_1_FINAL.pdf. Accessed May 30, 2003.

CDC. 2002d. Summary of October 2002 ACIP Smallpox Vaccination Recommendations. [Online] Available at http://www.bt.cdc.gov/agent/smallpox/ vaccination/acip-recs-oct2002.asp. Accessed January 9, 2003.

CDC. 2003a. CDC Recommends Smallpox Vaccination to Protect Persons Exposed to Monkeypox. [Online] Available at http://www.cdc.gov/od/oc/media/pressrel/r030611.htm. Accessed June 16, 2003.

CDC. 2003b. Continuation Guidance—Budget Year Four—Annex A: Summary of Smallpox Preparedness Activities. [Online] Available at http://www.bt.cdc.gov/planning/continuationguidance/pdf/annex_a.pdf. Accessed July 7, 2003.

CDC. 2003c. National Public Health Performance Standards Program. [Online] Available at http://www.phppo.cdc.gov/nphpsp/. Accessed June 20, 2003.

CDC. 2003d. Notice to readers: supplemental recommendations on adverse events following smallpox vaccine in the pre-event vaccination program: recommendations of the Advisory Committee on Immunization Practices. *Morbidity and Mortality Weekly Report* 52(13):282-284.

CDC. 2003e. Smallpox Emergency Personnel Protection Act of 2003: Benefits and Compensation for Smallpox Vaccine Injuries. [Online] Available at http://www.bt.cdc.gov/agent/smallpox/vaccination/bene-comp.asp. Accessed June 16, 2003.

CDC. 2003f. Smallpox Vaccine Information Statement (VIS). [Online] Available at http://www.bt.cdc.gov/agent/smallpox/vaccination/pdf/smallpox-vis.pdf. Accessed August 6, 2003.

CDC. 2003g. Unpublished. Smallpox Vaccination Program Plans for Phase 1 Evaluation and Research.

CDC. 2003h. Smallpox Vaccine Information Statement (VIS) Supplement E: Pregnancy and Breastfeeding Mean You Should Not Get Smallpox Vaccine. [Online] Available at http://www.bt.cdc.gov/agent/smallpox/vaccination/preg-contra.asp. Accessed June 17, 2003.

CDC. 2003i. CDC Telebriefing Transcript: Update on Monkeypox and Severe Acute Respiratory Syndrome (SARS) Investigations. [Online] Available at http://www.cdc.gov/od/oc/media/transcripts/t030619.htm. Accessed July 5, 2003.

CDC. 2003j. Update: cardiac-related events during the civilian smallpox vaccination program—United States, 2003. *Morbidity and Mortality Weekly Report* 52(21):492-496.

CDC. 2003k. Women with smallpox vaccine exposure during pregnancy reported to the national smallpox vaccine in pregnancy registry—United States, 2003. *Morbidity and Mortality Weekly Report* 52(17):386-388.

CDC. 2003l. Smallpox Vaccination Program Status by State, July 25, 2003. [Online] Available at http://www.cdc.gov/od/oc/media/spvaccin.htm. Accessed July 31, 2003.

CDC. 2003m. CDC Telebriefing Transcript: Safer, Healthier Summer. [Online] Available at http://www.cdc.gov/od/oc/media/transcripts/t030626.htm. Accessed July 6, 2003.

CDC. 2003n. Update: cardiac and other adverse events following civilian smallpox vaccination—United States, 2003. *Morbidity and Mortality Weekly Report* 52(27):639-642.

CDC. 2003o. Smallpox Vaccination Information for Women Who Are Pregnant or Breastfeeding. [Online] Available at http://www.bt.cdc.gov/agent/smallpox/vaccination/pdf/preg-factsheet.pdf. Accessed July 17, 2003.

CIDRAP (Center for Infectious Disease Research and Policy) News. 2002. Scope of Smallpox Vaccination Program Not Yet Decided, HHS Official Say. [Online] Available at http://www.cidrap.umn.edu/cidrap/content/bt/smallpox/news/pox2shots.html. Accessed August 1, 2003.

Columbia University School of Nursing. 2003. Project Public Health Ready. [Online] Available at http://www.nursing.hs.columbia.edu/institute-centers/chphsr/phready.html. Accessed July 1, 2003.

Committee on Smallpox Vaccination Program Implementation Study Staff. 2003. Unpublished. Conversations with Public Health Agencies About the Smallpox Vaccination Program and Smallpox Preparedness: Synthesis and Detailed Notes.

Connolly C. 2003a, April 15. Smallpox Vaccine on Verge of Spoiling. *Washington Post.*

Connolly C. 2003b, June 20. Panel Urges Caution on Smallpox Inoculation. *Washington Post*, A9.

Cook R. 2003, April 5. Smallpox Planning Detracts from Core Public Health, Officials Say. *Associated Press.*

Covert MH. 2001. Public Health System's Capacity to Respond to Bioterrorism. Testimony on Behalf of AHA (American Hospital Association) Before the Subcommittee on Technology and Procurement Policy, Committee on Government Reform, U.S. House of Representatives on December 14, 2001.

Das SK, Colfer HT, Pitt B. 1985. Long-term follow-up of patients with previous myocarditis using radionuclide ventriculography. *Heart Vessels* 1(Suppl.):195-198.

Dec GW, Fuster V. 1994. Idiopathic dilated cardiomyopathy. *New England Journal of Medicine* 331(23):1564-1575.

DiGiovanni C Jr., Reynolds B, Harwell R, Stonecipher EB, Burkle Jr. F. 2003. Community reaction to bioterrorism: prospective study of stimulated outbreak. *Emerging Infectious Diseases* 9(6):708-712.

DoD (Department of Defense). 2003. Smallpox Information. [Online] Available at http://www.smallpox.army.mil/media/pdf/Smallpoxinfo.pdf. Accessed June 17, 2003.

Drucker NA, Newburger JW. 1997. Viral myocarditis: diagnosis and management. *Advances in Pediatrics* 44:141-171.

Edmond M. 2003. Transcript from the IOM's Committee on Smallpox Vaccination Program Implementation Meeting Three on May 1, 2003, Washington, DC:231-251.

Elliott VS. 2002, April 22/29. Public Health Reporting Flaws Spell Trouble: Doctors Complain About Requirements That Appear to Lack Follow-Through. *American Medical News.*

Elliott VS. 2003, February 24. Public Health's Main Fear Over Bioterrorism: Surge Capacity. *American Medical News.*

ENA (Emergency Nurses Association). 2003. Status: U.S. Smallpox Vaccination Program. ENA Washington Update. May 2003.

English JF, Cundiff MY, Malone JD, Pfeiffer JA, Bell M, Steele L, Miller JM. 1999. Bioterrorism Readiness Plan: A Template for Healthcare Facilities. [Online] Available at http://www.ntis.gov/search/product.asp?ABBR=PB2002108954. Accessed July 7, 2003.

Fock R, Bergmann H, Bussmann H, Fell G, Finke EJ, Koch U, Niedrig M, Peters M, Riedmann K, Scholz D, Wirtz A. 2002. Influenza pandemic: preparedness planning in Germany. *Euro Surveillance* 7(1):1-5.

Fraser MR, Fisher VS. 2001. Elements of Effective Bioterrorism Preparedness: A Planning Primer for Local Public Health Agencies. Washington, DC: NACCHO.

Frelinger JA, Garba ML. 2002. Responses to smallpox vaccine. *New England Journal of Medicine* 347(9):689-690.

GAO (U.S. General Accounting Office). 2000. West Nile Virus Outbreak: Lessons for Public Health Preparedness. GAO/HEHS-00-180. Washington, DC: Health, Education, and Human Services Division.

GAO. 2003. Bioterrorism: Preparedness Varied Across State and Local Jurisdiction. GAO-03-373. Washington, DC: Health, Education, and Human Services Division.

Grabenstein JD. 2003. U.S. Military Smallpox Vaccination Program. Presented to the CDC Advisory Committee on Immunization Practices Meeting on June 18, 2003.

Halsell JS, Riddle JR, Atwood JE, Gardner P, Shope R, Poland GA, Gray GC, Ostroff S, Eckart RE, Hospenthal DR, Gibson RL, Grabenstein JD, Arness MK, Tornberg DN. 2003. Myopericarditis following smallpox vaccination among vaccinia-naive U.S. military personnel. *Journal of the American Medical Association* 289(24):3283-3289.

Hardy G. 2002. Transcript from the IOM's Committee on Smallpox Vaccination Program Implementation Meeting One on December 19, 2002, Washington, DC:284-291.

Hayakawa M, Inoh T, Yokota Y, Kawanishi H, Kumaki T, Takarada A, Seo T, Fukuzaki H. 1984. A long-term follow-up study of acute myocarditis: an electrocardiographic and echocardiographic study. *Japanese Circulation Journal* 48(12):1362-1367.

Heinrich J. 2001. Bioterrorism: Public Health and Medical Preparedness. Testimony on Behalf of GAO (United States General Accounting Office) Before the Subcommittee on Public Health, Committee on Health, Education, Labor, and Pensions, U.S. Senate on October 9, 2001.

Henderson J. 2003. Transcript from the IOM's Committee on Smallpox Vaccination Program Implementation Meeting Three on May 1, 2003, Washington, DC:54-82.

Hiroe M, Sekiguchi M, Take M, Kusakabe K, Shigeta A, Hirosawa K. 1985. Long follow-up study in patients with prior myocarditis by radionuclide methods. *Heart Vessels* 1(Suppl.):199-203.

Hupert N, Cuomo J, Callahan MA, Mushlin AL. 2003. Modeling Efficient Mass Vaccination Campaigns. Paper Presented June 26, 2003 at AcademyHealth's Public Health Systems Research Meeting in Nashville, TN.

IOM (Institute of Medicine). 2000. Ending Neglect: The Elimination of Tuberculosis in the United States. Washington, DC: National Academy Press.

IOM. 2002. The Future of the Public's Health in the 21st Century. Washington, DC: The National Academies Press.

IOM. 2003a. Microbial Threats to Health: Emergence, Detection, and Response. Washington, DC: The National Academies Press.

IOM. 2003b. Review of the Centers for Disease Control and Prevention's Smallpox Vaccination Program Implementation: Letter Report #1. Washington, DC: The National Academies Press.

IOM. 2003c. Review of the Centers for Disease Control and Prevention's Smallpox Vaccination Program Implementation: Letter Report #2. Washington, DC: The National Academies Press.

IOM. 2003d. Review of the Centers for Disease Control and Prevention's Smallpox Vaccination Program Implementation: Letter Report #3. Washington, DC: The National Academies Press.

IOM and NRC (National Research Council). 1999. Chemical and Biological Terrorism: Research and Development to Improve Civilian Medical Response. Washington, DC: National Academy Press.

Libbey PM. 2003. Testimony on Behalf of NACCHO (National Association of County and City Health Officials) Before the Subcommittee on Labor, Health, and Human Services, Education and Related Agencies, Committee on Appropriations, U.S. Senate on January 29, 2003.

Madlock Y. 2003. Transcript from the IOM's Committee on Smallpox Vaccination Program Implementation Meeting Three on May 1, 2003, Washington, DC:152-173.

Manning A. 2002, October 16. Advisory Panel Expands Smallpox Vaccine Plan. *USA Today*.

McNeil DG Jr. 2003, June 18. After the War: Biological Defenses; 2 Programs to Vaccinate for Smallpox Come to a Halt. *New York Times*, A13.

Mitchell S. 2003, June 12. Monkeypox Shows Gap in Bioterror Readiness. *United Press International*.

Mootrey G. 2003a. Adverse Events Following Smallpox Vaccination in Civilians. Presented to the IOM's Committee on Smallpox Vaccination Program Implementation on May 1, 2003.

Mootrey G. 2003b. Adverse Events (non-cardiac) Following Smallpox Vaccination in Civilians. Presented to the CDC Advisory Committee on Immunization Practices Meeting on June 18, 2003.

Mootrey G. 2003c. Transcript from the IOM's Committee on Smallpox Vaccination Program Implementation Meeting Three on May 1, 2003, Washington, DC:72-73.

Mulinare J, Broder K, Cano M, Seward J. 2003. Preventing Inadvertent Exposure of Pregnant Women to Smallpox Vaccine. Presented to the CDC Advisory Committee on Immunization Practices Meeting on June 18, 2003.

NACCHO (National Association of County and City Health Officials). 2001. West Nile Virus: Lessons Learned for State and Local Planning. [Online] Available at http://archive.naccho.org/documents/WestNileVirus.pdf. Accessed June 17, 2003.

NACCHO. 2003a. Bt CREATE: A Customizable Bioterrorism Tabletop Exercise Builder. [Online] Available at http://www.naccho.org.

NACCHO. 2003b. Impact of Smallpox Vaccination Program on Local Public Health Services. NACCHO Research Brief No. 9.

Neergaard L. 2003, May 12. SARS Battle Strains U.S. Health System. *The Kansas City Star*.

Neff J. 2003. Report for the Work Group on Smallpox Vaccine Safety. Presented to the CDC Advisory Committee on Immunization Practices Meeting on June 18, 2003.

Nikolai K. 2003. Transcript from the IOM's Committee on Smallpox Vaccination Program Implementation Meeting Three on May 1, 2003, Washington, DC:173-189.

NVAC (National Vaccine Advisory Committee). 2003. Letter from NVAC Chairman to Acting Assistant Secretary for Health and Director, National Vaccine Program. [Online] Available at http://www.cdc.gov/od/nvpo/meetings/ jun2003/letter.pdf. Accessed July 30, 2003.

Peters KE, Drabant E, Elster AB, Tierney M, Hatcher B. 2001. Cooperative Actions for Health Program: Lessons Learned in Medicine and Public Health Collaboration. Chicago, IL: American Medical Association; and Washington, DC: American Public Health Association.

Powers MJ, Ban J. 2002. Bioterrorism: threat and preparedness. *The Bridge* 32(1):29-33.

Russell S. 2003, January 18. Smallpox Vaccine Plan Starts Tuesday, Despite Concerns; Some Health Workers May Opt Out Over Risks, Compensation Issues. *San Francisco Chronicle*.

Salinsky E. 2002. Will the Nation Be Ready for the Next Bioterrorism Attack? Mending Gaps in the Public Health Infrastructure. NHPF Issue Brief No. 776.

Selecky MC. 2003. Transcript from the IOM's Committee on Smallpox Vaccination Program Implementation Meeting Three on May 1, 2003, Washington, DC:82-106.

Slifka, M. 2003. Is There Still Immunity to Smallpox? [Online] Available at http://www.asm.org/Media/index.asp?bid=17304. Accessed June 26, 2003.

Snowbeck C. 2003, July 4. Thousands of Smallpox Shots Unused. *Pittsburgh Post-Gazette*.

Solet D. 2003, February 19. Smallpox Pre-vaccinations Misdirect Resources. *Seattle Post-Intelligencer*.

Strikas R. 2002. Transcript from the IOM's Committee on Smallpox Vaccination Program Implementation Meeting One on December 19, 2002, Washington, DC:65-67.

Strikas R. 2003. National Smallpox Vaccination Program Update. Presented to the CDC Advisory Committee on Immunization Practices Meeting on June 18, 2003.

Teutsch SM, Churchill RE, eds. 1994. Principles and Practices of Public Health Surveillance. New York: Oxford University Press.

Thacker SB, Stroup DF. 1994. Future directions for comprehensive public health surveillance and health information systems in the United States. *American Journal of Epidemiology* 140(5):383-397.

Thompson T. 2003. Medical Reserve Corps (MRC): A Message from HHS Secretary Tommy G. Thompson. [Online] Available at http://www. medicalreservecorps.gov/. Accessed August 6, 2003.

Turning Point Public Health Statute Modernizing Collaborative. 2003. The Turning Point National Excellence Collaboratives—Draft Document. [Online] Available at http://www.turningpointprogram.org/Pages/MSPHA013103.pdf. Accessed June 17, 2003.

U.S. Congress. 2003. Smallpox Emergency Personnel Protection Act of 2003 (Public Law 108-20). [Online] Available at http://frwebgate.access.gpo.gov/cgi-bin/getdoc.cgi?dbname=108_cong_public_laws&docid=f:publ020.108.pdf. Accessed July 11, 2003.

White House. 2002. President Delivers Remarks on Smallpox. [Online] Available at http://www.whitehouse.gov/news/releases/2002/12/20021213-7.html. Accessed January 8, 2003.

LETTER REPORT #4, APPENDIX SUMMARY OF RECOMMENDATIONS: INTEGRATING SMALLPOX PREPAREDNESS INTO OVERALL PUBLIC HEALTH PREPAREDNESS

A Standard for Smallpox Preparedness

The committee recommends that CDC provide guidance to assist state public health agencies (and their partners,[6] as appropriate) in establishing a baseline level or a minimum standard of preparedness for a smallpox at-

[6]State partners may include, but not be limited to, emergency management agencies, law enforcement, fire and emergency medical services, hospital and other health care associations.

tack, after which, each state could individually assess its priorities and further expand its preparedness against smallpox and other threats to the public's health as needed.

Preparing Key Responders

The committee recommends that CDC support the establishment of state and/or local, and if appropriate, national, voluntary registries of individuals who have undergone vaccination to be mobilized, trained, and assigned as needed in the event of a smallpox attack. Such registries would include all willing vaccinated personnel not associated with a response team ranging from retired or relocated health care or public health workers to military reservists and former military personnel.

Using Scenarios to Test Preparedness

The committee recommends that CDC facilitate the development of a range of scenarios for potential smallpox attack(s), including one or more multithreat scenarios, and urge states to use these to expand and continuously improve their plans to respond to a wide range of possibilities.

VACCINATION OF MEMBERS OF THE GENERAL PUBLIC WHO INSIST ON RECEIVING SMALLPOX VACCINE

The committee recommends that CDC proceed with a deliberate and stepwise approach toward meeting the president's policy of offering vaccine to members of the general public who insist on receiving it by:

1. Conducting brief quantitative surveys to determine public interest and desire for smallpox vaccine. These surveys should include public and private health agencies as well as the general public, in order to understand the potential scope of public interest.
2. Determining the budgetary and other requirements that would meet the demand noted.
3. Identifying, monitoring, and referring people to existing or planned smallpox vaccine clinical research trials or other well-structured clinical arrangements that meet the basic requirements of medical and public health ethics, including assurances for safety of vaccinees and their contacts, acceptable balance between risk and benefit, and acceptable distribution of scarce public health resources to meet all preparedness as well as other public health goals. The committee encourages CDC to consider utilizing a pilot program or some other means of evaluating the initial experiences with this effort.

SELECTED ASPECTS OF SMALLPOX VACCINATION PROGRAM IMPLEMENTATION

Communicating About and Coordinating the Response to Adverse Events

To help ensure that the adverse event reporting and follow-up procedures work as seamlessly as possible, the committee recommends that CDC coordinate better with their state partners and provide feedback to local partners who reported the adverse event.

Streamlining Data Collection

The committee recommends that CDC pursue ways to streamline the data systems that are used in the smallpox vaccination program, improving user-friendliness and integrating the multiple systems to avoid duplicate data entry, especially considering that any future expansion of the vaccination program would require a larger number and greater diversity of data system users, some of whom may be using these systems for the first time.

Utility of the Active Surveillance System

Because the civilian smallpox vaccination program is a true partnership between CDC, states, and local jurisdictions, the committee recommends that CDC continue and expand their communication with states and local jurisdictions about the imperativeness of their participation in the Active Surveillance System, stressing that the safety of the vaccination program cannot be guaranteed without their full participation and cooperation.

Pregnancy Screening

Considering that the rate of inadvertent exposure to smallpox vaccine during pregnancy is lower than expected and it is impossible to detect all pregnancies at the time of vaccination, the committee does not recommend extra pregnancy screening efforts at this time.

Evaluation and Safety Studies

The committee recommends that CDC begin developing a structured, prioritized research agenda that can aid decision-making as the smallpox preparedness program moves forward.

The committee recommends that in the short term, studies of the serious adverse events should receive the highest priority. For safety-related questions, in the longer term, studies examining long-term outcomes for those who experienced both serious and mild adverse events and studies of how mild adverse events contributed to lost work or social function should be a high priority. For system-related questions, in the longer term, studies of cost and opportunity costs should be a high priority.

F

Review of the Centers for Disease Control and Prevention's Smallpox Vaccination Program Implementation, Letter Report #5

December 19, 2003
Dr. Julie Gerberding
Director
Centers for Disease Control and Prevention (CDC)
1600 Clifton Road, NE
Atlanta, GA 30333

Dear Dr. Gerberding:

The Committee on Smallpox Vaccination Program Implementation is pleased to offer you the fifth in a series of brief reports providing timely advice to assist CDC in preparing for a potential smallpox emergency. CDC asked the Institute of Medicine (IOM) committee to review CDC's smallpox readiness indicators, which are part of a larger set of public health emergency preparedness indicators being developed through the Public Health Preparedness Project.[1] The IOM committee reviewed the smallpox readiness indicators and heard from panelists representing public health, health care providers, health care institutions, and first responders at its

[1]CDC has used the terms "readiness" and "preparedness" relatively interchangeably in their description of the goals, purpose, and implementation of the Public Health Preparedness Project. Accordingly, the committee also has used both terms to describe essentially the same concept throughout this report.

November 6, 2003, meeting and offers this report based on the information gathered at that meeting and during its ongoing assessment of the smallpox vaccination program.

INTRODUCTION

The committee commends CDC for communicating more clearly that the focus of the smallpox preparedness effort is on all components of smallpox readiness (e.g., preparedness, detection, response,[2] containment, and recovery). Development of the smallpox readiness indicators—and the overall public health preparedness indicators—has helped to put preparedness for one hazard (e.g., smallpox) into the context of all-hazards public health preparedness. By planning to use the public health preparedness indicators to assess readiness and establish a baseline during the first year of their use, CDC has helped cast preparedness within the broader work of public health.

The committee also applauds CDC for responding to the needs of state and local public health agencies by beginning the development of smallpox—and overall public health emergency—preparedness indicators. CDC's state and local partners have stated that they need assistance in determining what constitutes a minimum level of preparedness (Selecky, 2003) and the most likely scenarios for which they should be preparing. The IOM committee echoed these concerns in its second report by encouraging CDC to define smallpox preparedness and to work with states to decide what more is needed to achieve smallpox preparedness (IOM, 2003a), and again in its fourth report by recommending that CDC assist states in establishing a baseline level or minimum standard of smallpox preparedness (IOM, 2003b). CDC has begun important work in this area by launching the Public Health Preparedness Project to ensure national preparedness for bioterrorism. The committee commends CDC for aiming toward indicators that will help state and local public health agencies document their progress on preparedness.

Description of the Public Health Preparedness Project

CDC has long recognized the importance of preparedness for bioterrorism and other public health threats. Prior to September 11, 2001,

[2]In this report, the committee uses the terms "response" and "respond" to mean all the activities that are necessary following identification of an infectious disease outbreak or bioterrorism event (e.g., epidemiologic investigation, activation of communication plans, implementing mass vaccination plans, enhanced surveillance, etc.).

CDC had awarded over $120 million to state and local public health agencies to support bioterrorism preparedness and response activities (CDC, 2003a). Through the Cooperative Agreement on Public Health Preparedness and Response for Bioterrorism (Program Announcement 99051) (hereafter, referred to as the "CDC cooperative agreement"), CDC awarded $918 million in fiscal year 2002 and $870 million in fiscal year 2003 (with an additional $100 million for smallpox preparedness) to support state and local agencies' bioterrorism preparedness activities.

In the past 6 months, CDC has launched the Public Health Preparedness Project to help define a baseline level of public health preparedness and to assess how states are using the funds received through the CDC cooperative agreement. The goals of the Public Health Preparedness Project are (Henderson, 2003b):

1. Define and establish a fundamental level of public health preparedness—initially associated with the CDC bioterrorism preparedness and response cooperative agreement program.
2. Serve as the basis of score-carding state and local preparedness.
3. Provide the framework for the fiscal year 2004 cooperative agreement guidance;.
4. Assist in identifying technical assistance needs of state and local public health agencies.

At the time of the November meeting, the score cards were intended to be used for identifying states' gaps in preparedness and areas where more resources are needed and were not intended to be used to reduce funding to states that are not performing as well as others (Henderson, 2003a). The committee endorses this view and believes that it is important that the score cards be used as opportunities for improvement.

In developing and implementing this project, CDC has made the following assumptions (Henderson, 2003a):

- It is important to focus first on bioterrorism and other infectious disease outbreaks, and then on chemical and radiological/nuclear terrorism.
- Flexibility is needed to address jurisdictional variability.
- Little science-based evidence exists for clear-cut criteria.
- Current resources may not be sufficient to fully address indicators.
- State and local health agencies have primary responsibility for assuring community capacity.

After an internal CDC workgroup, an external workgroup of national stakeholders, public health partners, and the IOM committee (through this report) provide feedback on the 4 goals, 22 objectives, and 127 indicators,

CDC will pilot test the indicators at five cooperative agreement recipient sites and some local health jurisdictions (Henderson, 2003a). Revisions will be made based on the pilot testing. In the summer of 2004, CDC will begin state and local assessments (based on the indicators) to establish a baseline, against which states will be assessed in subsequent years (Henderson, 2003b).

Committee Tasks

CDC asked that the IOM Committee on Smallpox Vaccination Program Implementation address the following tasks in their deliberations after the November 6, 2003 meeting (Henderson, 2003b):

1. Review the smallpox readiness indicators to determine if they are appropriate in assessing smallpox preparedness;
2. Develop/identify criteria or evidence that could be used to qualify a "Yes" response to a smallpox readiness indicator; and
3. Develop a smallpox case study/scenario (addressing jurisdictional variability) that can be used to test the relevance of the smallpox readiness indicators.

In the first task, the committee was asked to focus on a subset of 10 smallpox-specific indicators within the full set of 127 indicators and also to consider smallpox-related indicators from the larger set. In the report text, the committee makes some general observations about the entire set of all-hazards public health preparedness indicators. In Appendix 5-A, the committee offers specific comments about the 10 smallpox indicators and some criteria to aid in validating "yes" answers to the questions asked by the indicators (second task). The third task is addressed below.

GENERAL PARAMETERS OF FOUR SCENARIOS TO ASSESS SMALLPOX READINESS INDICATORS

Utility of Smallpox Scenarios

Learning from Real-Life Experiences and Hypothetical Scenarios

There are aspects of all-hazards public health preparedness that are hypothetical, because the nation has not experienced smallpox or certain other types of bioterror attacks, and the range of potential agents, extent of attack or outbreak, locations, and other variables are nearly limitless. Nevertheless, there are at least two ways to develop a useful framework for conceptualizing public health emergency response activities: designing scenarios that illustrate what could happen, and examining responses to real-life public health crises that have occurred already. Scenarios and real-life experiences help program planners consider the range of possibilities and complications that must be considered and addressed when responding to a public health emergency.

Some recent public health challenges highlight how real-life lessons can help inform future planning activities and the development of scenarios to test and improve planning (IOM, 2003b). The anthrax attacks of October 2001 underscored that successful mass prophylaxis activities are dependent upon clarity of mission, clear eligibility criteria for prophylaxis, well-defined lines of authority and responsibilities, effective communication, collaboration among all agencies involved in a response, and coordination of staffing and supplies (Blank et al., 2003). The emergence of Severe Acute Respiratory Syndrome (SARS) in early 2003 suggests that even though the modes of transmission of a virus may not be understood fully, health care workers will report to work if health care administrators institute procedures to maximize the safety of health care workers (Emanuel, 2003). The monkeypox outbreak in the summer of 2003—and the 2-week delay in reporting the first case to public health authorities—reminded the public health community that more work is needed to educate health care providers about when and how to report unexpected infectious diseases, and that overall communication between the health care and public health communities needs to be improved (Edmiston et al., 2003; MacKenzie, 2003). These recent public health challenges illustrate the range of issues that must be considered when designing detailed scenarios to help guide planning efforts.

Purpose, Development, and Use of Four Smallpox "Scenarios"

At the November 6, 2003, committee meeting, CDC asked the committee to develop a smallpox case study/scenario (addressing jurisdictional variability) that can be used to test the relevance of the smallpox readiness indicators (Henderson, 2003b). Accordingly, the committee developed four smallpox "scenarios" (described in detail below) that it used as an organizing framework for assessing the 10 draft smallpox readiness indicators and developing their subsequent evaluative criteria.

In developing these "scenarios," the committee recognized that these are not detailed scenarios that can be used for broad planning purposes but, rather, are general parameters of scenarios that are only meant to be used for the committee's purpose—to help test the draft smallpox readiness indicators. The simple descriptions of four smallpox contingencies that the committee has laid out below could be called many things—scenarios, case studies, vignettes. For the sake of simplicity, the committee decided to use the term "scenario," though recognizing that the descriptions below are mere sketches and at most can be called general parameters of smallpox scenarios.

Due to time limitations and their limited purpose, these particular scenarios are simply four possible situations, and the activities that would need to receive particular attention in each scenario. These scenarios were chosen because they represent a range of possible situations, without focusing on the extremes (i.e., assuming that there is zero risk of a smallpox attack or assuming that smallpox will infect every single person in the United States). Should CDC and its partners deem these four scenarios a useful starting point, providing an illustrative range of smallpox contingencies, more work would be needed to fill in the details to lead to more elaborate scenarios that are useful for conceptualizing the federal, state, and local response to a smallpox outbreak. As described in previous reports (IOM, 2003b), the committee believes that detailed smallpox planning scenarios are necessary to assist states in planning their response activities and evaluating their level of preparedness. **If CDC intends to use scenarios as a planning tool, the committee recommends that the scenarios represent a range of possible situations, be used to help guide state and local planning activities, and facilitate state and local assessment of their level of preparedness.**

Description of Smallpox "Scenarios" Used to Assess Readiness Indicators

Scenario #1: No smallpox case(s)/known presence of virus[3]

This scenario assumes that preparedness activities continue, with no new data on degree of risk (most recent statement from the President about risk: "no information that a smallpox attack is imminent" [White House, 2002]). This scenario can be thought of as the "maintenance state," and would also include any false alarms (i.e., pseudo-case). For this "no case" scenario, state and local public health agencies would need to focus, in particular, on training, vaccinating new members of response teams due to turnover, surveillance, planning, exercises, public information for false alarms, and clear lines of authority for decision-making.

[3]By "known presence of virus," the committee means the existence of the smallpox virus (i.e., in a vial or in the environment) outside of the two laboratories in the U.S. and Russia with known secured stocks of the smallpox virus.

Scenario #2: Limited number of confirmed smallpox case(s)/known presence of virus outside United States

This scenario assumes that one or a very limited number of confirmed smallpox cases have been identified somewhere in the world, but there is no immediate evidence of cases in the United States. For this scenario, state and local public health agencies would need to focus, in particular, on criteria for deciding if, when, and how strongly to encourage vaccination of the general public, communication with the public, risk communication, enhanced surveillance (including surveillance by clinicians), laboratory capacity, and plans for enhanced clinical capacity.

Scenario #3: Limited number of confirmed smallpox case(s)/known presence of virus in United States, outside of own jurisdiction

This scenario assumes that one or a very limited number of confirmed smallpox cases have been identified somewhere in the United States, but there is no immediate evidence of cases in the particular jurisdiction. For this scenario, state and local public health agencies would need to focus, in particular, on enhanced surveillance (particularly focusing on travel hubs), communication with the public, risk communication, decision-making about distribution and delivery of vaccine, enhanced clinical capacity, enhanced laboratory capacity, interjurisdictional issues, and anticipation of legal issues.

Scenario #4: Multiple confirmed smallpox case(s)/known presence of virus in multiple U.S. jurisdictions, with at least one case in one's own jurisdiction

This scenario assumes that multiple confirmed smallpox cases exist in multiple U.S. jurisdictions, with at least one confirmed case in the local jurisdiction. For this scenario, state and local public health agencies would need to focus, in particular, on frequent communication with the public, risk communication, close working relationships with the media, shifting legal authority among federal, state, and local entities, decision making about distribution and delivery of vaccine, clinical capacity, laboratory capacity, plans for disposal of human remains and coordination with Disaster Mortuary Operational Response Teams (DMORT), and recovery plans.

Caveats to Consider in Proposed "Scenarios"

Even though bioterror agents differ in important ways, many preparedness activities will be the same, no matter what the specific agent is. Whereas scenarios for different agents will require some activities unique to that particular agent, scenarios reflecting a continuum of possibilities for one agent (e.g., smallpox) will require escalating activities.

Detailed smallpox planning scenarios that represent the range of response activities that might be necessary could help state and local jurisdictions assess how this range of activities correlates to different levels of preparedness. It is important to recognize, however, that a real-life event probably is not going to proceed exactly according to any of the simple "scenarios" proposed by the committee, or more detailed scenarios yet to be developed. For planning purposes, communities will have to assess the pace at which they can respond to the different situations represented by each possible scenario.

The committee recognizes the value of also developing scenarios for other threats (e.g., anthrax, botulinum toxin, chemical attacks), but due to the scope of its charge, it only offers comments on smallpox scenarios that can be used for assessing the readiness indicators. The embedding of smallpox within an all-hazards approach also means that some of what might be considered smallpox preparedness (e.g., mass vaccination clinics) is really a specific example of a more general response (i.e., mass distribution of any vaccine, prophylaxis, or medication). Irrespective of specific scenarios that may be chosen eventually, the committee believes that the number used by state and local agencies should be relatively small, so that the multitude of specific details for the set of scenarios does not confuse planning activities and even detract from preparedness. Meta-scenarios that transcend individual bioterror agents—and address the possibility that two or more public health emergencies may occur at the same time—may be needed, and their use would reinforce the all-hazards approach to preparedness.

Applicability of Scenarios to Specific Local Circumstances

The committee used the general parameters of smallpox scenarios described above to evaluate the smallpox readiness indicators. If scenario parameters such as these are used as a starting point for developing detailed smallpox scenarios, state and local jurisdictions will have to use some judgment in determining to which scenario they want to apply their jurisdiction's limited resources. For example, some may say that it would be imprudent for jurisdictions that have already experienced a terrorist attack (e.g., New York City, Washington, DC, area) to assume that a smallpox attack in their community is not a possibility, whereas others may say that it would be ill-advised for a small, rural, Midwestern town with numerous other public health problems to assume that a smallpox attack in their community is a high probability and put all their resources into preparing for this scenario. A whole range of scenarios is possible for any community, but it will be the role of state and local health departments, local boards of health, and communities to assess the possible scenarios and decide how they want to allocate public health and bioterrorism preparedness funds. No matter where an attack initially occurs, it can spread to other areas, so communities will need to consider how they would respond to such an event.

Little Variability in Types of Planning Activities Across Scenarios

The general parameters of four scenarios that the committee used to assess the smallpox readiness indicators highlight key differences in the scope of response activities—the pace of the response, the overall timeline for accomplishing response activities, supplies and personnel that are readily available—but in terms of the planning activities that are required before the event, most of the same activities are needed.

By examining the 10 proposed smallpox indicators, the committee determined that most of the indicators deal with planning activities that would be required of any community should smallpox appear anywhere in the world (e.g., enhanced surveillance, preparations for increased laboratory capacity, more frequent and widespread communications, expanded education and training). Even the indicator addressing the activation of mass vaccination clinics shows little variability in terms of planning activities across the four scenarios (except for the "no cases" scenario) since CDC has stated that a case of smallpox anywhere in the world would lead to a decision to offer mass vaccination to the public (Henderson, 2003b). The main variability in planning that emerges across scenarios is for those indicators that are related to the response to a case in one's own jurisdiction (e.g., activation of quarantine and isolation procedures, designation of medical surge capacity sites).

Since it would not be prudent to only plan for the "no case" scenario, most communities will find that most of the readiness indicators are applicable to a majority of their *planning* activities. However, variability does exist in the *response* activities that would be required for different scenarios. If any of these scenarios occurs, the actions needed for that particular situation, the time frame in which those actions will need to be accomplished, and the resources that will be required for the response will be very different from what is required for another scenario.

Applicability of Scenarios to Decision-Making and Management Structure of a Smallpox Response

Although the four smallpox scenarios described above (or any range of scenarios) may be of limited utility for differentiating planning efforts that must take place prior to an event, scenarios are useful tools for designing a decision-making and management structure for a smallpox response. Scenarios provide a framework for characterizing the decisions that will need to be made once a smallpox case is identified and the range of decisions that will be necessary, depending upon the circumstances of the outbreak.

Since decisions will need to be made rapidly once there is evidence of a smallpox outbreak, a decision-making and management structure should be agreed upon by federal, state, and local entities before an event—when there is time to consider the options and generate support for the planned decision-making process—so that all parties involved understand how decisions will be made post-event and precious time will not be wasted on process issues. Such a decision-making and management structure should specify how the stages of the progression of the outbreak will be defined and, at each stage, who will make the key decisions, who will be the spokesperson, who will advise those decisions, who will be consulted, who will be informed of the decision, and what types of external validation and advice will be needed. A decision-making and management structure for a smallpox outbreak also should specify the criteria that will be used to decide: if, when, and how strongly to encourage vaccination of the general public; the necessary speed of vaccination activities; when to close social institutions (e.g., schools, public transportation, workplaces) for epidemic control; and when and how to institute isolation and quarantine procedures. By having these decision-making and management process issues specified a priori, the likelihood of confusion, public mistrust, delay, and rushed decision-making will be reduced.

Although it is outside state and local agencies' purview to plan for a nation-wide smallpox emergency that would affect all corners of the country and all segments of the national infrastructure (and the committee chose not to test the smallpox readiness indicators against such a catastrophic scenario), it is important for the federal government to create the necessary linkages across all federal agencies for such a possibility (this could be an extension of the Federal Response Plan coordination activities, with a focus on smallpox).

Pandemic influenza planning is characterized by many of the same decision-making challenges, and any work on these decision-making issues for pandemic influenza planning that could assist smallpox response planning should be utilized. The swine flu event of 1976 provided important lessons and insights into the complications and nuances of responding to an infectious disease outbreak. Since a smallpox outbreak would share many of the characteristics of an influenza pandemic (e.g., surprise emergence, need for vaccination, importance of communication to the public), many of the same guiding principles for decision-making would apply to both types of incidents. The swine flu incident underscored that decision-making during this type of infectious disease outbreak must be incremental and science-based, flexible, designed for efficiency and speed, show clear lines of authority, and have public acceptance (Neustadt and Fineberg, 1978).

Because it is impossible to foreshadow the exact circumstances of a smallpox outbreak, **the committee recommends that a flexible, incremental, science-based decision-making and management structure for smallpox response that includes all levels of government be developed and communicated to state and local agencies so that the consequences of a smallpox outbreak can be managed effectively.**

> Key message #1:
>
> Preparedness must include a greater emphasis on planning, management, and decision-making.

COMMENTS ABOUT THE DRAFT READINESS INDICATORS

The committee reviewed CDC's draft readiness indicators and at its November 2003 meeting received thoughtful input from representatives of the public health, health care, and first responder communities. A significant proportion of the testimony complemented many of the committee's own observations—that some readiness indicators seem unevenly matched (with some very broad and others too detailed and minor), that there is an unnecessarily large number of indicators, and that some indicators are redundant or could be condensed. Furthermore, the committee discussed the issue of score-carding vis-à-vis the greater principle of continuous quality improvement, the purpose of the indicators, a framework for the indicators, and several important elements of preparedness that are under-represented if not completely overlooked in the indicators.

Due to time limitations and because the broader set of all-hazards indicators was still under development, the committee chose not to conduct a "big picture" determination of whether the 10 smallpox indicators are true predictors of smallpox preparedness. The committee did not systematically discuss the full scope of what is required for smallpox and overall preparedness, except to acknowledge that measuring preparedness requires asking "prepared for what?" and hence implies the need for scenarios. Nevertheless, the committee had some detailed comments about each of the 10 smallpox indicators, as described in Appendix 5-A. Committee members also identified important areas initially included in the CDC planning materials and cooperative agreement guidance, but not evident within the larger set of indicators and offers these areas (described below) for consideration as CDC refines its readiness indicators. Furthermore, the committee outlined four scenarios (described above) and the various capabilities needed in each case—an exercise which helped the committee draft some criteria (see Appendix 5-A) to help document "yes" answers to the 10 smallpox indicators and ensure well-rounded assessment of jurisdictions' capabilities in areas identified by the current indicators.

Continuous Quality Improvement

Measuring preparedness should be characterized as a process of continuous quality improvement within the public health system (CDC, 2003c) rather than a way to focus on shortcomings in states' capacities. The readiness indicators themselves should be subject to the process of continuous quality improvement (in relevance and validity), as they are not static but could be expected to change with time as the Public Health Preparedness Project evolves.

Although CDC has stated that it does not intend that the indicators be used in a punitive fashion (Henderson, 2003a), some panelists perceived the notion of score-carding as potentially intimidating to jurisdictions and not necessarily reflective of quality performance and preparedness (Dunn, 2003; Schulman, 2003). Also, in a process of developing an entirely new measurement tool to be used in widely divergent settings and requiring many subjective judgments, using a reporting device (e.g., a red to green spectrum) that suggests precision is probably an error. Any version of a numeric or color-coded scale such as that illustrated in the CDC presentation to the committee seems premature. The use of Likert-type scales is probably appropriate, and the CDC is encouraged to look at the four-level scale already in use in the state and local public health performance indicators as a model (CDC, 2003b, 2003d). Any type of overall score should be similarly based on a common public health framework, which is discussed on subsequent pages.

The committee heard from panelists that yearly assessments of states' bioterrorism and infectious disease preparedness capacities could become a burden. Many assessment and accreditation programs acknowledge this in their routine use of reviews on a multiyear cycle (e.g., Joint Commission on Accreditation of Healthcare Organizations hospital accreditation, health professional education accreditation). In order to ease the resource strain on grantees and to more clearly separate measures of compliance from measures of preparedness, **the committee recommends that CDC consider conducting the preparedness assessments on a multiyear basis** (e.g., every 3 to 4 years).

Concise evaluations of grantee compliance with cooperative agreement requirements could be conducted yearly to provide more frequent assessments of grantee accountability to policy makers and communities.

Key message #2:

Readiness to respond to public health emergencies (including smallpox emergencies) should be part of overall continuous quality improvement of the public health system.

Purpose of the Indicators

A Dual Purpose in Developing Indicators

In its review of the readiness indicators, the committee noted (and also was informed by CDC [Henderson, 2003b]) that the purpose of the indicators is two-fold: to measure grantees' compliance with the CDC cooperative agreement guidance, and to measure grantees' preparedness to respond to public health threats. This duality of purpose is a cause of concern to the committee, as it may lead to having an overly large set of indicators and to using indicators that are not indicative of preparedness. Although the two purposes—compliance and preparedness—are valid and related, one addresses an immediate need, focused on line items to be met by grantees (e.g., meetings held, number of workers trained), while the other is a longer process, focused on outcomes.

The indicators developed to address the immediate need of measuring compliance with the CDC cooperative agreement will accomplish some, but not all, of what is needed for a longer, ongoing assessment of the scope of federal, state, and local preparedness activities. **The committee recommends that CDC address its immediate need of measuring cooperative agreement compliance with a concise and simple set of indicators, and then use this set of indicators as the foundation of a longer, deliberative, national process to develop measures that address the full range and appropriate balance of preparedness activities.**

Distinct Indicators Needed for Federal, State, and Local Jurisdictions

Further questions about the purpose of the indicators ask whose preparedness is being evaluated and whose accountability is being assessed. Most indicators refer to "local and/or state agency" but the committee was unsure whether "local" referred to the four local jurisdictions funded by CDC or to local public health agencies funded in turn by states. The public health panel that addressed the committee at its meeting recommended, and the committee agreed, that there should be separate indicators (or sets of indicators) for local and state jurisdictions (Plough, 2003; Williamson, 2003). It is imperative that the indicators distinguish among the roles of the federal government, states, or local jurisdictions. The indicators should distinctly identify the specific activities for which local jurisdictions are responsible and the specific activities for which states are responsible.

The federal government also needs to be held accountable for its preparedness activities. The federal government and CDC, specifically, are responsible not only for assisting state and local jurisdictions in their preparedness activities and monitoring their progress, but also for carrying out certain activities that must be accomplished at the federal level. The CDC has some unique responsibilities in national smallpox preparedness (e.g., developing a vaccination priority list for the nation, working with FDA for provisional use of smallpox vaccines still under Investigational New Drug protocols, and establishing decision-making and management processes). The role of CDC in national preparedness must be laid out clearly so that state and local jurisdictions have clear assurance of the federal public health resources that will be available in an emergency. **The committee recommends that federal agencies and CDC, specifically, be held accountable for their unique federal responsibilities in an emergency response and assessed on their progress in facilitating national public health emergency preparedness.**

Key message #3:

CDC should address its immediate need of measuring cooperative agreement compliance with a concise and simple set of indicators, and then use this set of indicators as the foundation of a longer, deliberative, national process to develop measures that address the full range and appropriate balance of preparedness activities.

Key message #4:

Federal agencies bear unique responsibilities in emergency response, and they should be held accountable and assessed on their progress, similar to their state and local counterparts.

BOX F-1
The Essential Public Health Services

1. **Monitor** health status to identify community health problems
2. **Diagnose and investigate** health problems and health hazards in the community
3. **Inform, educate, and empower** people about health issues
4. **Mobilize** community partnerships to identify and solve health problems
5. **Develop policies and plans** that support individual and community health efforts
6. **Enforce laws and regulations** that protect health and ensure safety
7. **Link** people to needed personal health services and assure the provision of health care when otherwise unavailable
8. **Assure** a competent public health and personal health care workforce
9. **Evaluate** effectiveness, accessibility, and quality of personal and population-based health services
10. **Research** for new insights and innovative solutions to health problems

SOURCE: CDC (2003c).

A Framework for Readiness Indicators

It was not apparent to the committee what framework was used to develop and structure the readiness indicators and to ensure that there are indicators identified for every major component of preparedness. CDC noted that it is moving away from the focus areas described in the CDC cooperative agreement guidance for FY 2003 (CDC, 2003a) but did not explain what, if any, new framework would be used, and one does not emerge from the indicators document, other than the four chronological goals (pre-event activities; detection and reporting; response and containment; recovery).

The committee recommends that CDC consider utilizing the Ten Essential Public Health Services as a framework for the readiness indicators (see Box F-1). There are several reasons for this recommendation. The 10 essential services are fundamental in identifying the core responsibilities of public health and, therefore, the capacities and resources a public health system needs to be effective. The importance of a strong public health infrastructure for preparedness has been emphasized repeatedly (GAO, 2000; IOM, 2002a; Salinsky, 2002), because preparedness for bioterrorism does not occur in a vacuum but is one component of a public health system capable of maintaining optimal population health against a wide range of current and potential threats. Also, the 10 essential services are a well-established framework widely used by local and state public health agencies in planning and evaluation, and they have served as the foundation for the Department of Justice/CDC Public Health Performance Assessment for Emergency Preparedness (DOJ, 2000), and most important, for the National Public Health Performance Standards (CDC, 2003c), which are used by many public health agencies to measure performance and ensure continuous quality improvement (NACCHO, 2002).

Other sets of indicators could be used to help refine CDC's readiness indicators process. To ensure reasonable alignment with global preparedness efforts, the World Health Organization's indicators effort should be reviewed (WHO, 2003). Also, the Department of Health and Human Services (DHHS) Metropolitan Medical Response System (MMRS) program conducted some pioneering work in the areas of multi-sectoral coordination for preparedness, bringing together public health, government, first responders, health care, and others. IOM's *Tools for Evaluating the Metropolitan Medical Response System Program: Phase I Report* (2001) highlighted the importance of placing the "emphasis on enhancing existing systems rather than building new, perhaps competing [ones]" as a principle of preparedness for chemical, biologic, and radiological terrorism. Using the 10 Essential Public Health Services as a framework for the indicators would reinforce these major structuring principles within the public health system. The IOM review of tools for evaluating the MMRS itself provides some examples of preparedness indicators as well as a comprehensive framework of 23 essential capabilities of preparedness (see Appendix 5-C) (IOM, 2001, 2002b).

Elements Not Reflected in the Readiness Indicators

At its November 6, 2003, meeting, the committee heard from four groups of stakeholders in public health and smallpox preparedness: first responders, health care providers, health care institutions, and the public health community. The panels presented findings from their review of the CDC readiness indicators and focused on areas they considered important to preparedness but were not sufficiently reflected in the indicators: communication, collaboration (in particular, between CDC and the Health Resources and Services Administration), and training and education.

Collaboration and Communication

A recurring theme in the panel presentations is the need for diverse collaborations and the engagement of all relevant stakeholders in the work of preparedness. A closely related theme is communication—among levels of government and the various partners in preparedness, with communities and the general public, and with the media—also an area panelists found missing or severely underrepresented among the indicators, despite the vital importance of effective communication channels and methods in most preparedness activities.

The committee found that, despite the fact that the pre-event guidance emphasized the need for intersectoral relationships among the public health system and the first responder communities (i.e., fire, emergency medical services, law enforcement), the indicators do not reflect this emphasis on collaboration and communication. They contain almost no mention of these important partners in preparedness and little mention of the cross-linkages with health care providers and professional organizations, health care institutions (including, but not limited to, hospitals), and health care insurers. With the exception of a few representatives of the public health community, other partners were not involved in the development of the readiness indicators, although their critical roles in responding to smallpox attack (and other public health crises) were acknowledged and described in earlier planning materials developed by CDC. To remedy these gaps, formal measures of the strength and effectiveness of collaboration could be added to the readiness indicators to assess jurisdictions' capacity in these important areas.

In recent years, the role of communities in the public health system has been increasingly recognized and supported. With their ethnically and culturally diverse populations, service and social organizations, opinion leaders, and faith groups, communities can contribute knowledge and other resources to the work of keeping the population healthy. Bioterrorism is just one of the threats to the public's health, and developing purposeful community engagement in preparedness should be part of the range of activities conducted by the public health agencies and their partners. Involving the community in planning and evaluation requires good communication, building partnerships with organizations and community leaders, and including community representatives in decision-making. This investment in counting communities among partners in preparedness also could lead to a better informed citizenry, which may help to decrease the potential for fear and panic in the course of a bioterror event or other emergency.

Risk communication is largely absent from the activities measured by the smallpox readiness indicators. As the committee has emphasized in previous reports, in particular its second report (IOM, 2003a), effective communication is key to preparedness and should include building relationships with the media, designating trained, trusted, knowledgeable spokesperson(s), developing uniform messages, relaying timely and accurate information to the public, and planning communication strategies and materials to respond to a range of contingencies. The response capacity of the public health system and its partners must include communication strategies and activities, and the readiness indicators should measure communication preparedness. If an event were to occur, would the jurisdiction being assessed have the necessary components of a good communication plan in place and ready to implement immediately, or will it appear unprepared, and thus leading to misinformation, panic, mistrust, and ultimately resulting in a failure to mount an effective emergency response? In a smallpox event (or other emergency), hospital communication capacity also may become overwhelmed by requests for information, and therefore would need readily available communication materials, well-known protocols, and well-established linkages to local and state public health agency spokespersons and resources.

Collaboration and Communication Among Federal Agencies with Health Responsibilities

The relationship between CDC and Health Resources and Services Administration (HRSA) parallels the connections between public health agencies at all levels and health care providers in hospitals, health centers, and communities. Although the CDC and HRSA cooperative agreement guidance documents are somewhat analogous, and make references to each other (and include an appendix about cross-cutting activities and benchmarks), it seemed to both the committee and the panelists that the agencies themselves have yet to fully coordinate their preparedness planning and their work on preparedness indicators. In addition to planning and collaboration at the administrative level, frequent and productive communication using efficient and redundant channels is needed to facilitate the exchange of information between the health care and public health communities, to clarify reporting requirements and technical assistance resources, to familiarize all health care providers and public health workers with each other's roles and capabilities in a smallpox or other emergency, to address unknowns and concerns, and to jointly implement various preparedness activities.

Strengthening surge capacity, discussed below, is an area that requires particular, joint attention from CDC and HRSA, given the interdependence of the public health and health care communities and the need for enhanced familiarity with each other's unique and interrelated responsibilities (e.g., public health to conduct surveillance, and health care to report suspected or confirmed cases), capabilities (e.g., public health to conduct mass vaccination or distribution of countermeasures, and health care to provide diagnosis and treatment), and resources.

Furthermore, the communication and collaboration between the health care and public health communities and relevant federal agencies should extend to the Centers for Medicare and Medicaid Services (CMS), the Department of Defense (DoD), the Department of Veterans Affairs (VA), the Indian Health Service (IHS), and the Substance Abuse and Mental Health Services Administration (SAMHSA). CMS coordinates the Medicaid and Medicare programs, including developing conditions of participation in the programs. If bioterrorism planning and exercises were included among the conditions of participation in Medicaid and Medicare, this could further hospital preparedness planning. DoD, VA, and IHS operate major health care facilities for specific populations and would likely play vital roles in the health care response to a smallpox attack or other emergency. SAMHSA would be responsible for addressing the need for mental health services arising from a bioterrorism event.

Preparedness indicators are needed to assess the strength, scope, stability, and sustainability of health care–public health linkages. **In addition to considering indicators that assess such linkages, the committee recommends that CDC collaborate with HRSA to integrate the preparedness indicators into one document, in order to help the health care and public health communities work hand-in-hand to plan, implement plans, and evaluate their readiness to respond to threats (including, but not limited to, a smallpox attack) and to avoid requiring duplicate reporting from states.**

Training and Education

Another component of preparedness not evident among the readiness indicators is the training and education of all workers (including first responders) expected to respond to a smallpox attack or other public health threat. Well-trained personnel are essential to mount an effective response, and training needs range widely depending on the type and functional responsibilities of personnel. This has been discussed extensively in other committee reports (IOM, 2003a). Several related comments about training and education were provided by meeting panelists (see below).

Issues Related to Surge Capacity

Several CDC readiness indicators focus on surge capacity—the ability to rapidly expand facilities (beds), workforce, and other capabilities (diagnostic, treatment, etc.) in response to a crisis, such as a smallpox attack or major infectious disease outbreak. All stakeholders who participated in the November meeting shared concerns about inadequate surge capacity in their respective health care, public health, and first response communities.

Although health care providers and emergency responders may be able to surge briefly in order to handle an acute event, their surge capacity may be limited if sustained effort is required over a longer period. Both the committee and the groups that provided their input at the committee's meeting identified the need to acknowledge the multiple obstacles to achieving surge capacity and the fact that existing systemic strains and limitations will not be resolved by the influx of bioterrorism funds. The emergency responder communities stated that in a crisis, they would be called upon to continue their usual duties and carry out other functions not necessarily related to public health response (Fischler, 2003). This could limit their ability to help enhance surge capacity for mass vaccination or in other areas. The health care institutions and providers who presented to the committee expressed concern about their ability to contribute to surge capacity when their current resources (e.g., hospital emergency departments, staff) are often overwhelmed by routine needs or even just seasonal spikes (e.g., cases of influenza) (Austin, 2003; GAO, 2003; Temte, 2003).

The surge capacity needs of public health laboratories also require careful consideration, as laboratories confirm diagnoses and conduct essential surveillance functions. It is important that federal and state public health agencies consider the possibility of weaponized smallpox and the need for environmental sampling, as well as the limiting factor of laboratory biosafety level. Furthermore, in a crisis, laboratories share some of the workforce and resource concerns of the public health agencies and health care entities.

Key message #5:

Public health readiness indicators need to address each of the distinct roles of federal, state, and local jurisdictions in the planning for and response to a public health or, specifically, smallpox emergency.

Key message #6:

The current set of readiness indicators provides a useful start to measuring preparedness, but many indicators seem too broad and redundant and not based on any evident framework, such as one common to the public health system.

Key message #7:

The draft readiness indicators do not reflect the significance of active and sustained collaboration and communication among the public health system, the health care system, first responders, and the community (conceived in the broadest sense).

Selected Gaps and Needs of Public Health Preparedness Identified by Stakeholders

The following bulleted list is a loosely structured summary of some of the important comments made by panelists—representatives of the public health, health care (providers and institutions), and first responder communities—invited to address the committee at its November 6, 2003, meeting. CDC has stated that the assessments that will be conducted through the Public Health Preparedness Project will help identify technical assistance needs and gaps in preparedness of state and local public health agencies (Henderson, 2003a). These assessments will be an important tool for gathering information about how preparedness activities across the country need to be improved. To provide some interim guidance, before the systematic assessments of needs and gaps are implemented, the committee summarizes suggestions, problems, and insights offered by panelists. Although these issues are not necessarily incorporated into formal recommendations based on the charge to the committee, CDC is encouraged to consider these issues as appropriate prior to conducting the formal state assessments.

Panelist Comments About Training and Education

- Fire, police, and Emergency Medical Services (EMS) personnel expressed a desire for a simple pocket card that they could keep in their wallets that would describe the symptoms of smallpox compared to other rash illnesses and whom they should call if they suspect they are responding to a case of smallpox (Fischler, 2003).
- There needs to be greater coordination with primary care clinicians. Many are untrained in how to diagnose a case of smallpox (or the manifestation of any other bioterror or chemical agent), as well as how to report a suspected case. Education needs include "just-in-time" information available in real-time to physicians and other health care providers in the event of a possible case (Temte, 2003).
- One way to encourage clinicians to educate themselves on bioterrorism preparedness could be to include some elements of clinical bioterrorism expertise in the regular certification and recertification processes (Hirshon, 2003; Roquemore, 2003).
- First responder personnel need to receive additional education. Any educational materials provided to first responders and health care personnel must be easily accessible, organized simply, and provide the necessary information succinctly (Dunn, 2003; Fischler, 2003; Temte, 2003).

Panelist Comments About Resources (e.g., human, equipment and supplies, communication)

- Many fire, police, and emergency medical services personnel do not have access to personal protective equipment in the case of a bioterror or chemical attack (Peterson, 2003).
- 911 centers should be considered important communication nodes in providing information to the public during an emergency (though these, of course, should not be considered the primary communication nodes) (Fischler, 2003; Maniscalco, 2003; Trimble, 2003).
- A census of emergency medical technicians and EMS agencies, describing how EMS services are organized across the country (and thus, where the connections need to be made for bioterrorism preparedness), has not been conducted since the 1970s (Maniscalco, 2003).
- Many health care professionals currently are not in active practice. They may be in administration, policy, academia, or other careers. It may be useful to work with related professional associations to determine if any of these nonpracticing health care professionals could be mobilized to serve in a clinical capacity in the event of an outbreak (Ricci, 2003).
- Lists of vaccinated and trained health care personnel could be updated using health care professional licensure lists (Peterson, 2003).
- Representatives of both health care and first responder personnel strongly suggested that these personnel and their immediate families receive priority vaccination should a smallpox outbreak occur. For some panelists, this problem could be addressed by increasing access to pre-event vaccination for responders and their families. Health care workers and first responders may be reluctant to report for duty, or be distracted during duty, if they are unsure that their families are protected. Consideration of these issues may be related to supporting surge capacity (Fischler, 2003; Peterson, 2003; Temte, 2003).

Panelist Comments About Surge Capacity

- Changes in the scope of practice of EMS providers for emergencies should be considered, since the health care training that these personnel have received could, where appropriate, contribute to surge capacity in mass vaccination clinics (Fischler, 2003).
- The surge capacity needs of public health laboratories also must be considered. A suspected or confirmed outbreak greatly will increase the number of environmental samples that must be tested by public health laboratories (e.g., testing for anthrax at post offices) (Kelley, 2003).
- Another area of surge capacity that should not be overlooked pertains to handling human remains in an event with significant mortality. The

role of DMORTS and whether their services can fulfill all the surge capacity needs in multiple communities are still unclear (Dunn, 2003).

Panelist Comments about Mental Health

- It is unclear how much federal coordination exists around mental health issues during a smallpox emergency. SAMHSA's role in a smallpox emergency should be characterized more clearly (Benjamin, 2003; Temte, 2003).

Panelist Comments about Populations with Special Needs

- Special issues and concerns of the uninsured and undocumented immigrants need to be considered to a greater extent, as well as the needs of those who are homeless or have disabilities (Benjamin, 2003; Peterson, 2003; Temte, 2003).

CONCLUDING REMARKS

The committee commends CDC for responding to the needs of state and local public health agencies by developing smallpox and overall public health readiness indicators. These indicators are an important step in ensuring that states receive clear guidance on how to become more prepared to respond to a public health emergency, understand how they will be held accountable, and are assured of the federal role in national preparedness for a public health emergency. By addressing the three tasks with which CDC asked for advice (reviewing the smallpox readiness indicators, identifying criteria that could be used for the smallpox indicators, and developing smallpox scenarios that could be used to test the smallpox indicators), the committee has attempted to assist CDC with the important work of assessing the nation's readiness to respond to a smallpox outbreak.

In closing, the committee will summarize the report's key messages:

1. Preparedness must include a greater emphasis on planning, management, and decision-making.
2. Readiness to respond to public health emergencies (including smallpox emergencies) should be part of overall continuous quality improvement of the public health system.
3. CDC should address its immediate need of measuring cooperative agreement compliance with a concise and simple set of indicators, and then use this set of indicators as the foundation of a longer, deliberative, national process to develop measures that address the full range and appropriate balance of preparedness activities.

4. Federal agencies bear unique responsibilities in emergency response, and they should be held accountable and assessed on their progress, similar to their state and local counterparts.

5. Public health readiness indicators need to address each of the distinct roles of federal, state, and local jurisdictions in the planning for and response to a public health or, specifically, smallpox emergency.

6. The current set of readiness indicators provides a useful start to measuring preparedness, but many indicators seem too broad and redundant, and not based on any evident framework, such as one common to the public health system.

7. The draft readiness indicators do not reflect the significance of active and sustained collaboration and communication among the public health system, the health care system, first responders, and the community (conceived in the broadest sense).

The committee wishes to thank you for the continuing opportunity to be of assistance to the Centers for Disease Control and Prevention and its partners as they work to protect the nation's health.

Brian L. Strom, *Committee Chair*
Kristine M. Gebbie, *Committee Vice Chair*
Robert B. Wallace, *Committee Vice Chair*
Committee on Smallpox Vaccination Program Implementation

REFERENCES

Austin B. 2003. Transcript from the IOM's Committee on Smallpox Vaccination Program Implementation Meeting Four on November 6, 2003, Washington, DC:9-11, 13.

Benjamin G. 2003. Transcript from the IOM's Committee on Smallpox Vaccination Program Implementation Meeting Four on November 6, 2003, Washington, DC:144.

Blank S, Moskin LC, Zucker JR. 2003. An ounce of prevention is a ton of work: mass antibiotic prophylaxis for anthrax, New York City, 2001. *Emerging Infectious Diseases* 9(6):615-622.

CDC (Centers for Disease Control and Prevention). 2003a. Unpublished. Information and Instructions on Review of CDC's Smallpox Readiness Indicators for the Institute of Medicine's Smallpox Committee.

CDC. 2003b. Local Public Health System Performance Assessment Instrument in National Public Health Performance Standards Program. [Online] Available at http://www.phppo.cdc.gov/nphpsp/Documents/Local_v_1_OMB_0920–0555.pdf. Accessed November 14, 2003.

CDC. 2003c. National Public Health Performance Standards Program. [Online] Available at http://www.phppo.cdc.gov/nphpsp/. Accessed November 14, 2003.

CDC. 2003d. State Public Health System Performance Assessment Instrument in National Public Health Performance Standards Program. [Online] Available at http://www.phppo.cdc.gov/nphpsp/Documents/State_v_1_OMB_0920–0557.pdf. Accessed November 14, 2003.

DOJ (U.S. Department of Justice). 2000. Fiscal Year 1999 State Domestic Preparedness Support Program. [Online] Available at http://www.ojp.usdoj.gov/odp/assessment.pdf. Accessed November 14, 2003.

Dunn V. 2003. Transcript from the IOM's Committee on Smallpox Vaccination Program Implementation Meeting Four on November 6, 2003, Washington, DC:195-196, 207, 220.

Edmiston CE, Graham MB, Wilson PJ, Grahn B. 2003. The monkeypox virus outbreak: reflections from the frontline. *American Journal of Infection Control* 31:382-384.

Emanuel EJ. 2003. The lessons of SARS. *Annals of Internal Medicine*. 139(7):589-591.

Fischler D. 2003. Transcript from the IOM's Committee on Smallpox Vaccination Program Implementation Meeting Four on November 6, 2003, Washington, DC: 228-239, 252.

GAO (U.S. General Accounting Office). 2000. West Nile Virus Outbreak: Lessons for Public Health Preparedness. GAO/HEHS-00-180. Washington, DC: Health, Education, and Human Services Division.

GAO. 2003. Infectious Diseases: Gaps Remain in Surveillance Capabilities of State and Local Agencies. GAO-03-1176T. Washington, DC: Health, Education, and Human Services Division.

Henderson J. 2003a. Transcript from the IOM's Committee on Smallpox Vaccination Program Implementation Meeting Four on November 6, 2003, Washington, DC:26-108.

Henderson J. 2003b. Update on National Smallpox Preparedness: Smallpox Preparedness Indicators. Presented to the IOM's Committee on Smallpox Vaccination Program Implementation on November 6, 2003.

Hirshon JM. 2003. Transcript from the IOM's Committee on Smallpox Vaccination Program Implementation Meeting Four on November 6, 2003, Washington, DC:180.

IOM (Institute of Medicine). 2001. Tools for Evaluating the Metropolitan Medical Response System Program: Phase I Report. Washington, DC: National Academy Press.

IOM. 2002a. The Future of the Public's Health in the 21st Century. Washington, DC: The National Academies Press.

IOM. 2002b. Preparing for Terrorism: Tools for Evaluating the Metropolitan Medical Response System Program. Washington, DC: The National Academies Press.

IOM. 2003a. Review of the Centers for Disease Control and Prevention's Smallpox Vaccination Program Implementation: Letter Report #2. Washington, DC: The National Academies Press.

IOM. 2003b. Review of the Centers for Disease Control and Prevention's Smallpox Vaccination Program Implementation: Letter Report #4. Washington, DC: The National Academies Press.

Kelley K. 2003. Transcript from the IOM's Committee on Smallpox Vaccination Program Implementation Meeting Four on November 6, 2003 in Washington, DC:141-142.

MacKenzie D. 2003, June 21. Slow Response to Monkeypox Reveals Glaring Gap in Bioterror Defenses. *New Scientist*, 12.

Maniscalco P. 2003. Transcript from the IOM's Committee on Smallpox Vaccination Program Implementation Meeting Four on November 6, 2003, Washington, DC:243-244, 260-261.

NACCHO (National Association of County and City Health Officials). 2002. Compendium of Resolutions. [Online] Available at http://www.naccho.org/files/documents/compendium-May-2002.pdf. Accessed November 14, 2003.

Neustadt RE, Fineberg HF. 1978. The Swine Flu Affair: Decision-Making on a Slippery Disease. U.S. Department of Health, Education, and Welfare.

Peterson C. 2003. Transcript from the IOM's Committee on Smallpox Vaccination Program Implementation Meeting Four on November 6, 2003, Washington, DC:151-157, 166.

Plough A. 2003. Transcript from the IOM's Committee on Smallpox Vaccination Program Implementation Meeting Four on November 6, 2003, Washington, DC:109-151.

Ricci K. 2003. Transcript from the IOM's Committee on Smallpox Vaccination Program Implementation Meeting Four on November 6, 2003, Washington, DC:190.
Roquemore J. 2003. Transcript from the IOM's Committee on Smallpox Vaccination Program Implementation Meeting Four on November 6, 2003, Washington, DC: 241-242.
Salinsky E. 2002. Will the Nation Be ready for the Next Bioterrorism Attack? Mending Gaps in the Public Health Infrastructure. NHPF Issue Brief No. 776. Washington, DC: National Health Policy Forum.
Selecky M. 2003. Transcript from the IOM's Committee on Smallpox Vaccination Program Implementation Meeting Three on May 1, 2003, Washington, DC:93-94.
Schulman R. 2003. Transcript from the IOM's Committee on Smallpox Vaccination Program Implementation Meeting Four on November 6, 2003, Washington, DC:213-214.
Temte J. 2003. Transcript from the IOM's Committee on Smallpox Vaccination Program Implementation Meeting Four on November 6, 2003, Washington, DC: 157-159, 165-166, 173-174, 186.
Trimble M. 2003. Transcript from the IOM's Committee on Smallpox Vaccination Program Implementation Meeting Four on November 6, 2003, Washington, DC.
White House. 2002. President Delivers Remarks on Smallpox. [Online] Available at http://www.whitehouse.gov/news/releases/2002/12/20021213-7.html. Accessed January 8, 2003.
WHO (World Health Organization). 2003. Unpublished. Strengthening National Health Preparedness and Response for Chemical and Biological Weapons Threats.
Williamson D. 2003. Transcript from the IOM's Committee on Smallpox Vaccination Program Implementation Meeting Four on November 6, 2003, Washington, DC:109-151.

APPENDIX 5-A
DRAFT SMALLPOX INDICATORS AND SUGGESTED CRITERIA

The committee reviewed the draft 10 smallpox indicators included in CDC's readiness indicators document. The committee's analysis does not reflect an endorsement of the current indicators as indicative of readiness for smallpox attack. In fact, some of the indicators seem narrow and unclear, whereas others seem to incorporate multiple activities, and it is not evident whether and how they could represent a carefully selected, concise set of the most relevant measures of smallpox preparedness.

The committee outlined four scenarios, discussed the indicators as they would operate in each scenario, and developed some examples of criteria that might help assess a jurisdiction's work in an area summarized by a given indicator. Unless otherwise noted, the committee believes that the criteria it developed would apply to all scenarios. The committee has also indicated, as appropriate, whether a criterion is applicable to state public health agencies, local public health agencies, or both.

Indicator 1.1.9.1: Legal issues related to smallpox vaccination (e.g., liability, compensation, licensure for administration of vaccine, investigational new drug issues) have been reviewed and addressed.

This indicator should be broadened to more fully reflect the wide range of legal issues pertaining not only to vaccination, but to smallpox preparedness in general. Such issues would include quarantine, isolation, access to medical records, legal authority to mandate employees to work, emergency medical technicians' scope of practice, etc.

Within the framework provided by the Ten Essential Public Health Services, this indicator corresponds to Essential Services 5 and 6.

Suggested Criteria

- Are appropriate consent forms available and in use? (most relevant for scenario 1, and less for 2-4) (either state or local level, as appropriate)
- Are copies of relevant public health law available in all appropriate agencies?
- Is there documentation of thorough legal review to ensure that the jurisdiction's law is current, including a record of changes and decisions made with policy-makers? (state level)
- Is information about relevant public health laws included in new employee orientation handbooks? (state and local levels)
- Is there documentation of legal authority for emergency licensing and credentialing?
- Are there information sheets describing the relevant legal issues in appropriate language to all relevant stakeholders, including the general public? (state or local, depending on the state's plan)
- What evidence is there of a review of federal legislation and decisions made? (most important in scenario 4)
- Have federal agencies provided state/local agencies with documentation of federal legal authority and described under what circumstances federal agencies would become involved and what they would do (or other material defining the transition from one level of authority to another)? (most important in scenario 4)

Indicator 1.3.3.1: Local and/or state public health has identified and secured governmental and nongovernmental agencies for surge capacity at mass distribution sites for medical countermeasures (e.g., vaccination).

Indicator 1.3.4.1: Local and/or state public health has trained governmental and nongovernmental agencies for surge capacity at mass distribution sites for medical countermeasures (e.g., vaccination).

Indicator 1.3.5.1: Local and/or state public health has identified and secured community resources for surge capacity as mass distribution for medical countermeasures (e.g., facilities).

The three indicators above can be easily grouped into one, because they are all related to preparation for mass distribution of vaccine (or other countermeasures). The new, joint indicator might read as follows: Local and/or state public health has identified, engaged, and trained governmental and nongovernmental agencies to participate in and taken the necessary steps to establish sites for mass distribution of vaccine (or other countermeasures).

Within the framework provided by the Ten Essential Public Health Services, these indicators correspond to Essential Service 7 and 8.

Suggested Criteria

- Does the agency have lists with contact information, addresses, and letters of agreement with all planned distribution sites in the community? (state or local, depending on which is managing the distribution process)
- Does the operational plan (which should be consistent with CDC guidelines) include rosters of staff, with contact information, functional role descriptions, and evidence of training for all personnel on the roster? (state or local, depending on which is managing the distribution process)
- Are there written collaborative agreements with all agencies that would be involved in some aspect of vaccination/distribution of countermeasures (school districts, EMS, law enforcement, etc.)? (state or local, depending on which is managing the distribution process)

Indicator 2.3.1.1: Local and/or state public health maintains core personnel who are trained to provide technical assistance in the differential diagnosis of smallpox syndrome.

Indicator 3.1.10.1: Local and/or state public health trains health care personnel to provide differential diagnosis of smallpox syndrome.

These indicators are closely related and should be integrated. "Differential diagnosis" is more clearly worded as "confirming the diagnosis of . . . ." The new, combined indicator might read as follows: Local and/or state public health agency has trained health care personnel and has core personnel available to provide technical assistance in confirming the diagnosis of smallpox syndrome.

Within the framework provided by the Ten Essential Public Health Services, these indicators correspond to Essential Service 2 and 8.

Suggested Criteria

- Is there a plan for ongoing education and training of health care providers and evidence of its implementation? (state or local, depending on specific state plan)
- Do local public health agencies have contact information at every

hospital and a communication method for immediately informing all hospital and community-based providers of a smallpox case?

- Is there a system for 24/7 two-way communication between the public health agency and health care providers (including what samples to get and where to send them)?
- Does the alert system include information on how a provider can immediately access "just-in-time" provider training on the diagnosis of smallpox?

All these criteria (except the first) would be evidenced by retrospective analysis of actual test cases (monkeypox, varicella) or a (unannounced) test case/drill.

Indicator 3.1.12.1: Local and/or state public health has secured community resources for surge capacity as sites for medical care and monitoring for potential victims of a smallpox outbreak (e.g. facilities).

Within the framework provided by the Ten Essential Public Health Services, this indicator corresponds to Essential Services 4 and 7.

Suggested Criteria

- Is there a community plan for the distribution of initial smallpox cases for medical care?
- Is there a triage plan for making space for an escalating number of cases?
- Are there resources (workforce, buildings, access to emergency funds) or plans to access resources to operationalize the triage plan?
- e.g., is there a current contact list for health care providers who have agreed to participate in the treatment of victims, including their vaccination status and multiple means to contact them?
- e.g., is there a list of all appropriate isolation rooms in the community?
- Is there a plan for the disposal of remains?
- Do facility/agency plans identify the other services or functions that would need to be maintained during the emergency (what *must* be provided and what can temporarily be suspended)?
- Are plans in place to support the environmental sampling surge capacity needs of public health laboratories?
- Is there a plan for the psychological management and general mental health issues of the worried well and of the families of health care providers and first responders?
- Is there a plan for the recovery of facilities after the epidemic is ended?

Indicator 3.1.3.1: Local and/or state public health identified members of epidemiology investigation and surveillance teams targeted for immediate smallpox vaccination.

This indicator is unclear in several ways. First, it should be clarified whether "immediate" means "pre-event," and whether "epidemiology investigation and surveillance teams" refers to the public health response teams commonly described in the CDC guidance. Second, the wording used implies three related tasks: the identification of teams, defining the qualifications required for teams, and the vaccination of teams. It should be made clear exactly which task(s) the indicator aims to evaluate. Because this indicator only applies to pre-event activities, it is only applicable to scenario 1; it is presumed under scenarios 2, 3, and 4.

Within the framework provided by the Ten Essential Public Health Services, this indicator corresponds to Essential Services 1 and 2.

Suggested Criteria

- Is there an updated list or registry for each locale with smallpox public health response team members' names, contact information, and vaccination status?
- Does the team possess the minimum public health bioterrorism response competencies appropriate to their role(s)?
- Is there an effective, efficient notification system for contacting team members?

Indicator 3.1.9.1: Local and/or state public health identifies members of epidemiology and investigation teams targeted for immediate smallpox vaccination following the notification of an outbreak.

The indicator wording should be clarified to explain what "notification of an outbreak" really means. Does this mean when an outbreak is officially declared? Immediately after a single case is identified? When an outbreak occurs anywhere in the world or in the United States? Also, as in 3.1.3.1, does "epidemiology investigation and surveillance teams" mean the public health response teams commonly described in the CDC guidance?

The indicator also implies three different tasks, and it is unclear which task is being evaluated, whether it is the identification of teams, the vaccination of teams, or the expansion of teams with functional role descriptions for needed expertise.

This indicator is not applicable to scenario 1, which is pre-event (i.e., before an outbreak), but it may apply to scenario 2 and is most relevant to scenarios 3 and 4 due to enhanced surveillance needs.

Within the framework provided by the Ten Essential Public Health Services, this indicator corresponds to Essential Services 1 and 2.

Suggested Criteria

- Is there an updated list/registry for each locale with smallpox emergency team members' names, contact information, and vaccination status?
- Does the team possess the minimum team competencies as described above? If not, is there a plan for acquiring members with those competencies immediately after notification of an outbreak?
- Has the notification system for contacting team members been tested and is it effective in mobilizing the team within the desired time frame (with a time parameter if that can be identified)?

Indicator 3.3.2.1: Local and/or state public health will stockpile at least 20 doses of smallpox vaccine per 100,000 population to be available at all times (or a minimum of 1,000 doses [=10 vials] for states with population <3 million) in order to respond initially to a smallpox outbreak using search and containment strategies.

It seems that the terms "search and containment" imply that this stockpile is meant for commencing ring vaccination and intended to be short-term and limited. It is unclear whether states are advised to have one or multiple storage sites. Furthermore, is there a plan (and ways to communicate it) for prioritizing access to the vaccine in the initial 24 hours post-event, including considering vaccinating the families of responders?

This indicator applies to all scenarios.

Within the framework provided by the Ten Essential Public Health Services, this indicator corresponds to Essential Service 7.

Suggested Criteria

- Is the stockpiled smallpox vaccine in an appropriate storage facility ("appropriate" to be defined by CDC)?
- Is there a distribution plan for the stockpile, with a timeline for distribution?

Possible Additional Indicators

The set of smallpox indicators, as well as that of overall readiness indicators, seems to lack several important measures. Some, such as measures to assess communication and collaboration, were discussed to a greater extend in the text of the report. As CDC moves forward in refining and pilot-testing the indicators, some additional areas should be considered to ensure that even a limited set of indicators provides a comprehensive assessment of readiness. Such additional measures include, but are not limited to:

- Sentinel indicators of diversion of effort, such as childhood immunization rates.
- The implementation of exercises and drills (which are both a way to test some of the criteria for various indicators, and an indicator on their own—does public health agency conduct drills/exercises and how does it do?).

APPENDIX 5-B
SUMMARY OF RECOMMENDATIONS

1. If CDC intends to use scenarios as a planning tool, the committee recommends that the scenarios represent a range of possible situations, be used to help guide state and local planning activities, and facilitate state and local assessment of their level of preparedness.
2. The committee recommends that a flexible, incremental, science-based decision-making and management structure for smallpox response that includes all levels of government be developed and communicated to state and local agencies so that the consequences of a smallpox outbreak can be managed effectively.
3. The committee recommends that CDC consider conducting the preparedness assessments on a multiyear basis.
4. The committee recommends that CDC address its immediate need of measuring cooperative agreement compliance with a concise and simple set of indicators, and then use this set of indicators as the foundation of a longer, deliberative, national process to develop measures that address the full range and appropriate balance of preparedness activities.
5. The committee recommends that federal agencies and CDC, specifically, be held accountable for their unique federal responsibilities in an emergency response and assessed on their progress in facilitating national public health emergency preparedness.
6. The committee recommends that CDC consider utilizing the Ten Essential Public Health Services as a framework for the readiness indicators.
7. The committee recommends that CDC collaborate with HRSA to integrate the preparedness indicators into one document, in order to help the health care and public health communities work hand-in-hand to plan, implement plans, and evaluate their readiness to respond to threats (includ-

ing, but not limited to, a smallpox attack) and to avoid requiring duplicate reporting from states.

APPENDIX 5-C
ESSENTIAL CAPABILITIES NEEDED FOR PREPAREDNESS

Source: IOM. 2002. Preparing for Terrorism: Tools for Evaluating the Metropolitan Medical Response System Program. Washington, DC: The National Academies Press, pp. 115-159.

1. Relationship development
2. Communication system development
3. Hazard assessment
4. Training
5. Equipment and supplies
6. Mass immunization and prophylaxis
7. Addressing the information needs of the public and the news media
8. First responder protection
9. Rescue and stabilization of victims
10. Diagnosis and agent identification
11. Decontamination of victims
12. Transportation of victims
13. Distribution of supplies, equipment, and pharmaceuticals
14. Shelter and feeding of evacuated and displaced persons
15. Definitive medical care (includes mass immunization or distribution of drugs or vaccines)
16. Mental health services for responders, victims, caregivers, and their families
17. Volunteer utilization and control
18. Crowd and traffic control
19. Evacuation and quarantine decisions and operations
20. Fatality management
21. Environmental cleanup, physical restoration of facilities, and certification of safety
22. Follow-up study of responder, caregiver, and victim health
23. Process for continuous evaluation of needs and resources

G

Review of the Centers for Disease Control and Prevention's Smallpox Vaccination Program Implementation, Letter Report #6

July 6, 2004
Dr. Julie Gerberding
Director
Centers for Disease Control and Prevention (CDC)
1600 Clifton Road, NE
Atlanta, GA 30333

Dear Dr. Gerberding:

The Institute of Medicine (IOM) Committee on Smallpox Vaccination Program Implementation is pleased to offer you the sixth in a series of brief reports.

This report may seem like a departure from the committee's previous work, which focused on smallpox vaccination as a part of public health preparedness. However, this report responds to a CDC request for guidance as the agency moves toward comprehensive preparedness for bioterrorism and other public health disasters and toward broad smallpox preparedness efforts. The committee was asked to look specifically at preparedness exercises, which are required by CDC grant guidance and are being conducted by public health agencies. In general, the public health community has somewhat limited experience with exercises, so the committee was asked to describe the state of the science in evaluation of exercises, to identify leadership and experience to build on, and to identify issues or concerns about the use of exercises as a means to performance measurement.

At its fifth meeting, on March 29, 2004, the committee heard presentations about: CDC's recent efforts in public health preparedness; the modeling workgroup of the Department of Health and Human Services (DHHS) Secretary's Council on Public Health Preparedness; the theory and science related to preparedness and exercises[1] from both a sociological and a disaster management and response perspective; the perspective of a Center for Public Health Preparedness; and the Department of Homeland Security's experience with planning, conducting, and evaluating exercises. This letter report contains the committee's findings and recommendations based on information from that meeting and additional though limited (given time constraints) review of what public health may learn from disaster research and from the practice of disaster response.

INTRODUCTION

Charge to the Committee

One way to measure public health agencies' performance in achieving preparedness is by performing and evaluating exercises.[2] Whereas exercises have been conducted and evaluated in the emergency management field for many years, public health has had less experience with exercises and is currently beginning to assess their value for relationship building, training, and performance measurement. To place the role of exercises appropriately into the broader definition of what it means to be prepared and to identify specific aspects for which measures can be developed, CDC asked the Committee on Smallpox Vaccination Program Implementation to:

1. Describe the state of the science in exercises and related preparedness strategies;
2. Identify leadership and experience to build upon, from other fields and other federal agencies; and
3. Identify issues or concerns about this approach to performance measurement (Sosin, 2004).

---

[1]The Federal Emergency Management Agency (FEMA) defines exercise as "a focused practice activity that places the participants in a simulated situation requiring them to function in the capacity that would be expected of them in a real event" (FEMA/EMI, 2003).

[2]Initially, the committee's discussion was concerned with both exercises and drills, as they are related categories along a spectrum of possible activities used for training, performance measurement, etc. However, since drills tend to be very narrowly focused and they typically take place within a single agency, their usefulness is more easily verified. Therefore, they are less relevant to the present broad discussion of preparedness exercises and evidence of their usefulness.

To meet the charge presented by CDC, the committee has endeavored to: (1) examine conceptual issues and challenges related to integrating public health into disaster preparedness and response; (2) review some of the evidence base from disaster research and practice that is germane to public health preparedness; (3) learn from the public health response to proxy events; (4) discuss the usefulness of modeling; and (5) discuss the usefulness of exercises, including a description of some of the exercise activities occurring in the federal government.

Summary of Recommendations

The report's recommendations revolve around the issues of interagency and intersectoral coordination, learning from experience and research, and continuously improving performance.

Recommendation 1:
The committee recommends that all federal entities concerned with bioterrorism preparedness (e.g., CDC, the Health Resources and Services Administration [HRSA], the Office of Domestic Preparedness [ODP]) should more actively coordinate guidance and funding activities. Federal agencies should also work together to develop mechanisms that facilitate coordination and collaboration among their grantees at the state and local levels. Such mechanisms may include, but are not limited to, regular meetings to familiarize CDC and ODP program staff with each other's program priorities and activities, a database for informing ODP and other partners of exercises planned by CDC grantees, etc. Federal coordination efforts should also include the clarification of primary responsibility and authority in bioterrorism events, to ensure that CDC can fulfill its unique role as the nation's public health agency.

Recommendation 2:
The committee recommends that CDC should collaborate with all of its partners to strengthen preparedness by applying research findings and experience in public health emergency response, bioterrorism preparedness, and disaster management. In order to strengthen the evidence base for public health preparedness, CDC should:

- **Strengthen the link between public health research and practice;**
- **Participate in and promote interdisciplinary research about preparedness;**
- **Support a system to assure the ongoing collection, synthesis, and sharing of lessons learned and best practices from public health preparedness exercises and public health response to proxy events; and**

- **In coordination with the appropriate federal-level partners, such as the Agency for Healthcare Research and Quality, evaluate the effectiveness, design, and opportunity costs of preparedness strategies, such as exercises.**

Recommendation 3:
The committee recommends that CDC should use the Evidence-Based Performance Goals for Public Health Disaster Preparedness to develop standards against which CDC, states, and localities may regularly measure their performance in exercises and in response to proxy events. Public health agency performance in exercises and proxy events should be used to identify gaps in preparedness and to improve planning, communication, and coordination at the agency and interagency levels, as part of a process of continuous quality improvement in preparedness planning and response. Preparedness drills and exercises should not be evaluated individually, but their cumulative and long-term impact on preparedness, such as generalizability to other potential hazards, must be considered in the evaluation process

INTEGRATING PUBLIC HEALTH INTO DISASTER PREPAREDNESS AND RESPONSE: CONCEPTUAL ISSUES

The public health community has become an active partner in the world of emergency and disaster preparedness and response, joining other members in the traditional emergency management and response field who have defined roles and established ways of doing work (Landesman et al., 2001). Although public health workers and agencies have played active roles after many emergency events (and in some states, the emergency medical services [EMS] entity is part of the state public health agency), public health workers have not necessarily counted themselves or been counted among emergency responders (Landesman et al., 2001; Kahsai and Kare, 2002).

Some important conceptual issues must be considered in the process of more effectively integrating public health into the disaster preparedness and response field. These issues include (1) the history of public health disaster response, and its relevance to contemporary public health preparedness; (2) the unique role of public health in disasters and primary role in disasters that involve biological agents; and (3) the heterogeneity that characterizes the field of emergency and disaster preparedness and response.

A History of Public Health Disaster Response

History provides myriad examples of public health emergencies and disasters (e.g., cholera outbreaks, toxic spills), that wreaked destruction akin to or greater than that of major natural disasters and to which the evolving discipline of public health responded. Epidemiologic and other public health skills and knowledge also have been advanced through lessons learned in such responses (Landesman et al., 2001).

The threat of bioterrorism has mobilized the engagement of many disciplines and government agencies both to prevent and to respond. The reemergence of infectious diseases in part related to demographic change and globalization has elevated interest in public health's role as both a responder to and a preventer of epidemics and infectious disease outbreaks. Public health agencies have the ongoing responsibility to prevent disease outbreaks and other emergencies through measures such as immunization, sanitation, and community education. In cases where preventive measures are not successful, or there are barriers to their implementation, or an unexpected threat causes disease, public health becomes a responder, conducting surveillance, controlling the spread of disease, conducting mass immunization, etc. At the same time, public health agencies continue prevention to limit secondary public health problems. The current integration of public health preparedness efforts with those of more traditional "responder" disciplines is based on a growing acknowledgement of public health's singular capabilities and importance in preparing for and responding to bioterrorism, as well as the health aspects of a range of disasters. These include deliberate attacks with nonbiological weapons, natural disasters that may result in the contamination of food or water supplies and lead to infectious diseases, and technological disasters that may endanger population health with radiation or chemical hazards.

Unique Role of Public Health in Disasters, and Primary Role in Response to Bioterrorism

Public health generally does not have a formal tradition of disaster preparedness and response. However, notable and instructive exceptions are found in the experience of the following types of public health agencies, some of which have developed varying levels of expertise in planning and exercising for disasters and in managing disasters (e.g., the experience of the state of Georgia described by Werner et al., 1998):

- Public health agencies located in the vicinity of nuclear facilities and involved in federally mandated training and exercise programs;
- Public health agencies located in areas with frequent natural disasters (hurricanes, floods, or tornadoes);
- Public health agencies at sites of one-time or recurring major events or entertainment venues (e.g., auto racing, Olympics, amusement parks); and

- State public health agencies in states where emergency medical services (EMS) are integrated into the public health agency.

The role of public health in disaster preparedness and response is unique and is not performed by any of the other disciplines that typically respond to disasters and that differ from public health in mission, services provided, and personnel training (e.g., EMS, clinical medicine). Therefore, the role of public health as a responder needs to be formalized and become an indispensable and recognizable part of comprehensive response to disasters. One common thread characterizes the work of public health agencies in relation to most types of disasters: they possess the knowledge and skills required to safeguard the health of the public by limiting morbidity and mortality, whether an event poses a threat to health from the outset (i.e., bioterrorism) or creates secondary threats to health, as in the case of natural disasters. The public health community's role before, during, and after the occurrence of disasters is to some extent anchored in its capacity to conduct routine, noncrisis activities, and is consistent with public health's assessment, policy development, and assurance functions, but varies with community resources and interagency agreements and service provision roles (Salinsky, 2002). Carrying out these functions requires public health agencies to collect, evaluate, and disseminate information; cooperate and collaborate with other disciplines (including, but not limited to, the health care sector); and to prevent disease and ensure the continuity of health care (Landesman et al., 2001; IOM, 2003d).

In addition to the public health effects of most other types of disasters, attacks with biologic agents, as exemplified by the anthrax attacks of 2001, require that governmental public health agencies serve as primary responders. Events that involve biologic agents are different from other types of disasters because their emergence is likely to go unnoticed for some time; biologic agents are microscopic and may be more likely to be introduced silently (e.g., through airborne droplets), rather than with explosions, and become evident over time. Also, the fallout from attacks with biologic agents may not remain confined to a specific physical space; in other words, there may not be a "scene" or a "ground zero" (Perry, 2003) and its impact may not be contained but may ripple outward for some time due to contagion. Preparedness for biologic agents therefore involves at least some different requirements from other types of agents and requires the unique knowledge and skills of trained public health personnel (e.g., case identification and containment) and the unique capabilities (e.g., laboratories, surveillance, communication, community education) and statutory responsibilities (e.g., quarantine) of public health agencies, as well as the complementary facilities, skills, and resources of the health care community (Perry, 2003).

	Nonbioterrorism disasters	Bioterrorism disasters
Public Health	Support role to limit morbidity and mortality due to secondary health effects	Primary role, given the direct and potentially immense health effect
Traditional First Responders	Primary role To mitigate the loss of life and property	Support role, multifaceted

FIGURE G-1 Contrasting roles of public health and traditional responders in bioterrorism and other disasters.

In order to integrate the preparedness and response efforts of public health most appropriately with those of the traditional emergency management and response field, some key differences need to be identified. For example, disaster preparedness and response is the central mission of local, state, and national civilian and military response organizations and they train and exercise regularly to test and maintain their response capabilities. They have the dual role of responding to disasters and to routine emergencies in their communities. For public health agencies, responding to major crises has been the exception from their usual work; therefore, conducting regular drills and training to prepare for disaster response has generally not been a common practice. Also, even when public health agencies have gained experience dealing with disease outbreaks, these events do not typically reach the scale of a disaster, and response is largely limited to the public health and health care communities.

Given the statutory responsibilities and special capabilities of public health, and CDC's leadership role in the provision of essential public health services under all circumstances, it is clear that CDC and the public health community must be ready to fulfill their primary role in responding to bioterrorism and their support roles in other types of disasters, including terrorism with chemical, nuclear, and other types of weapons (see Figure G-1).

The Diverse Field of Emergency and Disaster Preparedness and Response

Public health is not entering a monolithic or homogeneous field of emergency and disaster management. Disasters involve people, physical structures, and the broader environment, and they may be caused by a wide range of natural, technological, and deliberately introduced agents. This variety of factors explains the complex array of disciplines and organizations involved in the emergency and disaster response field. The category of first responders has typically included personnel from the firefighting, EMS, and law enforcement fields, along with state emergency management agencies and federal agencies (e.g., Federal Emergency Management Agency, Environmental Protection Agency), and nongovernmental organizations, such as the Red Cross and the Salvation Army. Other disciplines involved in preparedness include structural engineers, civic planners, public administrators, etc. Clearly, the set of contributors to emergency and disaster preparedness and response is vast and includes a patchwork of methods, cultures, and disciplines that are in some cases themselves struggling to integrate their activities (Kahsai and Kare, 2002; Tang and Fabbri, 2003). In addition to being multidisciplinary, the field of emergency and disaster preparedness and response is undergoing change toward increased professionalization and an all-hazards[3] approach, and is evaluating its assumptions and modes of practice, as discussed elsewhere in this report (Alexander, 2003; NRC, 2003).

CHALLENGES AND OPPORTUNITIES INHERENT IN INTEGRATING PUBLIC HEALTH INTO A BROADER FIELD

The integration of a relative newcomer into the large and complex field of emergency and disaster preparedness and response presents challenges and tensions. Disasters require rapid decisions and quick action, which may bring about cross-jurisdictional conflicts, professional differences, and questions about authority, expertise, and the appropriate chain of command.

Coordination Issues

In its fifth report (IOM, 2003a), the committee discussed at some length the importance of close collaboration between the public health and health care communities, from the level of federal agencies such as HRSA and CDC, to local public health agencies and their health care counterparts (health care organizations, hospitals, private providers, long-term care facilities, etc.). Previous reports by this committee also have called for public health and health care organizations and workers to coordinate and col-

[3]The term "all-hazards" refers to the full spectrum of causes of disasters, which now includes not only natural and technological, but also deliberate, that is, terrorist-induced (Landesman et al., 2001).

laborate with agencies, disciplines, and entities with which they were previously not well acquainted, including, but not limited to, fire authorities, law enforcement, EMS, voluntary organizations, and communities.

Research and practical experience show that coordination among all agencies involved is one of the fundamental requirements of effective disaster response and that the lack of adequate coordination is one of the major problems encountered in the field (Auf der Heide, 1989; Tierney et al., 2001). Given the large number of federal, state, and local agencies involved in preparedness efforts, establishing adequate coordination across federal, state, and local levels is proving to be a challenge (Advisory Panel to Assess Domestic Response Capabilities for Terrorism Involving Weapons of Mass Destruction, 2003; GAO, 2003a; Clements and Evans, 2004). Within the federal government, preparedness and response activities are coordinated through the Department of Homeland Security (DHS). Coordination at the top levels of the federal government occurs through the Homeland Security Council (HSC), which is charged with ensuring coordination of all homeland security related activities among executive departments and agencies and promoting the effective development and implementation of all homeland security policies (White House, 2001). Day-to-day coordination of homeland security issues—both within the federal government and among federal, state, and local government agencies—is meant to occur through the Policy Coordination Committees (PCCs) of the HSC (White House, 2001). There are eleven PCCs for different functional areas, including a Medical and Public Health Preparedness PCC. The committee was unable to obtain sufficient information to determine whether and how Medical and Public Health Preparedness PCC actions or policy decisions shape CDC's preparedness program and whether the PCC plays a role in strengthening CDC's relationship with DHS.

Despite the existence of mechanisms for coordination at the top departmental level, such as the PCCs, it is not evident to the committee that adequate coordination and information sharing are occurring formally at the level of federal program staff involved in the day-to-day work of public health preparedness (GAO, 2003b). Although the creation of DHS holds the promise of streamlined oversight and funding, there are concerns that coordination between DHS and key preparedness functions in DHHS remains a significant challenge (GAO, 2003a). At the committee's March 2004 meeting, conversation among presenters from federal agencies and the committee revealed that personal relationships and serendipity may be credited with some coordination and information sharing across agencies, but it was not immediately evident that there are sufficient and functioning formal mechanisms for coordination and collaboration between DHS and DHHS. Coordination must be planned with forethought and deliberation, not left simply to chance and the goodwill of program staff. Coordination also must be planned and implemented during the preparedness or pre-event phase, beginning with effective communication about funding objectives and activities. For example, it is important for CDC staff to be familiar with relevant activities occurring in DHS and its programs funded and/or administered through FEMA and ODP, and for DHS staff to be aware of CDC priorities and activities to ensure the best use of limited federal preparedness resources.

State and local public health agencies receive funding through CDC's Cooperative Agreement on Public Health Preparedness and Response for Bioterrorism, and health care entities are funded through HRSA's National Hospital Bioterrorism Preparedness Cooperative Agreements. These cooperative agreement programs require that grantees conduct exercises that test public health and health care preparedness (and the integration between them) for an attack with biologic or chemical agents. Through the DHS Office of Domestic Preparedness Fiscal Year (FY) 2004 Homeland Security Grant Program and FY 2004 Urban Area Security Initiative Grant Program, states and some local emergency management offices receive funding to conduct exercises that test many of the same capacities and interagency collaborations expected by HRSA and CDC (DHS, 2003). Furthermore, FEMA, which is now under DHS, although its activities seem not yet fully coordinated with those of ODP, also oversees exercises relevant to chemical and radiation emergencies, which include public health components. The committee learned that sometimes states pool different sets of resources to conduct a larger drill or exercise involving a larger number of state and local agencies and community partners, and in other cases, the different funding streams are used to fund separate exercises (Schweitzer, 2004).

ODP has released guidelines for exercises and their evaluation through the Homeland Security Exercise and Evaluation Program (HSEEP). Although the committee is not aware of the nature and extent of CDC's involvement in the development of the HSEEP guidelines, the committee believes it is important that both CDC and DHSODP work to ensure a reasonable level of compatibility and coordination. This is necessary because of the functional overlap between public health and other state agencies, and because some state public health agencies already plan and execute their bioterrorism preparedness exercises in conjunction with their state emergency management offices. While public health preparedness exercises are needed to assess the unique functions and goals of public health, they will ideally be coordinated with other types of exercises where appropriate. Since state emergency management offices will be following the HSEEP guidelines, and some state public health agencies may be participating in exercises that follow these guidelines, a certain level of coordination is necessary between CDC's public health preparedness exercise guidelines and the HSEEP guidelines. In order to maximize the knowledge, skills, and relationship building that states and local jurisdictions gain from participating in preparedness exercises supported by limited federal resources, the committee encourages CDC to work closely with ODP (as well as HRSA) to coordinate, where appropriate and consistent with agency goals, the funding and guidelines for exercises provided by all federal agencies to states, local jurisdictions, and to private sector entities, such as hospitals.

Responding to a public health disaster, such as a smallpox attack, will require coordination with other organizations in the private sector and within the health care community. At the March 2004 meeting, the committee heard about the initiatives of the Joint Commission on Accreditation of Healthcare Organizations (JCAHO) to engage communities in preparedness planning and exercises. The committee believes it is important that CDC identify other organizations that, like JCAHO, require and set standards for preparedness activities, including exercises, and interact with communities in the area of bioterrorism and disaster preparedness. This is needed to help avoid duplicative efforts as well as ensure the best coordination of preparedness efforts. The range of partners in preparedness should be conceived broadly, to include local community, health care institutions, voluntary organizations, and others.

The committee also heard that state grantees funded by the DHS ODP FY 2004 Homeland Security Grant Program are encouraged to share exercise calendars with other partners and to coordinate or integrate efforts with other state and local exercises (Schweitzer, 2004). The committee suggests that CDC develop and maintain a list or database of exercises funded under the current (and future) cycle of the Cooperative Agreement on Public Health Preparedness and Response for Bioterrorism and to share this resource with ODP. Also, regular communication between CDC and ODP would inform both about planned exercises and would provide opportunities for coordination of exercises within a state and between states.

CDC and DHS guidance to grantees makes some reference to the need for interdisciplinary and intersectoral coordination (CDC and ODP, 2003; CDC, 2003a, 2004a, 2004b; DHS, 2003). However, it is not clearly spelled out how these linkages function at the federal, state, and local levels, and it is unclear whether the need for coordination is more specifically confirmed with and reinforced with grantees. For example, the CDC guidance for FY 2004 calls for integrating efforts and closely coordinating with "activities funded by the Department of Homeland Security and/or other federal agencies" (CDC, 2004a, 2004b). The guidance does not specifically identify relevant programs funded by DHS, and the committee was unable to locate more detailed explication of the formal linkages and coordination mechanisms that exist or are desirable in the relationship between CDC and DHS grantees.

The committee was unable to find a comprehensive resource describing all of the funding streams available for emergency preparedness activities, their purpose, funding amounts, and intended recipients. Such a tool would aid coordination of funding at the state and local level and also would facilitate coordination of all-hazards preparedness activities among national, state, and local partners in the academic, nonprofit, and business sectors. The committee did find a useful matrix of federal all-hazards grants from the International Association of Emergency Managers (IAEM, 2003). If a similar federal resource exists, that has been verified for accuracy and timeliness by the relevant federal agencies, the committee encourages that such a document be shared widely to facilitate coordination among all participants in emergency preparedness.

The committee urges all federal agencies to plan for and implement adequate collaboration and communication to ensure the long-term sustainability and effectiveness of an interagency approach to funding, developing, implementing, and evaluating public health preparedness in general, and exercises in particular.

An Example of Intersectoral Tension and Collaboration

The relationship between public health and law enforcement in responding to bioterrorism illustrates some of the potential tensions inherent in the coming together of different cultures and approaches to address a crisis.

An attack with biologic agents would put into motion two major and divergent systems (in addition to many others): public health, which attempts to deal with consequences and spread of infectious disease, and law enforcement, which targets the commission of a crime implicit in a deliberate introduction of a biologic agent. In the anthrax attacks of 2001, differences between public health and law enforcement became apparent. These included different investigative approaches (inductive versus deductive, respectively), evidentiary standards (scientific versus legal), and communication objectives. Public health tried to share complete and accurate information with the public in a timely manner, while law enforcement sought to disclose little or nothing pertaining to an investigation in order to maintain the integrity of a potential legal case (Ornstein, 2001; Butler et al., 2002; Gerber, 2002). Given these very different objectives and approaches, bioterrorism events would challenge each set of responders to do its own work while allowing the other to carry out its responsibilities. Preparedness efforts must include discussion and clarification of roles and responsibilities in a way that meets the needs of both public health and law enforcement professionals and undermines neither the disease prevention goal of public health nor the evidentiary standard required by law enforcement (Butler et al., 2002; Richards, 2002).

In the wake of the anthrax attacks of 2001, the position of CDC liaison to the FBI was created (Butler et al., 2002; GAO, 2003c). This seems to be a step in the right direction, but it would be useful only as long as the liaison unit is considered a priority by both agencies and it is given an adequate scope of work and level of authority. The Forensic Epidemiology training program, a joint effort between CDC and Department of Justice to facilitate mutual understanding between law enforcement and public health, is an example of successful and productive collaboration between public health and law enforcement in the area of bioterrorism preparedness and response (CDC, 2003b).

Collaboration between seemingly disparate government agencies and disciplines is not a new need, and there is some history on which to draw to help clarify and streamline these relationships. In the early 1980s, the CDC and the Federal Bureau of Investigation (FBI) created an interagency bioterrorism unit, located at CDC with secure communication capacity in the wake of a botulinum hoax. Plans were developed for the defense of the civilian population in the event of a bioterrorism incident. This unit was later disbanded (personal communication, W. Foege, Bill and Melinda Gates Foundation, March 30, 2004). This is an example of the type of collaboration that must be initiated and sustained to help address deliberate threats with health consequences.

Common Definitions and Terminology Are Needed

The emergency and disaster management field and federal agencies associated with it have developed a great deal of experience planning for disaster response and designing and conducting exercises to promote relationship building and training (GAO, 2001; Kuhr and Hauer, 2001; Landesman, 2001; FEMA, 2003). As disaster response becomes increasingly interdisciplinary, a common language is needed for good communication and interagency coordination in preparing for and responding to a chemical, biologic, radiological, nuclear, or explosive incident.

The committee found that similar terms do not always have the same meaning in documents created by different federal agencies (e.g., CDC, HRSA, FEMA, and ODP) or in the way they are used by the many disciplines conducting disaster research (CBACI, 2002; Hilhorst, 2003). The terms "exercise," "drill," and "simulation" in particular can mean different things to different agencies and disciplines.

Language differences go beyond practical terms used to describe specific activities. Definitions for fundamental concepts such as preparedness and response also are not unambiguous and certainly not universally shared across the disciplines that employ them (Advisory Panel to Assess Domestic Response Capabilities for Terrorism Involving Weapons of Mass Destruction, 2003). Effective communication and coordination are only possible when concepts and terms are used and understood in the same way by all participants. As is the case with any cross-cultural encounter, however, language is only one potential barrier. A more comprehensive kind of harmonization will require a great deal of effort on the part of each federal, state, and local agency, and of all disciplines involved in preparedness to understand each other's perspective, assumptions, biases, culture, and goals. Meetings between high-level officials will not suffice to bring this about. Regular, institutionalized, and sustained interaction among program staff will be needed, and all preparedness planning would benefit from applying the values and strategies of cultural competence at the interface between the many disciplines and agencies involved.

Speaking the Same Language: the Lexicon Project

The DHS has already recognized the need for a baseline understanding of the terms, acronyms, and phrases regularly used by different federal agencies that are involved in preparedness activities. For example, there are often very different understandings of the terms "first responder" and "surveillance." The Homeland Security Advisory Council has created a report for the secretary of Homeland Security on the Lexicon Project—a project that would create a homeland security lexicon by identifying the terms, acronyms, and phrases (and their associated definitions) used most commonly by agencies involved in homeland security activities (Moscoso, 2004). The goal is to develop a baseline level of understanding of all the terms and acronyms that are commonly used by different agencies so that communication can be improved (DHS, 2004c). The council has recommended the creation of an electronic database that would be accessible to all federal agencies, Capitol Hill staffers, lawmakers, and state and local agencies as they draft legislation, submit grant proposals, or prepare emergency plans (Moscoso, 2004). The council also has recognized the value in making such a database accessible to the media and other partners so that standard terminology also would be conveyed to the public at large (DHS, 2004c).

Part of the Lexicon Project at DHS involves assembling "foundational documents" from federal agencies that include the terms commonly used when discussing homeland security activities. To the extent that it is not involved already, the committee encourages CDC to work with the DHS to ensure that the commonly used public health preparedness terms and the relevant CDC documents are incorporated into the Lexicon Project and that knowledge of this effort is shared broadly across CDC and DHHS.

In the preceding pages, the committee has outlined challenges and opportunities inherent in integrating public health into a broader field. In order to address the challenges and maximize the opportunities, **the committee recommends that all federal entities concerned with bioterrorism preparedness (e.g., CDC, HRSA, ODP) more actively coordinate guidance and funding activities. Federal agencies should also work together to develop mechanisms that facilitate coordination and collaboration among their grantees at the state and local levels. Such mechanisms may include, but are not limited to, regular meetings to familiarize CDC and ODP program staff with each other's program priorities and activities, a database for informing ODP and other partners of exercises planned by CDC grantees, etc. Federal coordination efforts should also include the clarification of primary responsibility and authority in bioterrorism events, to ensure that CDC can fulfill its unique role as the nation's public health agency.**

THE EVIDENCE BASE FROM DISASTER RESEARCH AND PRACTICE

Nature of the Evidence

Although quantitative evidence (with randomized controlled trials as the gold standard) is extremely important in public health and medicine, this level of evidence may be difficult or impossible to obtain in research pertaining to public health disasters. While endeavoring to conduct quantitative, empirical research whenever possible, public health professionals also value other types of knowledge that contribute to decision-making and research methodologies that provide alternate routes to usable evidence. For example, the Task Force on Community Preventive Services, which is a major contributor to evidence-based public health, evaluates population-based health interventions through systematic and rigorous reviews that are not restricted to empirical and quantitative evidence (Briss et al., 2004). Methodologies for research used in public health are drawn from the social sciences, statistics, and epidemiology rather than solely from the biologic sciences.

Disaster research is in a position somewhat similar to public health research; there is some disconnectedness between academic research and practice (i.e., bringing research to bear on practice, and practice to inform and be validated by research), researchers come from diverse disciplines, there are challenges in translating research to practice, and it has been difficult to develop and secure funding for a comprehensive research agenda (Tierney, 1993; Quarantelli, 1994; Peters et al., 2001). Being aware of these similarities may help public health better understand and interpret disaster research and practice and their potential contributions to public health preparedness.

What Has Been Learned from Disaster Research

The following are some examples of major findings identified in two systematic surveys of the disaster and emergency management literature, two literature reviews on the subject of interorganizational coordination in disasters, and several theoretical articles (Auf der Heide, 1989; Tierney, 1993; Quarantelli, 1994; Granot, 1999; Tierney et al., 2001; Drabek and McEntire, 2002). These concise summaries of findings and research gaps are not provided in any specific order or priority. A general observation emphasized in the literature (and reiterated below) is that a comprehensive, systematic research agenda is needed in disaster research, and the committee would add, analogously, in public health preparedness.

Some Key Research Findings and Recurring Themes

- Human behavior in disasters is continuous with predisaster behavior patterns; individuals will generally behave adaptively, altruistically, and will not panic (except for rare situations characterized by an identified set of factors[4]) (Tierney et al., 2001; Auf der Heide, 1989; Drabek and McEntire, 2002). This finding is relevant to every aspect of planning for and responding to disaster, such as defining a role for communities in disaster response, developing communication plans and messages, and allocating resources based on what is likely to happen, rather than on inaccurate assumptions (Quarantelli, 1994).
- Collaborative interorganizational planning and preparedness are essential to successful response (Tierney, 1993; Granot, 1999; Burkle and Hayden, 2001; Tierney et al., 2001; Drabek and McEntire, 2002). Contact and coordination must be established pre-event among government agencies, between public and private entities, and among all entities likely to respond to a disaster.
- Studies of the preparedness activities of local emergency management agencies show that they are diverse in structure and operate in ways that make them well adapted to local conditions (Quarantelli, 1994). This demonstrates the importance of focusing on local needs and developing local response capacity, within the context of regional and national coordination and standards.
- The level of perceived risk among organization leaders is positively correlated with emergency preparedness (Tierney et al., 2001). This would

[4]Examples include: when people believe that certain situations lead to panic, where crisis management is ineffective and people feel abandoned, when people begin to believe they must flee to save themselves, when people feel socially isolated in a disaster, etc. (Tierney et al., 2001).

indicate that conducting regular, accurate risk assessments and communicating this information to all responder agencies would help strengthen the rationale for preparedness.[5]

- Severe disasters lead to the creation of impromptu community organizations that mobilize to address gaps in response capacity or failure of existing systems to surge adequately in situations where their resources are strained excessively (Tierney et al., 2001). This phenomenon, sometimes called "emergence," is noteworthy because it underscores the tremendous capacity of communities and their social networks and formal associations to respond to crises. Communities are likely to know themselves better than most outside agencies or organizations, and their knowledge and resources should be part of public health preparedness, including planning for bioterrorism and other public health crises (IOM, 2003d). The evidence about inadequacies in certain aspects of postdisaster response, or in addressing the needs of special populations may be helpful in anticipating and planning to correct such inefficiencies in future responses (Quarantelli, 1994; Kreps and Bosworth, 1999; Tierney et al., 2001).
- Studies of disasters have shown that when plans exist simply for compliance with administrative requirements but are not part of a dynamic process of learning, planning, and preparing, responders involved are likely to ignore all or most of the plan (Quarantelli, 1988). In some cases, plans have been found to be irrelevant, inaccurate, or simply unfamiliar to responders who did not know the plan or their role in it (Auf der Heide, 1989). An emergency response plan does little good if the participants in the plan have not developed a relationship with their partners, have not practiced the plan, or have not updated the plan as circumstances have changed (Auf der Heide, 1989; Perry, 2003). The importance of an emergency response plan lies in the process of developing, exercising, and improving it rather than in the document itself, for it is the process that allows relationships to be built, understanding of different disciplines to be fostered, and communication barriers to be broken down.

Examples of Gaps in Disaster Research

- There is a need to expand what is known about preparedness, since there is more evidence about how first responders respond to a disaster than how they prepare and how preparedness relates to ability to respond (Auf der Heide, 1989; Tierney et al., 2001). "Large-scale studies are needed

[5]The committee's first two reports repeatedly emphasized that government is responsible for updating the smallpox threat assessment and communicating this information to the public (IOM, 2003b, 2003c).

to systematically examine the impact of emergency preparedness on the effectiveness of emergency response activities while controlling for differences in disaster impacts and community characteristics" (Tierney et al., 2001).

- More research is needed to identify the planning assumptions that result in effective organizational performance (Tierney et al., 2001). Although disaster practice has benefited from research, it is still common for emergency responders and organizations to adopt certain concepts not based on scientific evidence, but on convenience, a concept's popularity among peers, and perhaps, anecdotal evidence (Quarantelli, 1995). More research is needed to substantiate or discredit the effectiveness of practices and concepts used in disaster planning (NRC, 2003).
- Little is known about what makes local emergency management agencies effective and successful (Tierney et al., 2001).
- Research is needed to determine what preparedness and response strategies or models are most useful, under what circumstances, and to what extent they should be implemented for optimal results. For example, more research on the Incident Command System (ICS) is needed (Tierney, 1993; NRC, 2003). Although its value has been questioned by some disaster researchers, and there is limited empirical evidence documenting its effectiveness, ICS has been widely embraced by the emergency management field and even in health care and other areas, and forms the foundation of the National Incident Management System adopted by DHS (Tierney, 1993; Quarantelli, 1995; Drabek and McEntire, 2002; NRC, 2003).
- Research on police and fire department preparedness was conducted mainly in the 1970s, so it is out of date (Tierney et al., 2001).
- Not enough is known about local emergency preparedness networks, their composition, and the relationships among responder agencies (Tierney et al., 2001).
- Little is known about the resources or community characteristics that are related to better levels of preparedness (Tierney et al., 2001).
- More effort needs to focus on translating research into the practice of emergency and disaster management, for example, identifying the elements of emergency management applicable to all-hazard preparedness (NRC, 2003).
- The emergency management field has frequently grappled with the question of whether to ensure generic or specific preparedness capabilities and processes (NRC, 2003). For example, should the training of first responders center on a set of generic capabilities, or should more attention be paid to specific types of disasters? The field of emergency management has moved to an all-hazards approach in the past decade, and although this approach has certain strengths, it also may have limitations and present challenges. During the planning phase, however, research findings support

a greater focus on generic approaches rather than agent-specific ones. Reasons for this may include: the fact that it is impossible, for practical and resource reasons, to plan for every possible contingency; most disasters share a core of common elements; and disasters cause temporary changes in organizational structure and functioning that require flexibility in planning (Tierney, 1993; Kiel, 1995; Quarantelli, 2004). As the public health community joins other emergency and disaster responders, the question of generic versus specific deserves renewed consideration for its implications to public health preparedness. Should public health preparedness be generic, or should it, for instance, focus on specific biologic agents, like smallpox or botulinum toxin? Or is there a way to strike an ideal balance between generic and specific preparedness?

What Has Been Learned from Disaster Practice

Key Lessons Learned in Disaster Practice

Although many of the lessons learned in disaster practice are not in areas clearly relevant to public health preparedness, certain broad themes may translate relatively well.

- Technology may fail in disasters; therefore, planning and training should include "low-tech" alternatives for communication and other activities (Tierney et al., 2001).
- Communication among responding agencies is essential during a disaster. The experience of disaster responders across the country contains numerous examples of situations where communications equipment or frequencies were not compatible and responder agencies were unable to communicate with each other (fire to law enforcement, EMS to hospitals, etc.). This can present enormous challenges to all involved (Auf der Heide, 1989).
- Ongoing needs assessment is needed over the course of a disaster for efficient distribution of resources and prioritization of activities (Auf der Heide, 1989).
- Emergency response is sometimes based on myths that research has disproved, with consequences for the success and effectiveness of the response (Auf der Heide, 1989; Tierney et al., 2001). This also underscores the need to better link research and practice.

A Resource for Learning from Past Experience

It has been observed that a great deal of the knowledge available in the disaster management field and in terrorism preparedness reflects a failure to learn from the past (actual events or exercises); the same mistakes are made again and again both within and across responder organizations (CBACI, 2002; Auf der Heide, 1989). This is partly due to the fact that what is learned is often not shared. One way to ensure that what is learned is disseminated widely is to create a database or other centralized repository of such information. Recently, the National Memorial Institute for the Prevention of Terrorism and the DHS Office of Domestic Preparedness jointly launched a website devoted to sharing lessons learned from exercises, www.LLIS.gov (LLIS stands for Lessons Learned Information Shared). This site summarizes a large amount of information, including lessons learned, best practices, reports, guidelines, and stories from a wide range of what it terms emergency disciplines (e.g., law enforcement, fire, HazMat, veterinary, search and rescue, public health, and medical), and pertaining to a variety of actual events and exercises. It must be noted, however, that certain aspects of preparedness and response are unique to bioterrorism preparedness, so lessons gathered by emergency responders in other areas may not be applicable in their entirety or at all.

The DHS and LLIS MIPT searchable database will undoubtedly prove helpful to government agencies and their partners as they work together to strengthen their capacity to respond to deliberately inflicted and other types of disasters. The architecture of the LLIS database includes public health among emergency disciplines and functions and seems to provide opportunity for entering material relevant to public health preparedness. Given the importance of disseminating knowledge, and the currently limited avenues that exist to facilitate such sharing, CDC and its state and local public health partners may wish to consider the DHS mechanism for sharing lessons learned and develop a similar and connected mechanism to support public health preparedness goals. Such a database may involve, but not be limited to the following activities: developing and gathering after action reports based on public health preparedness exercises and responses to actual events that tested the capacity of the public health system; conducting a retrospective analysis of public health agencies' responses to infectious disease and other relevant events in the past 2-3 years; and increasing the emphasis on studying the responses to proxy events and the effect of exercises and publishing findings in the peer-reviewed literature.

LEARNING FROM THE PUBLIC HEALTH RESPONSE TO PROXY EVENTS

Studying the Response to Public Health Challenges

Thus far, the committee has highlighted some key points from disaster research and practice that may be useful to CDC and the public health community. However, public health has its own rich knowledge base, which includes lessons from recent public health emergencies such as food-borne disease outbreaks, emerging infectious diseases, and the anthrax attack of 2001. Unfortunately, there is no systematic, comprehensive agenda for public health preparedness research to provide a structure for public health emergency preparedness and response research. Such an agenda would be a part of the broader public health research agenda that has recently begun to take shape, but it still requires infrastructure and funding (Council on Linkages between Academia and Public Health Practice, 2004). Systematic public health and interdisciplinary research is essential to inform preparedness against bioterrorism and other threats.

In general, the knowledge gathered from recent outbreaks and other public health emergencies is available predominantly in reports (e.g., from GAO, from nongovernmental organizations) or anecdotal assessments (e.g., in media reports). The peer-reviewed literature seems to offer little research on this subject. Recent anecdotal reports about the ways in which bioterrorism planning and training improved response to a crisis are encouraging, but it is important that such observations are documented and somewhat more quantitative and objective studies are undertaken to determine whether the public health system's performance (and therefore, response capacity) has indeed been enhanced by expanded resources, surveillance and information systems, and linkages with other partners.

In a study of 12 nationally representative communities, respondents acknowledged general improvements made possible by public health preparedness funding and requirements, including more training of personnel and the development of relationships to first responder and other local agencies and organizations (Staiti et al., 2003). Also, state officials in Massachusetts and Virginia attributed their states' rapid response to Severe Acute Respiratory Syndrome (SARS) to their public health preparedness efforts supported by funding for bio-terrorism (Staiti et al., 2003; Stoll and Lee, 2003). A GAO report (GAO, 2004) also found that some states have increased laboratory capacity and that the coverage by HAN, CDC's Health Alert Network, has increased to 90 percent of the nation, which can be assumed, would result in improved rapid notification of health care providers and other health personnel. However, the effect of HAN's expansion is yet to be determined. In 2003, the executive director of the American Public Health Association and former director of the Maryland Department of Health and Mental Hygiene asserted that previous experience with West Nile virus and anthrax taught the state public health agency in Maryland valuable lessons about communication and cross-jurisdictional coordination—lessons which paid dividends during Maryland's encounter with SARS (Benjamin, 2003). In April 2004, bioterrorism preparedness efforts were credited with the swift response to two measles outbreaks by state and federal public health agencies (Elliott, 2004).

Though the examples provided suggest that public health preparedness has been improved, more systematic research is needed to examine the link between the application of lessons learned and improvements in performance, the effect of preparedness on routine public health practice and the delivery of the Ten Essential Public Health Services, and the state of the formal and informal collaboration and communication between the health care and public health communities.

Evaluating Performance in a Proxy Event

Some disease outbreaks (e.g., monkeypox, West Nile virus, SARS) that can serve as proxy events for a bioterrorism disaster (such as a smallpox attack) may be valuable in testing preparedness activities because they are likely to possess some of the same characteristics, especially if they are of significant magnitude. These characteristics include:

- No prior planning or announcement (unlike most exercises), therefore placing increased stress on human and other resources;
- Unpredictability;
- Increased mobilization of resources;
- Enhanced surveillance activities;
- Frequent communication among all parties involved; and
- Increased scrutiny from the media.

Using the "What if?" Scenario Approach

Given that public health disasters such as attacks with biologic weapons or widespread epidemics are infrequent, plans must be put into place to capture important information and facilitate performance measurement during and after a proxy event. However, the magnitude of a public health emergency determines its potential usefulness as a proxy event for measuring bioterrorism preparedness. In significant proxy events, public health agencies should constantly ask themselves: what if the lead in drinking water, the monkeypox cases traced back to exotic pets, the appearance of SARS, or the occurrence of hepatitis A virus in restaurant food were the result of deliberate, ill-intentioned introduction? What if the number of cases of an unusual new disease was not a handful, but a few thousand? What if not one emergency occurred, but three? Would our response have been adequate, sufficiently rapid, or sufficiently well coordinated? Using various health threats as proxies for evaluating public health agency performance and identifying the requirements for an adequate response would support continuous quality improvement over time. Components of the evaluation of proxy events may include, but not be limited to: formal debriefings after an event; discussion of what went well, what went wrong, and what was learned (i.e., after-action report); and deciding what changes will be made in communication, staffing, training, equipment, facilities, and interagency/intersectoral coordination (i.e., improvement plan).

The committee believes that it is important to evaluate performance during proxy events at the local, state, and federal levels of the governmental public health infrastructure. CDC is the lead public health agency, not only as a standard setter and funder, but also as an important part of public health practice and of public health response to emergencies and disasters. Proxy events test CDC's resources and ability to respond to crises rapidly, expertly, and in coordination with state and local agencies. CDC may become a limiting factor during a disease outbreak or a deliberate attack with a biologic agent if the agency is the major or sole source of information or supplies. For example, CDC's Laboratory Response Network is the source of many reagents for laboratories around the country, and state distribution networks are ultimately dependent on CDC. Therefore, CDC's role in responding to a proxy event must be considered one of the major aspects of a response, the agency's own performance must be evaluated, and plans for improvement must be developed and implemented.

One way to use proxy events as a means of performance evaluation for states and CDC in particular is to conduct a systematic and careful review of Epidemic Assistance Investigations, or Epi-Aids. Epi-Aids are a mechanism through which CDC provides collaborative assistance to state, national, and international health officials in investigating disease outbreaks and other epidemiologic emergencies (Office of the Federal Register, 2003). The review of Epi-Aids, which are one form of after-action reports, may provide an additional window on public health performance in public health emergencies and disasters. In reviewing Epi-Aids or other types of after-action reports, it may be most useful to focus on incidents that involved infectious agents with bioterror potential and to review them as if the event had been a deliberate introduction. The questions that must be asked in the course of review include:

- How was the outbreak detected?
- How much time elapsed between the event and detection? How could that time have been reduced?
- Who was exposed and how?
- How could numbers of exposed have been reduced?
- Did the response to the event follow CDC guidelines?
- How quick was the response?

- How could the response be improved in the future? Based on the experience what would be the lessons for the next time?

As noted above, the research literature is limited in the area of public health emergency response, and much of what is known about the influence of preparedness on responses to recent outbreaks is based on subjective factors. Any proxy event, such as reoccurrences of West Nile virus, food-borne disease outbreaks, or other public health events of note, should be seen as an opportunity to measure progress toward preparedness goals and competent performance as another milestone in a continuing process. As CDC's Evidence-Based Performance Goals for Public Health Disaster Preparedness, currently under development, are disseminated and implemented, it is important that CDC and its state and local partners take steps to link these with a system for capturing lessons learned from the response to proxy events.

The committee has described some of the knowledge available from the practice of disaster response and from disaster research and the need to strengthen public health preparedness research. **The committee recommends that CDC should collaborate with all of its partners to strengthen preparedness by applying research findings and experience in public health emergency response, bioterrorism preparedness, and disaster management. In order to strengthen the evidence base for public health preparedness, CDC should:**

- **Strengthen the link between public health research and practice.**
- **Participate in and promote interdisciplinary research about preparedness.**
- **Support a system to assure the ongoing collection, synthesis, and sharing of lessons learned and best practices from public health preparedness exercises and public health response to proxy events.**
- **In coordination with the appropriate federal-level partners, such as AHRQ, evaluate the effectiveness, design, and opportunity costs of preparedness strategies, such as exercises.**

USEFULNESS OF MODELING

Role of Modeling in Policy Decisions

For public health preparedness, models can be useful tools to assist in decision-making, focusing preparedness efforts, and analyzing different response options. Though there sometimes can be a tendency to want to use models to predict outcomes, models have limitations and should not be relied upon for this purpose. Models should be used as "an aid to understanding, rather than being an end in themselves" (Taylor, 2003).

Modeling can be a useful tool to assist in assessing different policy options, but only with a clear understanding of the limitations of modeling. Models are only as good as the data that are used to develop them. The accuracy and generalizability of models depend on which components are included or excluded, the validity of any assumptions made about them, and the accuracy of modeling of the interactions between them (Taylor, 2003). If the data are timely, accurate, and appropriate, and the model includes all the relevant input parameters and appropriately portrays all the relationships among the input parameters, then models can serve as useful tools in making policy decisions. A good model can assist decision-making before an event by helping policy makers decide where to focus preparedness efforts, or while an event is occurring as current data can be added to the model to fine-tune the model for the particular situation.

For models to have utility, sensitivity analyses should be conducted for each input parameter, to assess which factor has the greatest effect on the outcome or outcomes of interest. Once it is determined how sensitive the outcome is to the different input parameters, preparedness efforts can be focused on the factor that is estimated to have the greatest effect on the outcome. This also will help policymakers determine the factors for which indicators should be developed. Considering the limited resources currently available for public health preparedness activities, knowing which factors potentially have the greatest influence on the course of an outbreak will be extremely valuable to those who decide how to allocate limited resources. Without sensitivity analyses, models are of limited value to policymakers.

Role of Modeling in Exercise Development

Modeling can help inform planning for exercises by elucidating the critical factors that affect the outcome, which in turn helps in designing exercises that stress that particular part of the system. For an exercise testing the response to smallpox, findings from some of the models described below could help inform the focus that should be placed on vaccination of the public compared to contact tracing and containment, the number of staff in mass vaccination clinics, and the need for post-event vaccination of health care workers.

A number of models created in the past few years have examined the potential spread of smallpox under varying scenarios (Meltzer et al., 2001; Halloran et al., 2002; Bozzette et al., 2003; Kaplan et al., 2003). These models used slightly different assumptions for most of the key input parameters, resulting in different conclusions. Meltzer et al. found from their model that a combination of quarantine and vaccination would be the best option for stopping a smallpox epidemic (2001). Mass vaccination is found to be the best option for limiting mortality and reducing the time it takes to end a smallpox epidemic in the model produced by Kaplan et al. (2003). In the Halloran et al. model, mass vaccination could produce better outcomes than targeted vaccination, and vice versa, depending upon specific components of the particular outbreak, such as preexisting immunity, rate of transmission to contacts, and vaccine supply (2002). Bozzette et al. found that the net benefits of vaccination depend upon the probability of an attack, with prior vaccination of health care workers being favored unless the probability of an attack is very low, and mass vaccination being favored only if the probability of a national attack or multiple attacks is high (2003). Ferguson et al. (2003) compared these four different models and offered reasons why the conclusions that could be drawn from each model were different.

Models have been used to examine different aspects of a smallpox outbreak. Some models have examined the speed of different components of a response to a bioterrorism incident and how this affects outcomes (Giovachino and Carey, 2001; Hupert et al., 2002). Other models have examined an individual's risk-benefit profile for pre-or postexposure smallpox vaccination (Meltzer, 2003), estimates of historical transmission rates (Gani and Leach, 2001), the course of historical smallpox epidemics (Duncan et al., 1994; Eichner and Dietz, 2003), and the effect of isolation of overt cases of smallpox and surveillance of contacts on the progression of a smallpox epidemic (Eichner and Dietz, 2003).

Each of these models has utility in examining particular aspects of a smallpox outbreak and the corresponding response options, but before a model is used to help make important decisions about a smallpox exercise or a smallpox response, the model's assumptions and input parameters must be deemed reliable and realistic. This also is another important reason why sensitivity analyses are necessary. They are used to study the effect of varying the range of assumptions that have been made. This is the importance of the model—not its overall conclusion.

There also may be opportunities to learn from other modeling efforts. The military has extensive experience with modeling, potentially providing a rich knowledge base that could aid smallpox modeling. Knowledge gained from modeling other communicable diseases (e.g., measles) also could inform the population dynamics and transmission aspect of modeling smallpox, West Nile virus, and SARS outbreaks, in particular. Recent efforts to model an intentional release of anthrax could shed light on factors that are unique to modeling a bioterrorism event. The committee encourages CDC to draw upon the knowledge and experience of other modeling efforts when developing models for smallpox or any other biologic agent.

Smallpox Modeling Working Group

Recognizing the potential value of modeling in informing policy decisions, the DHHS Secretary's Council on Public Health Preparedness recently formed a Smallpox Modeling Working Group (Borio, 2004). The Smallpox Modeling Working Group was created to "explore a range of policy options related to smallpox preparedness and response" (Borio, 2004). Three modeling groups were selected to model the effects of different response strategies. To overcome some of the reasons for differing conclusions of previous models (Ferguson et al., 2003), the Smallpox Modeling Working Group decided that a standardized set of biologically realistic input parameters for smallpox natural history and transmission needed to be agreed upon (Borio, 2004). In addition to the standardized input parameters, the working group also developed outbreak scenarios, policy options regarding outbreak containment measures, and outcome measures of interest to DHHS (Borio, 2004).

The three modeling groups ran their models using the agreed-upon parameters. Based on the results of these models, the Smallpox Modeling Working Group reached the following interim conclusions:

1. Surveillance and containment alone is sufficient to effectively contain an intentional smallpox release.
2. There is relatively small marginal benefit in prevaccination of hospital workers or mass vaccination of the population after an outbreak begins. Reactive mass vaccination may have additional value in bringing an epidemic under control.
3. In the absence of any interventions, the strongest controlling factor is people withdrawing to the home when they become "ill" (Borio, 2004).

As was mentioned earlier, models can offer illustrative guidance as to the factors that have the greatest influence on the outcomes of interest, but models have their limitations and should not be used alone for making policy decisions. Of the three models created under the aegis of the Smallpox Modeling Working Group, one is a deterministic model, since it uses single point estimates for each of the input parameters, whereas the other two are stochastic models, using probability estimates for the different input parameters (Borio, 2004). Since recent data on smallpox transmission rates, incubation period, case fatality rate, vaccine efficacy, vaccination adverse event rates, and population dynamics of the current U.S. population are limited, stochastic models may be more illustrative of the range of outcomes that are possible due to a smallpox outbreak. However, to accurately portray the role of modeling in policy decision-making, the sensitivity of particular input parameters on the model's outcomes must be provided, and the limitations of the model and uncertainties in the data must be conveyed (Ferguson et al., 2003).

USEFULNESS OF EXERCISES

The Use of and Rationale for Exercises

Exercises are believed to be effective in enhancing preparedness and are widely used by local, state, and national disaster response agencies (GAO, 2001). The emergency and disaster response field's assumptions that exercises work to improve preparedness have been reinforced by experience that has suggested a link between exercises and good performance in an emergency or disaster (FEMA/EMI, 2003). According to FEMA's Emergency Management Institute (2003), exercising reveals flaws in planning, clarifies roles, improves individual performance, and tests and evaluates plans, policies, and procedures. Moreover, exercises have become an institutionalized strategy for planning in homeland security. In fact, the DHS HSEEP materials assert that exercises "provide a risk-free environment for jurisdictions to assess if they have the plans, policies, procedures, resources, and agreements in place to enable homeland security personnel to perform critical tasks required to prevent, respond to, or recover from a terrorist attack" (DHS/ODP, 2003).

Exercises contribute to preparedness by fostering relationship building; by providing a context and tool for training; and by providing a method for evaluating performance. The use of exercises for training may originate in the military experience, but they are conducted as part of preparedness in a variety of contexts, from the nuclear plants required by the Department of Energy to use exercises to prepare for the possibility of an accident, to local firefighters training to deal with major fires or with natural disasters, to regional exercises required by FEMA to respond to hazardous materials (HazMat) and natural disasters.

When exercises are conducted in order to educate, train, or develop interorganizational and interjurisdictional relationships, the underlying assumptions may be easily validated. Disasters are complex events that require many different types of responders; therefore, having partnerships is preferable to working in isolation. Furthermore, some level of organization and coordination is essential to help avoid chaos; rehearsing processes may lead to smoother functioning of complex response systems, and in the event of an emergency, for example, a smallpox attack, having personnel that possess certain knowledge and skills (e.g., smallpox diagnosis, vaccination, and search and containment) is better than having personnel that did not receive such education and training. Exercises that test communication across jurisdictions or test certain skills and processes may provide some indication that certain things are likely to work well in a disaster.

Research on Exercises

Although the assumptions made about exercises are reasonable, and exercises seem like a practical strategy in many circumstances, there are at least two reasons to seek more objective study: the need to compare multiple types of exercises for more targeted use and the potential costs posed by exercises.

As noted above, more research is needed on preparedness (Tierney et al., 2001), but exercises and other means for evaluating performance (and for improving preparedness) form a particularly neglected subset of preparedness. The overall effectiveness of exercises as a preparedness strategy has not been well demonstrated, and research is needed to determine, for example, whether exercises could be considered predictors of successful response, what type of exercise would have the greatest positive influence on preparedness, what exercises are most cost-effective, and the best way to assess opportunity costs posed by conducting exercises (NRC, 2003). The use of scenarios, which may serve as a component of exercises, for training and planning purposes has not been well researched either, but there are "indications that they are an excellent method of teaching rapid response-style thinking, decision-making and the development of managerial skills" (Alexander, 2000; Simpson, 2002:56). Potential research questions would include: how do reality-based scenarios compare with entirely fictional scenarios, and under what circumstances would the use of one be preferable to the other?

In the disaster literature, mention of exercises seems limited to descriptions of how they were utilized by responder agencies and disciplines (EMS, emergency departments, fire departments, etc.), the lessons learned, and changes in operations made as a result (Tierney et al., 2001). A brief review of the medical and health peer-reviewed literature (using the National Library of Medicine's PubMed search engine) shows that hospitals and public health agencies conduct exercises and find them useful in evaluating the quality of training, the smoothness of emergency operations, and other aspects of disaster response, but there seems to be little or no empirical study of the validity or effectiveness of exercises themselves as a strategy for public health and health care preparedness. The Agency for Healthcare Research and Quality (AHRQ) Evidence-based Practice Center recently conducted a review of the literature on hospital exercises and drills and concluded that "the evidence was insufficient to support firm conclusions about the effectiveness of specific training methods because of the marked heterogeneity of studies, weaknesses in study design, and the limited number of exercises that have been reported in the literature" (AHRQ, 2004). The committee hopes that the experience of public health agencies with exercises and drills will not only be reported to CDC, but that there will be increased emphasis on more in-depth studies of the effectiveness of public health preparedness exercises, and more frequent publication of such studies in the literature. The growing partnerships between public health agencies and schools of public health (i.e., the Academic Centers for Public Health Preparedness) would certainly contribute to such an effort.

At the committee's March 2004, meeting, DHS ODP speakers presented a graphic describing a cyclical or building block approach to planning and training (see Figure G-2). This graphic outlines an incremental set of techniques or methods for preparedness planning and training, from the minimal complexity of a seminar to the significant complexity of functional or full-scale approaches. On the one hand, this building-block approach seems logical, and it is reasonable to select a training and capability testing method based on and scaled to match the complexity of the objective (e.g., a workshop to train for a particular role and then to test it; a functional exercise to rehearse and evaluate a complex interagency process). However, the committee believes this approach requires evaluation. For example, by what means are games determined to be more or less complex than tabletops, and in what circumstances is one method preferable to another? This type of evaluation research would help ensure the implementation of the most effective, evidence-based means for strengthening preparedness.

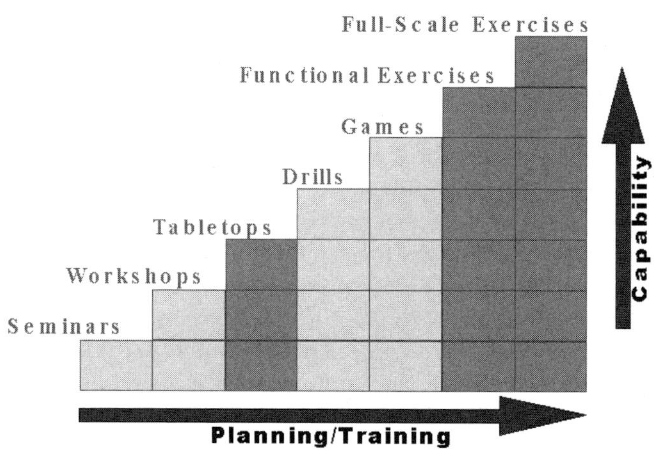

FIGURE G-2 HSEEP's Building block approach to planning and training.
SOURCE: DHS/ODP (2004b).

Exercise-Related Activities of the Department of Homeland Security (DHS)

To help ensure that the country is prepared for a possible terrorist attack or other emergency, DHS has primary responsibility in the federal government for organizing and evaluating preparedness exercises and drills. In DHS, the ODP is responsible for providing training, funds for the purchase of equipment, support for the planning and execution of exercises, technical assistance, and other support to assist states and local jurisdictions in preventing, planning for, and responding to acts of terrorism (DHS, 2004a). In addition to ODP, FEMA also has been incorporated into DHS, and it has brought over its expertise in the area of exercises. Together, ODP and FEMA are responsible for HSEEP, Radiological Emergency Preparedness (REP) Program, Community Hazards Emergency Response Capability Assurance Program (CHER-CAP), and the Chemical Stockpile Emergency Preparedness Program (CSEPP). These programs and others offer a rich history of exercise experience that could inform public health preparedness.

HSEEP, mentioned in preceding pages, details DHS's comprehensive exercise doctrine and is "a program of financial and direct support designed to assist state and local governments with the development and implementation of a state exercise and evaluation program to assess and enhance domestic preparedness" (DHS/ODP, 2004a). HSEEP resources include four volumes of reference materials to assist state and local jurisdictions with the design, development, conduct, and evaluation of exercises. The first volume of HSEEP includes a uniform approach for exercise design, development, conduct, and evaluation (DHS/ODP, 2004a). The second volume includes a methodology for conducting evaluation of homeland security exercises and implementing an improvement program (DHS, 2004b). The third volume is an exercise development manual, outlining a standardized planning process, adaptable to any type of exercise or scenario (Schweitzer, 2004). The fourth volume consists of sample exercise documents (DHS/ODP, 2004a).

As the committee learned at its March meeting, FEMA has extensive experience with executing and evaluating exercises as part of the agency's mission to prepare the country for disasters, and its work contributes to the practical knowledge base on exercises and drills (FEMA/EMI, 1995; FEMA, 2004; Kelkenberg, 2004). For example, FEMA has been involved with the REP program, which was established as a direct result of the Three-Mile Island incident and ensures adequacy of emergency plans and preparedness for areas near commercial nuclear power plants (Kelkenberg, 2004). Whereas the Nuclear Regulatory Commission is responsible for ensuring the adequacy of emergency plans onsite, FEMA is responsible for reviewing and evaluating offsite radiological emergency response plans developed by state and local governments and for evaluating exercises conducted by state and local governments to determine if radiological emergency plans can be implemented (Kelkenberg, 2004). FEMA also plays the significant role of educating the public about radiological emergency preparedness (Kelkenberg, 2004).

FEMA has a memorandum of agreement with the U.S. Army for the CSEPP program. Similar to REP, the Army is responsible for onsite preparedness and response, and FEMA is responsible for offsite preparedness and response in the surrounding community (Kelkenberg, 2004). Some useful documents have been created through this program and may be applicable to other preparedness programs. For example, Oak Ridge National Laboratories has developed training materials on sheltering in place that would be applicable to other emergency preparedness scenarios (Kelkenberg, 2004). CSEPP also includes an exercise component, which involves both the site itself and the surrounding community (e.g., emergency management agency, health department, hospitals). FEMA evaluates the local community's performance in the exercise and, based on the findings, recommends how the community partners' emergency response plans should be improved (Kelkenberg, 2004).

FEMA's Community Hazards Emergency Response Capability Assurance Program (CHER-CAP) consists of a planning, training assessment, and exercise process for all-hazards response operations (Kelkenberg, 2004). It consists of looking at a community's emergency response plans, coupling the plan with a risk assessment, identifying training to fill in the gaps in the plan, and then doing a tabletop exercise and peer-evaluated full-scale exercise to identify areas for improvement (Kelkenberg, 2004).

Sample Questions, Strategies, and Methodologies for Evaluation Research on Public Health Preparedness Exercises and Proxy Events

The committee has identified several possible questions, strategies, and methodologies that could be considered by CDC in evaluation and experimental research in public health preparedness. These include:

- Examining the effect of a proxy event on two similar communities with different public health infrastructure and capabilities.
- Conducting "placebo-controlled" trials comparing the response of two similar communities to a proxy event, false alarm, or to an unannounced exercise. One community previously conducted one or more exercises (or employed other methods) to test its preparedness, while the other did not. Compare response times, smoothness of interagency coordination, functionality of communication channels, and other aspects of their response.

- Conducting an unannounced exercise and comparing the performance of three different groups of personnel (with the same qualifications and functional roles) who have undergone one of the following: (1) preparedness-related training only; (2) training and a tabletop exercise only; (3) training and participation in a comprehensive functional exercise.
- Randomly assigning educational materials to various types of health personnel to determine whether the type and quality of educational materials have an effect on exercise outcomes.
- Randomizing the method of preparing responders and the community at large before an exercise is conducted in order to determine the best way to conduct them. Outcomes to be measured would include professional participation rates, community participation, and major desired outcomes of the activity.

The committee also suggests several areas for further study:

- A systematic assessment of all lessons learned in the course of the smallpox vaccination program (which could be considered a national-level, multisite, months-long preparedness meta-exercise);
- Determine what knowledge is available about public health preparedness and about conducting exercises (and drills) in public health agencies with experience in this area (history of working with EMS, preparing for nuclear accidents, etc.). Many lines of questioning could be followed in gathering information from public health agencies with a variety of linkages to emergency and disaster response. For example, it may be instructive to compare the engagement of public health in emergency and disaster response in states where EMS is part of public health to states where the two agencies are separate.
- Systematically assess the lessons learned by state and local public health agencies (perhaps organized by type according to characteristics such as size, urban or rural location, structure and governance) that have conducted exercises and drills. Such an assessment also must include an examination of any evidence that is available or is becoming available in the literature or in the reporting of public health agencies, of the effectiveness of exercises and drills conducted by public health agencies (similar to AHRQ's recent work [AHRQ, 2004]).
- A systematic and comprehensive research agenda for studying the response to public health emergencies and disasters be developed.
- An evaluation of patient safety literature to consider the pre- and posthandling of sentinel events.

A Framework for Performance Evaluation Using Exercises

Major outcomes in public health typically involve decreasing mortality and disease rates and progress is measured periodically (e.g., Healthy People 2010 process). Performance measurement in public health is, however, a relatively new field. In the case of public health preparedness for bioterrorism and other events with significant public health impact, outcomes are occasioned by actual events themselves, and the infrequency and huge variation among these events (including the proxy events discussed in preceding pages of this report) make it difficult or nearly impossible to gauge, for example, a decrease in rate of disease from contaminated water or other reductions in mortality and morbidity attributable to the disaster. Due to the nature of disaster-related public health problems, performance measurement in this area is by necessity more process-oriented. When CDC and its state and local partners identify exercise objectives that will be used in evaluating the exercise, these objectives will be most helpful if they are linked with the Evidence-Based Performance Goals for Public Health Disaster Preparedness developed by CDC.

Exercises offer an alternative way to measure performance and fine-tune preparedness before a crisis occurs. Public health preparedness exercises take place at national, state, and local levels, and it is important that evaluation of exercises take place at all levels. The committee believes it is essential to design and conduct exercises that stress and test CDC's own performance. As noted in the preceding discussion of proxy events, CDC is a vital part of preparedness and response and it is itself a limiting factor in terms of the resources it provides (e.g., laboratory reagents, information, technical assistance) to state and local counterparts. In asking "what if" questions in a proxy event or in an exercise, the limits of availability of such resources must be probed. In addition, modeling could be used to estimate such things as the rate of producing and renewing the supply of needed laboratory reagents, or the speed with which needed field experts could be moved from place to place. In a more dramatic type of exercise, questions could be asked about the potential effect if CDC itself was the target of an attack and critical facilities destroyed.

After-action reports will play an important role in facilitating continuous quality improvement. They provide an overview of agency or interagency performance in an exercise and identify areas where there are gaps in planning, unforeseen circumstances that are poorly managed, or areas where communication or the flow of information break down, among other issues.

Various types of methods for measuring performance will eventually be determined to be effective and even to have some predictive value (e.g., of future successful response). The link between research and practice requires strengthening, so that as research validates certain practices, such as types of exercises, and the most effective techniques to communicate to or evacuate the public, they may be rapidly translated into practice. The practices demonstrated to be most effective (e.g., specific types of exercises) need to then be institutionalized and adapted to local circumstances, with particular attention to maintaining and updating staff competence and sustaining readiness. Staff turnover itself, which requires regularly updating training and conducting exercises, could be used to create new cohorts for performance evaluation.

CDC might wish to consider describing the breadth and depth of exercises needed for public health. The HSEEP Building Block Approach illustrates one typology of training and capacity-building methods, including exercises. CDC could develop a similar representation with specific applications to public health. For example, in the area of exercises, some exercises may be external, conducted in coordination with other agencies at the federal, state, and local level (refer to the section on Coordination Issues), while others will be strictly internal exercises on such issues as how to move from normal to emergency operations, including decisions about closing or curtailing planned clinics, outreach, or investigation; decisions about and use of personal protective equipment under various circumstances; establishment of databases for unexpected investigations or unusual outbreaks.

One of the challenges in developing and implementing exercises is to make the mock disaster approximate as closely as possible a real-life one, including as much complexity and unpredictability as possible, and basing scenarios on what is likely to happen according to the microbiological, immunological, epidemiologic, and disaster literature, not on myths or on widely embraced assumptions.

Ensuring Compatibility Between the DHS Exercise Doctrine and Public Health Preparedness Exercises

The DHS HSEEP describes a yearly cycle of planning and development, followed by training, exercises, and the development and implementation of an improvement plan. The committee has learned that CDC intends to implement a similar cyclical process (target goals → exercise → target goals, etc.) with its grantees (Sosin, 2004). The goals of public health preparedness are a distinct subset of overall preparedness, and public health, as noted elsewhere in this report, has its unique capabilities, responsibilities, and information needs. The use of exercises to measure performance and public health preparedness will differ from their use in other fields in the processes being evaluated, in the skills and knowledge being assessed, in the specific relationships and coordination being tested. However, there will be areas of overlap with other disciplines and programs, and there will be some commonalities in structure and operations (e.g., a type of emergency operations center and/or other mechanisms for interagency collaboration and coordination, communication activities, information infrastructure). It is important to ensure that planning, conduct, and evaluation of public health exercises at the federal, state, and local levels are compatible with those of DHS activities under the HSEEP. For example, HSEEP describes three levels of performance evaluation: task level performance (individual); agency/discipline/function-level performance; and mission-level performance (interagency, interorganizational, and community) (DHS/ODP, 2003).

The HSEEP Exercise Evaluation Guides for tabletop and operational exercises include public health personnel/agencies under the "response element" heading in addition to EMS, law enforcement, fire department, HazMat, hospitals, and others, and though the exercise methodology indicates that public health is one of the agencies/disciplines/functions to be evaluated in HSEEP, it understandably does not go into detail. If CDC intends to coordinate with or make its public health exercise evaluation compatible with the HSEEP model, the committee suggests that existing resources, such as the Public Health Competencies for Bioterrorism and Emergency Preparedness be utilized in customizing the individual-level evaluation and that the Local and State Public Health Preparedness and Response Capacity Inventories be included in customizing the agency-level evaluation.

In preceding pages, the committee has explored the potential of proxy events and exercises as means to performance measurement. **The committee recommends that CDC should use the Evidence-Based Performance Goals for Public Health Disaster Preparedness to develop standards against which CDC, states, and localities may regularly measure their performance in exercises and in response to proxy events. Public health agency performance in exercises and proxy events should be used to identify gaps in preparedness and to improve planning, communication, and coordination at the agency and inter-agency levels, as part of a process of continuous quality improvement in preparedness planning and response. Preparedness drills and exercises should not be evaluated individually, but their cumulative and long-term impact on preparedness, such as generalizability to other potential hazards, must be considered in the evaluation process.**

CONCLUDING REMARKS

In closing, the committee encourages CDC to learn from the experience and research available from other fields, including, but not limited to disaster research and emergency and disaster response, and to develop the evidence base specific to public health preparedness; strengthen and sustain active coordination and communication with all relevant entities and government agencies at the federal, state, and local levels; and focus on continuous improvement in planning and performance to further the process and the goal of preparedness. The committee wishes to thank you for the continuing opportunity to be of assistance to the Centers for Disease Control and Prevention and its partners as they work to protect the nation's health.

Brian L. Strom, *Committee Chair*
Kristine M. Gebbie, *Committee Vice Chair*
Robert B. Wallace, *Committee Vice Chair*
Committee on Smallpox Vaccination Program Implementation

REFERENCES

Advisory Panel to Assess Domestic Response Capabilities for Terrorism Involving Weapons of Mass Destruction. 2003. Fifth Annual Report to the President and the Congress. Arlington, VA: The RAND Corporation.

AHRQ (Agency for Healthcare Research and Quality). 2004. Training of Hospital Staff to Respond to a Mass Casualty Incident. AHRQ Evidence Report/Technology Assessment Number 95. [Online] Available at http://www.ahrq.gov/clinic/epcsums/hospmcisum.pdf. Accessed June 10, 2004.

Alexander D. 2000. Scenario methodology for teaching principles of emergency management. *Disaster Prevention and Management* 9(2):89-97.

Alexander D. 2003. Towards the development of standards in emergency management training and education. *Disaster Prevention and Management* 12(2):113-123.

Auf der Heide E. 1989. Disaster Response: Principles of Preparation and Coordination. St. Louis, MO: CV Mosby.

Benjamin G. 2003. SARS: How Effective Is the State and Local Response? Testimony on Behalf of the American Public Health Association Submitted to the Senate Government Affairs Committee, Permanent Committee on Investigations. [Online] Available at http://www.apha.org/legislative/testimonies/sars52103.htm. Accessed May 11, 2004.

Borio L. 2004. Transcript from the IOM's Committee on Smallpox Vaccination Program Implementation Meeting Five on March 29, 2004, Washington, DC.

Bozzette S, Boer R, Bhatnagar V, Brower J, Keeler E, Morton S, Stoto M. 2003. A model for a smallpox-vaccination policy. *New England Journal of Medicine* 348(5):416-425.

Burkle F, Hayden R. 2001. The concept of assisted management of large-scale disasters by horizontal organizations. *Prehospital and Disaster Medicine* 16(3):87-96.

Butler J, Cohen M, Friedman C, Scripp R, Watz C. 2002. Collaboration between public health and law enforcement: new paradigms and partnerships for bioterrorism planning and response. *Emerging Infectious Diseases* 8(10):1152-1156.

CBACI (Chemical and Biological Arms Control Institute). 2002. What Should We Know? Whom Should We Tell?: Leveraging Communication and Information to Counter Terrorism and Its Consequences. [Online] Available at http://www.cbaci.org/summary.pdf and http://www.mipt.org/cbacilevcomm.asp. Accessed May 11, 2004.

CDC (Centers for Disease Control and Prevention). 2003a. Continuation Guidance for Cooperative Agreement on Public Health Preparedness and Response for Bioterrorism—Budget Year Four Program Announcement 99051.

CDC. 2003b. Forensic Epidemiology: Joint Training for Law Enforcement and Public Health Officials on Concurrent Investigative Responses to Bioterrorism Threats and Attacks. [Online] Available at http://www.phppo.cdc.gov/od/phlp/docs/For%20Epi%20Factsheet.pdf. Accessed May 25, 2004.

CDC. 2004a. Continuation Guidance for Cooperative Agreement on Public Health Preparedness and Response for Bioterrorism—Budget Year Five. Program Announcement 99051, p. 5. [Online] Available at http://www.bt.cdc.gov/planning/continuationguidance/index.asp. Accessed June 29, 2004.

CDC. 2004b. Continuation Guidance for Cooperative Agreement on Public Health Preparedness and Response for Bioterrorism—Budget Year Five. Attachment H: Cross-cutting Benchmarks and Activities, p. 1. [Online] Available at http://www.bt.cdc.gov/planning/continuationguidance/index.asp. Accessed June 29, 2004.

CDC and ODP. 2003. 2003 Statewide Homeland Security Grants Program: Frequently Asked Questions. [Online] Available at www.phppo.cdc.gov/HomelandSecGrants/index.asp. Accessed May 11, 2004.

Clements B, Evans R. 2004. Bioterrorism preparedness coordination: an ataxic saga continues. *Public Health Reports* 119:16-18.

Council on Linkages between Academia and Public Health Practice. 2004. National Public Health Systems Research Agenda. [Online] Available at http://www.phf.org/Link/projects.htm#NationalPHSRAgenda. Accessed May 25, 2004.

DHS (Department of Homeland Security). 2003. FY 2004 ODP Homeland Security Grant Program. [Online] Available at http://www.ojp.usdoj.gov/docs/fy04hsgp.pdf and http://www.dhs.gov/dhspublic/interapp/editorial/editorial_0356.xml. Accessed May 11, 2004.

DHS. 2004a. Office for Domestic Preparedness. [Online] Available at http://www.ojp.usdoj.gov/odp. Accessed on June 9, 2004.

DHS. 2004b. Office of Domestic Preparedness: A Better Prepared America Through Practice and Preparation. [Online] Available at http://www.ojp.usdoj.gov/odp/exercises.htm. Accessed June 9, 2004.

DHS. 2004c. Summary of Meeting #4—Public Session (U.S. Department of Homeland Security, Homeland Security Advisory Council). [Online] Available at http://www.dhs.gov/interweb/assetlibrary/HSAC_Minutes033104.pdf. Accessed June 1, 2004.

DHS/ODP (DHS/Office of Domestic Preparedness). 2003. HSEEP, Volume II: Exercise Evaluation and Improvement. [Online] Available at http://www.ojp.usdoj.gov/odp/docs/hseep.htm. Accessed April 2, 2004.

DHS/ODP. 2004a. Homeland Security Exercise and Evaluation Program (HSEEP), Volume I (Revised May 2004). [Online] Available at http://www.ojp.usdoj.gov/odp/docs/hseep.htm. Accessed May 25, 2004.

DHS/ODP. 2004b. Homeland Security Exercise and Evaluation Program. Presented at the Meeting of the IOM Committee on Smallpox Vaccination Program Implementation on March 29, 2004.

Drabek T, McEntire D. 2002. Emergent phenomena and multiorganizational coordination in disasters: lessons from the research literature. *International Journal of Mass Emergencies and Disasters* 20(2):197-224.

Duncan S, Scott S, Duncan C. 1994. Modeling the different smallpox epidemics in England. *Philosophical Transactions: Biological Sciences* 346(1318):407-419.

Eichner M and Dietz K. 2003. Transmission potential of smallpox: estimates based on detailed data from an outbreak. *American Journal of Epidemiology* 158:110-117.

Elliott V. 2004. Measles Cases Trigger Actions in 9 States. AMNews, April 26, 2004. [Online] Available at http://www.ama-assn.org/amednews/2004/04/26/hlsb0426.htm. Accessed May 1, 2004.

FEMA/EMI (Federal Emergency Management Agency/Emergency Management Institute). 2003. IS 139: Exercises Design. Unit 1: Introduction to Exercise Design. [Online] Available at http://training.fema.gov/EMIWeb/IS/is139lst.asp. Accessed April 1, 2004.

Ferguson N, Keeling M, Edmunds W, Gani R, Grenfell B, Anderson R, Leach S. 2003. Planning for smallpox outbreaks. *Nature* 425:681-685.

Gani R, Leach S. 2001. Transmission potential of smallpox in contemporary populations [Letter]. *Nature* 414(6865):748-751.

GAO (U.S. General Accounting Office). 2001. Combating Terrorism: Selected Challenges and Related Recommendations. GAO-01-822. Washington, DC.

GAO. 2003a. Major Management Challenges and Program Risks—Department of Homeland Security (Performance and Accountability Series). GAO-03-102. Washington, DC.

GAO. 2003b. Major Management Challenges and Program Risks—Department of Health and Human Services (Performance and Accountability Series), Report No. GAO-03-101. Washington, DC.

GAO. 2003c. Bioterrorism: Public Health Response to Anthrax Incidents of 2001. GAO-04-152. Washington, DC.

Gerber M. 2002, April. Anthrax Delay Blamed on Lack of Ties. *The Hill.*

Giovachino M, Carey N. 2001. Modeling the consequences of bioterrorism response. *Military Medicine* 166(11):925-930.

Granot H. 1999. Emergency inter-organizational relationships. *Disaster Prevention and Management* 8(1):21-26.

Halloran M, Longini I, Nizam A, Yang Y. 2002. Containing bioterrorist smallpox. *Science* 298:1428-1432.

Hilhorst D. 2003. Responding to Disasters: Diversity of Bureaucrats, Technocrats and Local People. *International Journal of Mass Emergencies and Disasters* 21(1):37-55.

Hupert N, Mushlin A, Callahan M. 2002. Modeling the public health response to bioterrorism: using discrete event simulation to design antibiotic distribution centers. *Medical Decision Making* 22(5 Suppl):S17-S25.

IAEM (International Association of Emergency Managers). 2003. Matrix of Federal All-Hazards Grants. [Online] Available at www.iaem.com/grantmatrix.pdf. Accessed June 17, 2003.

IOM (Institute of Medicine). 2003a. Review of the Centers for Disease Control and Prevention's Smallpox Vaccination Program Implementation: Letter Report #5. Washington, DC: The National Academies Press.

IOM. 2003b. Review of the Centers for Disease Control and Prevention's Smallpox Vaccination Program Implementation: Letter Report #1. Washington, DC: The National Academies Press.

IOM. 2003c. Review of the Centers for Disease Control and Prevention's Smallpox Vaccination Program Implementation: Letter Report #2. Washington, DC: The National Academies Press.

IOM. 2003d. The Future of the Public's Health in the 21st Century. Washington, DC: The National Academies Press.

Kahsai D, Kare J. 2002. Prehospital disaster management: implications for weapons of mass destruction. *Topics in Emergency Medicine* 24(3):37-43.

Kaplan E, Craft D, Wein L. 2003. Analyzing bioterror response logistics: the case of smallpox. *Mathematical Biosciences* 185:33-72.

Kelkenberg K. 2004. Transcript from the IOM's Committee on Smallpox Vaccination Program Implementation Meeting Five, March 29, 2004, Washington, DC:221-253.

Kiel D. 1995. Chaos Theory and Disaster Response Management: Lessons for Managing Periods of Extreme Instability. What Disaster Response Management Can Learn from Chaos Theory. In Koehler, GA, ed. California Research Bureau Conference Proceedings. May 18-19, 1995.

Kreps G, Bosworth S. 1999. Disaster, organizing, and role enactment: a structural approach. *American Journal of Sociology* 99(2):428-463.

Kuhr S, Hauer J. 2001. Intergovernmental Preparedness and Response to Potential Catastrophic Biological Terrorism. In Novick LF, Marr JS, eds. *Public Health Issues in Disaster Preparedness: Focus on Bioterrorism*, pp. 104-110. Gaithersburg, MD: Aspen Publishers Inc.

Landesman LY. 2001. Public Health Management of Disasters: The Practice Guide. Washington, DC: American Public Health Association.

Landesman L, Malilay J, Bissell R, Becker S, Roberts L, Ascher M. 2001. Roles and Responsibilities of Public Health in Disaster Preparedness and Response. In Novick LF, Marr JS, eds. *Public Health Issues in Disaster Preparedness: Focus on Bioterrorism*, pp. 1-56. Gaithersburg, MD: Aspen Publishers Inc.

Meltzer M. 2003. Risks and benefits of preexposure and postexposure smallpox vaccination. *Emerging Infectious Diseases* 9(11):1363-1370.

Meltzer M, Damon I, LeDuc J, Millar J. 2001. Modeling potential responses to smallpox as a bioterrorist weapon. *Emerging Infectious Diseases* 7(6):959-969.

Moscoso E. 2004, April 23. Terror Threat: Bureaucratic Babble. *Atlanta Journal-Constitution*, 1A.

NRC (National Research Council). 2003. The Emergency Manager of the Future: Summary of a Workshop—June 13, 2003, Washington, DC. Washington, DC: The National Academies Press.

Office of the Federal Register. 2003. Smallpox Vaccine Injury Compensation Program: Smallpox (Vacccinia) Vaccine Injury Table. Federal Register 68(166):51492-51499.

Ornstein C. 2001, November 11. FBI, Public Health Agencies Often at Odds Over Anthrax. Houston Chronicle (reprint from Los Angeles Times). [Online] Available at http://www.chron.com/cs/CDA/printstory.mpl/special/terror/front/1127841. Accessed May 20, 2004.

Perry R. 2003. Municipal terrorism management in the United States. *Disaster Prevention and Management* 12(3):190-202.

Peters KE, Drabant E, Elster AB, Tierney M, Hatcher B. 2001. Cooperative Actions for Health Program: Lessons Learned in Medicine and Public Health Collaboration. Chicago, IL, and Washington, DC: American Medical Association and American Public Health Association.

Quarantelli E. 1988. Local Emergency Management Agencies: Research Findings on Their Progress and Problems in the Last Two Decades. University of Delaware Disaster Research Center.

Quarantelli E. 1994. Draft of a Sociological Disaster Agenda for the Future: Theoretical, Methodological and Empirical Issues. University of Delaware Disaster Research Center Preliminary Papers (#228). [Online] Available at http://www.udel.edu/DRC/preliminary/228.pdf.

Quarantelli E. 1995. Disaster Planning, Emergency Management, and Civil Protection: The Historical Development and Current Characteristics of Organized Efforts to Prevent and to Respond to Disasters. Available at http://www.udel.edu/DRC/prepapers.html.

Quarantelli E. 2004. Transcript from the IOM's Committee on Smallpox Vaccination Program Implementation Meeting Five on March 29, 2004, Washington, DC.

Richards E. 2002. Collaboration between public health and law enforcement: the constitutional challenge. *Emerging Infectious Diseases* 8(10):1157-1159.

Salinsky E. 2002. Will the Nation Be Ready for the Next Bioterrorism Attack? Mending Gaps in the Public Health Infrastructure. NHPF Issue Brief No. 776.

Schweitzer R. 2004. Transcript from the IOM's Committee on Smallpox Vaccination Program Implementation Meeting Five on March 29, 2004, Washington, DC:265.

Simpson D. 2002. Earthquake drills and simulations in community-based training and preparedness programmes. *Disasters* 26(1):55-69.

Sosin D. 2004. Transcript from the IOM's Committee on Smallpox Vaccination Program Implementation Meeting Five on March 29, 2004, Washington, DC.

Staiti A, Katz A, Hoadley J. 2003. Has bioterrorism preparedness improved public health? Issue Brief: Findings from HSC, No. 65.

Stoll M, Lee H. 2003. State health department develops SARS emergency response plan. Virginia Department of Health News Release, June 23, 2003.

Tang N, Fabbri W. 2003. Medical direction and integration with existing EMS infrastructure. *Topics in Emergency Medicine* 25(4):326-332.

Taylor N. 2003. Review of the Use of Models in Informing Disease Control Policy Development and Adjustment. Reading, UK: University of Reading, School of Agriculture, Policy and Development. [Online] Available at http://www.defra.gov.uk/science/Publications/2003/UseofModelsinDiseaseControlPolicy.pdf. Accessed April 1, 2004.

Tierney K. 1993. Disaster Preparedness and Response: Research Findings and Guidance from the Social Science Literature. University of Delaware Disaster Research Center Preliminary Paper #193. [Online] Available at http://www.udel.edu/DRC/preliminary/193.pdf. Accessed April 25, 2004.

Tierney K, Lindell M, Perry R. 2001. Facing the Unexpected: Disaster Preparedness and Response in the United States. Washington, DC: Joseph Henry Press.

WADEM (World Association of Disaster and Emergency Medicine). 2001. Conceptual Framework of Disasters (Part III, Chapters 3-7). In Health Disaster Management: Guidelines for Evaluation and Research in the Utstein Style. [Online] Available at http://wadem.medicine.wisc.edu. Accessed June 1, 2004.

Werner L, Naud M, Kellogg A. 1998. Quick Response Report #11—Public Health Emergency Response: Evaluation of Implementation of a New Emergency Management System for Public Health in the State of Georgia. University of Colorado Natural Hazards Center. [Online]. Available at http://www.colorado.edu/hazards/qr/qr111/qr111.html. Accessed May 12, 2004.

White House. 2001. Fact Sheet: Homeland Security Council. [Online] Available at www.whitehouse.gov/news/releases/2001/10/print/20011029-16.html. Accessed April 10, 2004.

LETTER REPORT #6, APPENDIX 6-A SUMMARY OF RECOMMENDATIONS

Recommendation 1:
The committee recommends that all federal entities concerned with bioterrorism preparedness (e.g., CDC, the Health Resources and Services Administration, the Office of Domestic Preparedness [ODP]) should more actively coordinate guidance and funding activities. Federal agencies should also work together to develop mechanisms that facilitate coordination and collaboration among their grantees at the state and local levels. Such mechanisms may include, but are not lim-

ited to, regular meetings to familiarize CDC and ODP program staff with each other's program priorities and activities, a database for informing ODP and other partners of exercises planned by CDC grantees, etc. Federal coordination efforts should also include the clarification of primary responsibility and authority in bioterrorism events, to ensure that CDC can fulfill its unique role as the nation's public health agency.

Recommendation 2:
The committee recommends that CDC should collaborate with all of its partners to strengthen preparedness by applying research findings and experience in public health emergency response, bioterrorism preparedness, and disaster management. In order to strengthen the evidence base for public health preparedness, CDC should:

- Strengthen the link between public health research and practice;
- Participate in and promote interdisciplinary research about preparedness;
- Support a system to assure the ongoing collection, synthesis, and sharing of lessons learned and best practices from public health preparedness exercises and public health response to proxy events; and
- In coordination with the appropriate federal-level partners, such as the Agency for Healthcare Research and Quality, evaluate the effectiveness, design, and opportunity costs of preparedness strategies, such as exercises.

Recommendation 3:
The committee recommends that CDC should use the Evidence-Based Performance Goals for Public Health Disaster Preparedness to develop standards against which CDC, states, and localities may regularly measure their performance in exercises and in response to proxy events. Public health agency performance in exercises and proxy events should be used to identify gaps in preparedness and to improve planning, communication, and coordination at the agency and interagency levels, as part of a process of continuous quality improvement in preparedness planning and response. Preparedness drills and exercises should not be evaluated individually, but their cumulative and long-term impact on preparedness, such as generalizability to other potential hazards, must be considered in the evaluation process.

LETTER REPORT #6, APPENDIX 6-B ACRONYMS AND GLOSSARY

Acronyms

CDC Centers for Disease Control and Prevention
CHER-CAP Community Hazards Emergency Response Capability Assurance Program
CSEPP Chemical Stockpile Emergency Preparedness Program
DHHS Department of Health and Human Services
DHS Department of Homeland Security
EMS Emergency Medical Services
Epi-Aid Epidemic Assistance Investigation
FBI Federal Bureau of Investigations
FEMA Federal Emergency Management Agency
GAO General Accounting Office
HAN Health Alert Network
HSAC Homeland Security Advisory Council
HSC Homeland Security Council
HRSA Health Resources and Services Administration
HSEEP Homeland Security Exercise Evaluation Program
ICS Incident Command System
LLIS Lessons Learned Information Sharing (www.llis.org)
MIPT Memorial Institute for the Prevention of Terrorism
ODP Office of Domestic Preparedness
PCC Policy Coordination Committee (of the HSC)
REP Radiological Emergency Preparedness Program
WMD Weapons of Mass Destruction

Glossary

All-hazards: generally contrasted with "agent-specific," refers to a broad preparedness and response approach to all possible hazards to population health and safety, whether the complete range of known disasters, or specifically the complete range of public health disasters (from naturally occurring to deliberately introduced).

Disaster: phenomena caused by natural, technological, or deliberate causes. Term is sometimes used interchangeably with emergency, although the two are not only quantitatively but also qualitatively different. A key difference is that while emergencies call upon largely local resources and response, disasters are of sufficient magnitude to require external resources and personnel for response and recovery (Mothershead, 2003).

Drill: similar to exercises, but more narrowly focused activities used for training, testing, and refining capacities, and frequently involving a specific area of preparedness within only one agency rather than more complex processes and relationships at an interagency level.

Emergency manager: a title used for increasingly professionalized personnel in local or state government who are charged with coordinating or overseeing the jurisdiction's multiagency response to an emergency or disaster.

Emergency responder/first responder/traditional emergency responder: term refers to a set of disciplines and responsibilities, including, but not limited to Emergency Medical Services (EMS), fire, law enforcement, hazardous materials specialists, etc. Personnel in such agencies and the practitioners of such disciplines prepare for emergencies and disasters and are responsible for carrying out response when emergencies and disasters occur.

H

Agendas for Committee Information-Gathering Meetings

Meeting One
December 19, 2002
500 Fifth Street, NW
Washington, DC
Room 100

8:00 a.m.	Welcome *Harvey V. Fineberg, M.D., Ph.D., President, IOM* *Brian Strom, M.D., M.P.H., Chair*
8:15 a.m.	DHHS Bioterrorism Effort and the Role of the IOM Committee *William Raub, Ph.D., Deputy Director of the Office of Public Health Preparedness, Department of Health and Human Services*
8:30 a.m.	Charge to the IOM *David Fleming, M.D., Deputy Director for Science and Public Health, Office of the Director, CDC*

8:45 a.m.	Centers for Disease Control Progress Report on Smallpox Immunization Program and ACIP Recommendations *Larry Anderson, M.D., Senior Advisor for Smallpox, Office of Terrorism Preparedness and Response, Office of the Director, CDC* *Ray Strikas, M.D., Director, Smallpox Preparedness and Response Activity, National Immunization Program (NIP), CDC*
9:30 a.m.	Discussion
10:00 a.m.	Break
10:15 a.m.	Safety System Overview *Gina Mootrey, D.O., M.P.H., Senior Research Officer, Immunization Safety Branch, NIP, CDC*
11:00 a.m.	Clinical Operations/Screening Overview *Lisa Rotz, M.D., Chief of the Emergency Surveillance and Response Branch of the Bioterrorism Preparedness and Response Program, National Center for Infectious Diseases, CDC*
11:45 a.m.	Lunch
12:45 p.m.	Training and Education Overview *Linda Quick, M.D., M.P.H, Medical Epidemiologist, National Immunization Program, CDC*
1:30 p.m.	Communications Overview *Glen Nowak, Ph.D., Associate Director for Communication, NIP, CDC*
2:15 p.m.	Smallpox Vaccination in Israel *Yehuda L. Danon, M.D., Professor of Pediatrics, Tel Aviv University and Director, Schneider Children's Medical Center of Israel (invited)*
3:00 p.m.	Break

3:15 p.m. Department of Defense Smallpox Experience and Update
The Honorable William Winkenwerder, Jr., M.D., M.B.A.
Assistant Secretary of Defense for Health Affairs, DoD
LTC John Grabenstein, R.P.H., Ph.D., Deputy Director for Military Vaccines at the Army Surgeon General's Office, DoD

4:00 p.m. Solicited Comments
American College of Emergency Physicians
American Hospital Association
American Nurses Association
Association of State and Territorial Health Officials
National Association of County and City Health Officials

4:50 p.m. Discussion

5:30 p.m. Public Comment

6:00 p.m. Adjourn

Meeting Two
February 13, 2003
National Academy of Sciences
2101 Constitution Avenue, NW
Washington, DC
Lecture Room

9:00 a.m. Welcome and Introductions
Brian Strom, M.D., M.P.H.
Committee Chair

9:15 a.m. Overall Program Progress
Joe Henderson, Associate Director of Terrorism Preparedness and Response, CDC

9:45 a.m. Questions from the Committee

10:15 a.m. Update from State Programs
Eddy Bresnitz, M.D., M.S.
State Epidemiologist/Assistant Commissioner
Smallpox Vaccination Program Coordinator
State of New Jersey Department of Health and Senior Services

By phone:
Kathleen Toomey, M.D., M.P.H.
Director, Division of Public Health
Georgia Department of Human Resources

10:45 a.m. Questions from the Committee

11:00 a.m. The Department of Defense Experience
COL John Grabenstein, R.Ph., Ph.D.
Deputy Director for Military Vaccines at the Army Surgeon General's Office Department of Defense

11:30 a.m. Questions from the Committee

12:00 p.m. Lunch

1:00 p.m. Discussion of the Pre-event Vaccination System
Vicky Kipreos, PMP
Lead IT Specialist
Information Resource Management Office, CDC

1:20 p.m. Questions from the Committee

1:30 p.m. CDC Update—Safety System (active surveillance, etc.)
Gina Mootrey, D.O., M.P.H.
Senior Research Officer
Immunization Safety Branch
NIP, CDC

1:45 p.m.	ACIP Working Group on Smallpox Vaccine Adverse Events By phone: *John Neff, M.D.* *Vice-Chair of the ACIP Working Group*
2:00 p.m.	Questions from the Committee about Safety System and the ACIP Working Group
2:30 p.m.	CDC Update—Training and Education *Lynn Steele, M.S.* *Senior Advisor for Education and Training* *Office of Terrorism Preparedness and Response, CDC*
2:45 p.m.	Questions from the Committee
3:00 p.m.	Break
3:15 p.m.	CDC UpdateCommunication Strategy *Glen Nowak, Ph.D.* *Associate Director for Communication* *NIP, CDC*
3:45 p.m.	Questions from the Committee
4:15 p.m.	Smallpox Vaccine Risk Communication Activities at Walter Reed Army Medical Center *Renata J. M. Engler, COL, MC* *Chief, Allergy-Immunology Department* *Allergy-Immunology-Immunization Specialty Consultant to the Army OTSG* *DoD Ex-Officio Representative to the National Vaccine Advisory Committee* *Director, Walter Reed National Vaccine Healthcare Center* *Walter Reed Army Medical Center*
4:45 p.m.	Questions from the Committee
5:15 p.m.	Public Comment
5:45 p.m.	Meeting Adjourned

Meeting Three
May 1, 2003
Academy for Educational Development
1825 Connecticut Avenue, NW, 8th Floor
Washington, DC

8:00 a.m. Registration and Coffee

8:30 a.m. Welcome and Opening Statement
Brian Strom, M.D., M.P.H.
Committee Chair

8:45 a.m. Overview of CDC Activities to Date
Joe Henderson, Associate Director of Terrorism Preparedness and Response, CDC

Gina Mootrey, D.O., M.P.H., Senior Research Officer, Immunization Safety Branch, NIP, CDC

9:30 a.m. The ACIP Smallpox Vaccine Safety Working Group and the Vaccine Safety System
John M. Neff, M.D.
Director, Center for Children with Special Needs, Children's Hospital and Regional Medical Center (Seattle, WA)
Vice Chair, Advisory Committee on Immunization Practices (ACIP) Smallpox Vaccine Safety Working Group

10:00 a.m. Questions from the Committee

10:30 a.m. The State Perspective
Mary C. Selecky
Secretary of Health, Washington State Department of Health and President, Association of State and Territorial Health Officials

Gianfranco Pezzino, M..D, M.P.H.
State Epidemiologist, Kansas Department of Health and Environment and President, Council of State and Territorial Epidemiologists

11:30 a.m.	Questions from the Committee
11:45 a.m.	Lunch
1:00 p.m.	The Local Perspective *Yvonne Madlock, MAT* *Director, Memphis and Shelby County Health Department, Shelby County Government, Division of Health Services (Tennessee)* *Karen Nikolai, M.P.H., M.C.P.* *Program Supervisor, Immunization Services, Hennepin County Community Health Department (Minnesota)*
2:00 p.m.	The Hospital/Health System Perspective *Ron J. Anderson, M.D.* *President & CEO, Parkland Health & Hospital System (Texas)* *Franklyn Judson, M.D.* *Director of Public Health, Denver Health (Colorado)*
3:00 p.m.	Questions from the Committee
3:15 p.m.	Break
3:30 p.m.	Perspective of a Hospital/Health System NOT Participating in the Smallpox Vaccination Program *Michael Edmond, M.D., M.P.A.* *Hospital Epidemiologist, Virginia Commonwealth University Health System Authority*
4:00 p.m.	The Health Plan Perspective *David J. Witt, M.D.* *Chair of Infectious Diseases, Northern California Kaiser Permanente* *Skip Skivington, M.B.A.* *National Director, Healthcare Continuity, Kaiser Permanente*

4:30 p.m. Questions from the Committee

4:45 p.m. Additional Committee Questions for All Speakers

5:00 p.m. Public Comment

5:30 p.m. Adjourn

Meeting Four
November 6, 2003
The Wyndham Washington Hotel
Vista Ballroom BC
1400 M Street, NW
Washington, DC

9:00 a.m. Welcome and Introductions
Brian Strom, M.D., M.P.H.
Committee Chair

9:15 a.m. HRSA Cooperative Agreement Guidance
Commander Brad Austin
Senior Program Specialist, National Bioterrorism Hospital Preparedness Program, Office of Special Programs, HRSA

9:30 a.m. Update on National Smallpox Vaccination Program
Defining Smallpox Preparedness
Joseph Henderson
Associate Director of Terrorism Preparedness and Response, CDC

Draft Smallpox Preparedness Measures
Ray Strikas, M.D., Director, Smallpox Preparedness and Response Activity, National Immunization Program (NIP), CDC
Linda J. Neff, Ph.D., Senior Epidemiologist, Smallpox Preparedness and Response Activity, National Immunization Program (NIP), CDC

10:30 a.m. Questions from the Committee

11:15 a.m.	Adjourn for lunch
	• committee lunch in private • panel lunches in 4 separate meeting rooms *State and Local Public Health (Belle Air Room)* *Health Care Providers (Sherwood Room)* *Health Care Institutions (Westover Room)* *First Responders (Berkeley Room)* • liaison lunch (Ashlawn North Room)
12:30 p.m.	Panel 1: State and Local Public Health
	American Public Health Association *(Dr. Georges Benjamin)* *Association of Public Health Laboratories* *(Dr. Katherine Kelley)* *Association of State and Territorial Health Officials* *(Dr. Donald Williamson)* *Council of State and Territorial Epidemiologists* *(Dr. Gianfranco Pezzino)* *National Association of County and City Health Officials* *(Dr. Alonzo Plough)* *National Association of Local Boards of Health* *(Mr. Shepard Cohen)*
12:45 p.m.	Questions from the Committee
1:30 p.m.	Panel 2: Health Care Providers
	American Academy of Family Physicians *(Dr. Jonathan Temte)* *American College of Emergency Physicians* *(Dr. Jon Mark Hirshon)* *American Nurses Association* *(Ms. Cheryl Peterson)* *National Association of Emergency Medical System Physicians* *(Dr. Robert O'Connor)*
1:45 p.m.	Questions from the Committee
2:30 p.m.	Break

2:45 p.m.	Panel 3: Health Care Institutions
	American Association of Health Plans *(Mr. Bob Rehm)* *American Hospital Association* *(Ms. Roslyne Schulman)* *National Association of Public Hospitals and Health Systems* *(Dr. Van Dunn)*
3:00 p.m.	Questions from the Committee
3:45 p.m.	Panel 4: First Responders
	International Association of Chiefs of Police *(Dr. Kris Arnold)* *International Association of Fire Chiefs* *(Commissioner David Fischler)* *National Association of Emergency Medical Technicians* *(Mr. John Roquemore)* *National Association of State Emergency Medical System Directors* *(Ms. Margaret Trimble)*
4:00 p.m.	Questions from the Committee
4:45 p.m.	Public Comment and Discussion
5:30 p.m.	Adjourn

Meeting Five
March 29, 2004
National Academy of Sciences Building
2101 Constitution Avenue, NW
Washington, DC
Lecture Room

8:00–8:30 a.m.	Registration and Coffee

8:30–8:45 a.m.	Welcome and Opening Statement *Brian Strom* *Committee Chair*
8:45–9:15 a.m.	CDC's Next Steps for Public Health Preparedness *Dan Sosin* *Associate Director for Science* *Office of Terrorism Preparedness and Emergency Response* *Centers for Disease Control and Prevention* *Department of Health and Human Services*
9:15–9:45 a.m.	Questions from the Committee
9:45–10:05 a.m.	Presentation on the Modeling Workgroup of Secretary's Council on Public Health Preparedness *Luciana Borio* *Senior Health Advisor* *Office of Research and Development Coordination* *Office of the Assistant Secretary for Public Health Emergency Preparedness* *Department of Health and Human Services*
10:05–10:25 a.m.	Questions from the Committee
10:25–10:40 a.m.	Break
10:40–11:10 a.m.	The experience of local and state public health agencies *Patrick Libbey* *Executive Director* *National Association of County and City Health Officials* *George E. Hardy, Jr.* *Executive Director* *Association of State and Territorial Health Officials*
11:10–11:30 a.m.	Questions from the Committee

11:30 a.m.–12:00 p.m.	Theory and science behind scenarios, exercises, and drills—a disaster management and response perspective *Erik Auf der Heide* *Disaster Planning and Training Specialist* *Agency for Toxic Substances and Disease Registry* *Department of Health and Human Services*
12:00–12:20 p.m.	Questions from the Committee
12:20–1:20 p.m.	Lunch
1:20–1:50 p.m.	Theory and science behind scenarios, exercises, and drills—a sociological perspective *E.L. (Henry) Quarantelli* *Research Professor, Founding Director* *Disaster Research Center* *University of Delaware*
1:50–2:20 p.m.	Questions from the Committee
2:20–2:40 p.m.	Lessons learned from exercises and drills conducted by health care organizations for JCAHO accreditation *Margaret VanAmringe* *Vice President for External Relations* *Joint Commission on Accreditation of Healthcare Organizations*
2:40–3:00 p.m.	Questions from the Committee
3:00–3:15 p.m.	Break
3:15–3:45 p.m.	Regional FEMA experience with exercises and drills *Kelvin Kelkenberg* *Director, National Preparedness Division* *Emergency Preparedness and Response Directorate* *Department of Homeland Security*
3:45–4:10 p.m.	Questions from the Committee

4:10–4:30 p.m. The Homeland Security Exercise and Evaluation Program (HSEEP) of the DHS Office of Domestic Preparedness
Robert Schweitzer
Exercise Program Manager
Office of Domestic Preparedness
Department of Homeland Security

Sandra Santa
Exercise Program Manager
Office of Domestic Preparedness
Department of Homeland Security

4:30–4:50 p.m. Questions from the Committee

4:50–5:10 p.m. Perspective of an Academic Center for Public Health Preparedness
Maggie Potter
Associate Dean and Director, Center for Public Health Practice
Principal Investigator, Center for Public Health Preparedness
Graduate School of Public Health
University of Pittsburgh

5:10–5:30 p.m. Questions from the Committee

5:30–5:45 p.m. Public comment

5:45 p.m. Closing remarks

I

Committee Biosketches

Brian Strom (Chair) is Associate Vice Dean, University of Pennsylvania School of Medicine, Chair and Professor, Department of Biostatistics and Epidemiology, George S. Pepper Professor of Public Health and Preventive Medicine, Professor of medicine, Professor of pharmacology, and Director of the Center for Clinical Epidemiology and Biostatistics at the University of Pennsylvania. Internationally known for multiple areas of clinical epidemiology, Dr. Strom's major career interest is pharmacoepidemiology, specifically looking at adverse drug reactions and medical errors. He received his medical degree from Johns Hopkins University School of Medicine and his master's of public health from the University of California, Berkeley. He is an Institute of Medicine member and served as a member of the Committee to Review the CDC Anthrax Vaccine Safety and Efficacy Research Program. He was Chair of the Institute's Committee to Assess the Safety and Efficacy of the Anthrax Vaccine.

Kristine M. Gebbie (Vice Chair) is the Elizabeth Standish Gill Associate Professor of Nursing, Director of the Center for Health Policy, and Director of the Doctor of Nursing Science program at Columbia University School of Nursing. Her teaching and research focus is on health policy and health services, with particular attention to population-based public health services. Prior to Columbia, she was the first White House National AIDS Policy Coordinator (1993-1994) and served 4 years as a Senior Consultant on Public Health Initiatives to the Office of Public Health and Science for the U.S. Department of Health and Human Services. Dr. Gebbie is active in many professional organizations and has served as a member of the Executive Board of the American Public Health Association. Most recently, her completed research includes the first enumeration of the public health workforce in 20 years and the development of core competencies in emergency preparedness for public health workers. Dr. Gebbie received her master's in nursing from the University of California, Los Angeles, and her doctorate in public health from the University of Michigan School of Public Health. She is a member of the Institute of Medicine. Dr. Gebbie co-chaired the Institute's Committee on Educating Public Health Professionals for the 21st Century, and is currently chairing the Committee on Establishing a National Cord Blood Stem Cell Bank Program.

Robert Wallace (Vice Chair) is Professor of epidemiology and internal medicine at the University of Iowa Colleges of Public Health and Medicine. He received the Irene Ensminger Stecher Professorship in April 1999 for cancer and heart disease-related research. He was formerly Head of the department of preventive medicine at the University of Iowa College of Medicine and the Director of the University of Iowa Cancer Center. Dr. Wallace's research interests include cancer epidemiology and prevention; the causes and prevention of chronic, disabling diseases among older persons; women's health issues; and risk factors for cardiovascular disease. He is a Principal Investigator of several large clinical trials. He received his medical degree from Northwestern University School of Medicine. He is an Institute of Medicine member and currently serves as Chair of the Institute of Medicine's Medical Follow-up Agency Board.

E. Russell Alexander is Professor Emeritus of epidemiology at the University of Washington School of Public Health, where he has spent much of his career and was the first Chair of the Department of Epidemiology. His prior position was Chief of epidemiology for the Seattle-King County Department of Public Health (1990-1998). Dr. Alexander worked from 1983 to 1989 at the Centers for Disease Control and Prevention in the area of control and prevention of sexually-transmitted diseases. He received his medical degree from the University of Chicago with a clinical specialization in infectious diseases and is certified by the American Board of Pediatrics. Dr. Alexander is a member of the American Epidemiological Society, the Infectious Disease Society of America, and Pediatric Infectious Disease Society. He is also a fellow of the American Public Health Association. Dr. Alexander has participated in an Institute of Medicine (IOM) forum on vaccine safety, and has been a member of four IOM committees, including the Committee on Immunization Finance Policies and Practices and the committee on vaccine safety.

Ronald Bayer is a Professor of sociomedical sciences at the Joseph L. Mailman School of Public Health at Columbia University. His work focuses on ethical issues and public health policy, specifically centered on AIDS, as well as tuberculosis policy and tobacco regulations in liberal democracies. Prior to Columbia, Dr. Bayer was Associate for policy studies at The Hastings Center, a research center focused on medical ethics. Dr. Bayer received his Ph.D. at the University of Chicago. He is a member of the Institute of Medicine and serves on the Institute of Medicine's Board on Health Promotion and Disease Prevention. He has participated in the Institute of Medicine's Committee on Immunization Safety Review and the committee on the Ryan White CARE Act: Data for Allocation, Planning and Evaluation. In the past, he was a member of the Institute's Committee on the Elimination of Tuberculosis in the United States.

R. Alta Charo is Associate Dean of the University of Wisconsin Law School, and Professor of law and bioethics at the University of Wisconsin's law and medical schools. She offers courses on health law, bioethics and biotechnology law, food and drug law, medical ethics, reproductive rights, torts, and legislative drafting. In addition, she sits on the University's internal bioethics advisory committee and its Institutional Review Board for the protection of human subjects in medical research. Ms. Charo serves on the editorial boards of the *Journal of Law, Medicine, and Ethics*; *Cloning: Science and Policy*; and the *Monash Bioethics Review*. Ms. Charo received her law degree from Columbia University School of Law and was a member of the steering committee that founded the International Association for Bioethics. From 1996 to 2001 she served on the National Bioethics Advisory Commission, and she currently serves on the National Academy of Sciences' Board on Life Sciences.

Thomas Coates is Professor of infectious diseases at the David Geffen School of Medicine, University of California, Los Angeles. He was formerly Director and Principal Investigator of Center for AIDS Prevention Studies, Professor of medicine and Director of the behavioral medicine unit at University of California, San Francisco (UCSF), and Executive Director of the AIDS Research Institute at UCSF. Dr. Coates came to UCSF from Johns Hopkins in 1982. Before that, he was on the faculty of the Stanford Heart Disease Prevention program. His interests and experience focus on the study of disease-related behavior, with an emphasis on interventions to modify behaviors. He is the author of many publications on the effects of antibody testing on high-risk behavior, the efficacy of strategies to modify high-risk behavior, the relationship between psychosocial variables and AIDS-related immune dysfunction, and clinical illness and interventions to reduce high-risk behaviors among seropositive men. Dr. Coates has conducted large-scale clinical trials in the United States, Africa, and South America and has trained both domestic and international postdoctoral fellows. Dr. Coates received his Ph.D. from Stanford University. He is a member of the Institute of Medicine.

Penelope Dennehy is Professor of pediatrics at Brown Medical School and is Director of the division of pediatric infectious diseases at Hasbro Children's Hospital. She is the Chairperson for the committee on the protection of human subjects at Rhode Island Hospital and is a member of the infection control committee. She is a reviewer for many publications, such as *Clinical Infectious Diseases*, *The Pediatric Infectious Disease Journal*, and *Lancet*. She is a fellow of the Infectious Diseases Society of America and the Pediatric Infectious Diseases Society and holds memberships in organizations such as the International Society for Vaccines and American Society for Microbiology. She received her medical degree at Tufts University School of Medicine and is board certified in pediatric infectious diseases. Dr. Dennehy is active in the American Academy of Pediatrics Committee on Infectious Diseases, as well as the National Institutes of Health Collaborative Antiviral Study Group pediatric enterovirus subcommittee. Her research has included many clinical trials of vaccine and immunobiologics.

Vince Fulginiti is Professor Emeritus of pediatrics at the University of Arizona, as well as Professor Emeritus of pediatrics and Chancellor Emeritus for University of Colorado School of Medicine. While at the University of Colorado, Dr. Fulginiti also worked with the department of preventive medicine and biometrics in the Program in Ethics, Humanities, and Law. One of his major research contributions included running a large clinical program documenting the range of normal and adverse consequences of the smallpox (vaccinia) vaccine. He has held various committee positions, such as: President of the Western Society for Pediatric Research for the American Pediatric Society, member and Chair of the Academy of Pediatrics "Red Book" committee (Committee on Infectious Diseases), and member and Chair of the National Vaccine Advisory Committee for the U.S. Public Health Service. Dr. Fulginiti received both his medical degree and master's degree from Temple University.

Jay Harper is Medical Director of Employee Health Services at University of Pittsburgh Medical Center. His clinical activities involve job placement, medical surveillance and injury evaluations for hospital and university workers, and included providing smallpox vaccinations for lab workers using vaccinia in their research. He was previously Clinical Assistant Professor of Environmental and Occupational Health at the University of Pittsburgh

Graduate School of Public Health. Dr. Harper was also the associate program director for the occupational medicine residency program at the University of Pittsburgh and the clinical director for the program. He is a Fellow of the American College of Occupational and Environmental Medicine. He worked as a chemical engineer before medical school. Dr. Harper received his medical degree from West Virginia University and his M.B.A. and M.P.H. from the University of Pittsburgh.

Coleen Kivlahan is Medical Director of Ambulatory Primary Care at Fantus Health Center, Bureau of Health Services, Cook County, Illinois. She was formerly a Professor of family and community medicine at the University of Missouri School of Medicine. She also served as Assistant to the Dean for health policy and as an active clinician at the Family Health Center in Boone County. She was the Associate Chief of Staff of the University of Missouri Health Sciences Center (UMHSC), as well as the Director of the Office of Clinical Outcomes and Medical Management. She has also directed the UMHSC efforts to improve clinical quality at all levels of care. From 1993 to 1996, she was Director of the Missouri Department of Health. Her priorities while Director involved increasing access to effective primary and preventative services and improving the health status of minority populations. From 1989 to 1993, Dr. Kivlahan served as Medical Director of the Missouri Department of Social Services, where she devoted her time to increasing access for the uninsured and developed a statewide network of professionals to ensure high-quality child abuse examinations and child fatality investigations. In addition to her work at the state, Dr. Kivlahan has served as a public health leader at the national and local levels. She received her medical degree from Medical College of Ohio at Toledo.

Jeff Levine is Health Communications Director at American Institutes for Research in Silver Spring, Maryland. Mr. Levine was previously Vice President for Health Media at Ketchum Washington, DC's health-care practice, where he provided strategic counsel, media training and crisis management services to a variety of clients in the pharmaceutical and medical field. Mr. Levine's prior work experience includes 10 years as a CNN medical correspondent, where he covered numerous stories on federal health care policy, government regulations, and medical research. Mr. Levine also served as the Washington, DC, bureau chief for WebMD, preparing daily stories on health care and public policy, as well as managing news staff for this large physician and consumer internet health news service. At Porter Novelli, he developed broadcast releases and media strategies for clients in the health industry. Mr. Levine recently served as a consultant to the Institute of Medicine, executing an in-depth analysis to assess the organization's report writing process. He holds a master's degree in journalism from the University of California at Berkeley and a bachelor's degree in English literature from the University of Colorado.

Kenneth McIntosh is Professor of pediatrics at Harvard Medical School, as well as Professor of immunology and infectious diseases at the Harvard School of Public Health. Dr. McIntosh, who works in the Division of Infectious Disease at Children's Hospital in Boston, MA, has coauthored studies on the safety and immunologic response to the standard and attenuated smallpox vaccines. His current interest is in the pathogenesis of HIV disease in children and the treatment of HIV infected infants and children. Dr. McIntosh received his medical degree from Harvard University and is certified by the American Board of Internal Medicine. He is currently Vice Chair of the National Institute of Allergy and Infectious Diseases' HIV Vaccine and Prevention Data and Safety Monitoring Board and served on the Institute of Medicine's Vaccine Safety Committee.

Elizabeth Murane recently retired from being Director of nurses for the Shasta County Public Health Department in Redding, CA. As Director, she was responsible for immunization, tuberculosis, infectious diseases, and maternal, child, and adolescent health programs. Previously, she was a public health nurse for Shasta County Public Health Department and an evening charge nurse for the Shasta Convalescent Hospital. She is a licensed registered nurse in California, as well as being certified in California as a public health nurse. Ms. Murane received her nursing degree from Case Western Reserve University and her master's degree in nursing education, specializing in maternal child health, at Columbia University's Teachers' College.

Peter Rosen is a Professor Emeritus of clinical medicine and surgery and former Director of education in the department of emergency medicine at the University of California, San Diego. He currently also serves as Senior Lecturer in Medicine at the Harvard University School of Medicine and attending emergency physician at the Beth Israel/Deaconess Medical Center, and as Visiting Professor of Emergency Medicine at the University of Arizona School of Medicine. He is editor-in-chief of the *Journal of Emergency Medicine* and a consulting editor to *Emergindex Microindex*. Dr. Rosen received his medical degree from Washington University Medical School. He is a fellow in the American College of Surgeons, a senior board member and consultant with the American Board of Emergency Medicine, and a member of the Institute of Medicine. He served on the National Research Council's Committee on Science and Technology for Counter Terrorism: Biological Panel. He also chaired the Institute of Medicine's

Committee on Research and Development Needs for Improved Civilian Medical Response to Chemical or Biological Terrorism Incidents.

William Weston is Professor of dermatology and pediatrics at University of Colorado School of Medicine and Chief of dermatology at The Children's Hospital in Denver. Dr. Weston ended his 25 year tenure as Chair of the University of Colorado School of Medicine's dermatology department in 2001. In addition, Dr. Weston received the University of Colorado's Florence Rena Sabin Award in appreciation for national recognition as a medical educator and public health advocate. He serves as a reviewer for many medical journals including *Journal of Clinical Investigation*, *Journal of Pediatrics*, and the *Journal of American Academy of Dermatology*. He is board certified in dermatology and pediatrics with research interests in cutaneous immunology and virology and pediatric dermatology. Dr. Weston received his medical degree from the University of Colorado School of Medicine.

Robert Woolson is Professor of biostatistics and epidemiology at the Medical University of South Carolina as well as Professor Emeritus of biostatistics at the University of Iowa. He has served as Professor of biostatistics and Associate Dean for research at the University of Iowa's College of Public Health. Dr. Woolson has been as a member of the FDA Antiviral Drugs Advisory Committee, the NIAID AIDS Data Safety and Monitoring Committee and is currently serving on a data safety and monitoring board for the Department of Veterans Affairs Cooperative Studies Program. He is a member of Delta Omega, the National Honorary Public Health Society and is a fellow in The Royal Statistical Society and of the American Statistical Association. Dr. Woolson's research interest areas are as follows: analysis and design of longitudinal studies, statistical methods for categorical data, statistical methods in survival data analysis, psychiatric epidemiology/biometry, and clinical trials. He has been Associate Editor for *Controlled Clinical Trials* and is a member of the editorial board of *Statistics in Medicine*. Dr. Woolson received his doctorate from the University of North Carolina, Chapel Hill.

Index

A

D

E

H

I

M

P

S

T

W